Nurses and Work Satisfaction: An Index for Measurement

Second Edition

Nurses and Work Satisfaction:
An Index for Measurement

Paula L. Stamps

Second Edition

Health Administration Press
Chicago, Illinois

Library of Congress Cataloging-in-Publication Data

Stamps, Paula L.
   Nurses and work satisfaction : an index for measurement /
   Paula L. Stamps. — 2nd ed.
       p.   cm.
   Includes bibliographical references and index.
   ISBN 1-56793-061-1
   1. Nurses—Job satisfaction.   2. Index of Work Satisfaction.   3. Job enrichment.   I. Title.
   [DNLM: 1. Job Satisfaction.   2. Nursing Staff—psychology.   3. Data Collection—methods.   WY 87 S783n 1997]
   RT82.S73   1997
   610.73'06'9—dc21
   DNLM/DLC
   for Library of Congress   97-18700
                                                                              CIP

The paper used in this publication meets the minimum requirements of American National Standards for Information Sciences—Permanente of Paper for Printed Library Materials, ANSI Z39.48–1984. ∞™

Health Administration Press
A division of the Foundation of the
   American College of Healthcare Executives
One North Franklin Street
Chicago, IL 60606
312/424-2800

May the robin and the eagle fly together

CONTENTS

ACKNOWLEDGMENTS

There are always many people who provide assistance in an undertaking such as this. The list of both personal and professional acknowledgments could fill several pages. First of all, even though this second edition represents new work on the Index of Work Satisfaction, I want to remember two colleagues who provided critical assistance to the early part of the scale development process. The single major impetus for the continuation of this work came from Edward J. Rising, Professor of Industrial Engineering. As always, he was the ringleader in obtaining several grants from the National Center for Health Services Research and Development. Without this financial support, the whole line of investigation would not have continued. My colleague, the late Eugene B. Piedmonte, Associate Professor of Sociology and Associate Dean of the Graduate School, was the one who designed the first version of the IWS, including the idea of using paired comparisons to obtain information about expectations of nurses.

Special thanks go to several graduate students, each of whom made significant contributions to the early scale development phase. These include Dinah Slavitt, Howard Bond, Barry Shopnick, Pat Palmieri-Shea, and Mary Kit. Gretchen Ramirez-Sosa's dissertation led me to expand my thinking in the direction of applying this measure of satisfaction to the area of job redesign. Three other graduate students, Brad Penney, Don Allen, and Robin Bossi, provided important analytic services at various times during the early scale-development process.

Several people have been especially helpful in the continuation of the scale-development process, which has culminated in this second edition. Graduate students Alicia Doherty and Diane Scherr contributed significantly to my thought process on the relationship of satisfaction and empowerment. They both wrote master's theses that helped my progress on this project, and both shared numerous articles, saving me hours at the library. Liz Denny of Market Street Research had unfailing enthusiasm for this project beginning with our first conversation about the IWS. She provided financial support for a graduate student who assisted in the survey of users of the IWS, which is described in Chapter 4. I especially appreciate the many conversations we had while in the process of trying to "get down to business." I would also like to acknowledge the hard work and good humor of Susan Keyes, who provided enormous assistance in the survey of users of the IWS, as well as in finding so many examples of empirical research on nurse satisfaction.

Preparing this manuscript has been an awesome job. Clara Camilo remained calm and cheerful throughout, in spite of short deadlines and long pages of references. Dottie Knightly makes all the other parts of my job manageable, allowing me to concentrate on this work.

I fondly acknowledge the patience and support of my family, especially my husband Tom and daughter Jessie, both of whom heard the phrase "when my book is done" too often. A special note of thanks goes to my son Christopher, who had to give up his beloved computer far too often. I really appreciate his computer assistance, especially for the charts in Chapter 4. My family have all been supportive in many different ways, especially during the last month, when finishing this book became almost an obsession.

I want to thank all of the people using the IWS who have contacted me, either personally or by responding to the survey I sent out. The investigators using the IWS have provided me with the biggest reason for continuing to work on this scale. Their level of commitment to increasing nurse satisfaction has been an inspiration to me. If the IWS is useful, it is primarily due to these people. Some of them took the time to make a contribution to this book: I really appreciate this, and my only regret is that I could not give as much space to each one as I wanted.

Finally, I would like to acknowledge the support of Health Administration Press throughout the publication of both editions of this book. The staff were extremely supportive during the long process of completing this second edition. Their suggestions, as well as those of the external reviewers, encouraged me to consider the satisfaction of nurses from several different perspectives. Also, the Press's editorial staff enhanced the quality of this edition.

Obviously, a lot of people contributed to this project. If it is successful, they share much of the credit. As always, however, I must acknowledge my primary responsibility for this work, and hope the best for it. This second edition brings a real sense of closure to two decades of work in developing a measure for level of satisfaction for nurses that can also be used to improve communication within an organization. I hope this volume is helpful to others who wish to understand better the nurses who are such an important resource for the healthcare delivery system.

Paula L. Stamps
Amherst, Massachusetts
1997

1

A BEGINNING WORD ABOUT THIS BOOK

This second edition of *Nurses and Work Satisfaction: An Index for Measurement* presents an opportunity highly desired by anyone who has ever written anything down on a piece of paper: the chance to go back and not only make corrections, but also revise and complete previous thoughts on a topic. In this case, there are so many changes that this second edition is far more than a revision; it is more like the second volume of a continuing and evolving work. This edition was made possible by the people who have used the Index of Work Satisfaction (IWS) over the decade since the publication of the first edition. Their interest in finding a good measure for work satisfaction and their willingness to communicate their feedback—both good and bad—provided a rich and most unusual resource for someone primarily interested in developing solid quantitative measurements. My communication with these investigators involved technical matters, such as wording of scale items, scoring of both parts of the questionnaire, reversal of scoring on items, and statistical analyses of the structure of the scale. However, they have also consistently asked to be connected to others with similar research interests, or to engage in discussions related to organizational changes resulting from the use of the IWS. Because of the consistent interest of investigators using the IWS, I decided to undertake the work leading to this second edition. In this first chapter, I would like to share a bit of philosophy about measuring satisfaction and then provide an overview of this book.

A Bit of Philosophy

The first edition of this book, published in 1986, had two major goals, which have also provided general direction for this second edition. The first goal was to address a theoretical problem, the development of a statistically valid and reliable scale for use as a measure of the level of satisfaction of nurses. The second goal was to translate the scale into an information-gathering tool for managers and administrators to use in redesigning jobs or organizations so that the level of satisfaction will be improved. A decade later, pursuit of the first goal remains rare. Social scientists tend, understandably, to shy away from scale development. The initial development of the IWS took ten years, with some minor revisions suggested again here in this book based on ten years of use in the field. (The new version of the IWS appears in Appendix A.) Developing a statistically valid and reliable measurement tool is not a process that is ever complete, as will be noted time and again in this volume.

The second goal, ironically enough, is also not often accomplished. Few investigators have the inclination or time to convert a theoretical scale into an applicable one. This is perhaps because of an organizational and philosophical schism: academic researchers are more interested in scale development than in application. Managers and administrators lack the time and expertise to develop statistically valid scales. This conflict has been the framework against which much of the scale-development process occurred. One of the most rewarding aspects of doing this second edition is to see the increased integration of the academic and professional perspectives, which has strengthened the overall knowledge base in the area of nurse satisfaction.

Within the framework of these two large goals, work on the IWS was further guided by three objectives. The first was to develop a reliable and valid measurement instrument. Most of our work during the decade that led to the publication of the first edition focused on this objective, primarily because any other objectives depend on the accomplishment of this one. The second objective was related to practicality: to make the measurement instrument easy to understand and use. Initially, this required repeated revisions of both the scale and the scoring procedures. This also led to the inclusion of a standardized approach to the scoring and analysis, as well as computer instructions for scoring. This objective has received the most comments during the last ten years: it is obvious that the desire to have an easy-to-use scale was only partially met. This edition should solve remaining problems associated with applicability.

The third objective was to provide a mechanism and incentive for the measurement instrument to be used routinely for the benefit of nursing staff. This objective clearly differentiated our work from that of all others who have attempted to measure satisfaction. In some ways, of course, this is not a very academic approach. However, the group of people working on this scale always felt very strongly that, if a measure that could assess satisfaction was to be useful, it had to be able to do more than just measure satisfaction. It also had to be able to provide targeted information that managers and administrators could use to change the jobs or organizations in which nurses work. We designed the IWS to provide a mechanism by which organizations could change work environments to increase the satisfaction of the nurses (as discussed in Appendix C). Based on the use of the IWS in the field, it is obvious that a frequent use of the whole survey process has been to begin the communication process that is necessary for such redesign work. Without this emphasis, the other two objectives—having a valid and reliable measurement tool, a tool that is applicable in a wide variety of settings— would be of primarily academic importance. The instrument would have little value in the practice-based world.

It is important for those who use this scale to appreciate the ethical implications involved in a study of nurse satisfaction. The broader purpose of this scale is to facilitate communication, thereby permitting both measuring *and* changing of levels of satisfaction. As with any management tool, its success depends on the integrity and motivation of the administrators using it. This scale contains the potential for administrative manipulation to the extent that it provides insight into the needs and expectations of the nursing staff. These insights should be used to create new or changed work environments for the nursing staff. This is not only in the interest of the nursing staff; it is also in the interest of the organization. A lower turnover rate will save hospitals a great deal of money. Although the empirical documentation has been hard to develop, most research—and all intuition—suggests that improved patient care will also result.

Occupational satisfaction embraces not only the workers' adaptation to the organization, but also what their work means to them and ways in which the organization might adapt to their needs. This scale is designed to gather data on workers' expectations as well as their current level of satisfaction, so that priorities for the application of the information can be developed. Managers using the IWS gain not a generalized sense of work dissatisfaction but knowledge that can be used to create more meaningful and more satisfying jobs.

About the Book

This book is organized so that the technical information is separate from both the more application-oriented information and the conceptual framework. In this way, those who are interested in the scale-development process can find enough information, without overwhelming those who are less interested in this aspect of the instrument. The technical information is contained in three appendixes. The first, Appendix B, gives the history of the scale-development process prior to the publication of the first edition, as well as information related to the revision suggested by this current edition. Also included here are details about the structure of the IWS as a scale, including several statistical analyses done by other investigators. The second technical appendix, Appendix C, contains several important guidelines for using and interpreting the IWS. This appendix underscores some of the philosophical points discussed earlier, especially in terms of the use to be made of the information. Finally, Appendix D describes what will, I hope, solve the problems associated with scoring the IWS. As those who have used the IWS know, the measurement tool is unique in that it not only measures current level of satisfaction, but also assesses level of expectations, consistent with what most theories of motivation encourage. Although theoretically sound, this has caused the scoring to be tedious, which has somewhat decreased applicability. An important part of the work leading up to this edition (described in Chapter 4), was finding an organization that would provide technical support without affecting the easy availability of the IWS to researchers. Appendix D describes the services available from Market Street Research, located in Northampton, Massachusetts, to users of the IWS who desire this aid. This appendix also describes the new process by which investigators may gain permission to use the IWS questionnaire in their research.

The book itself begins where all academicians do: with theory. Chapter 2 of this edition, which is completely different from the theoretical chapter of the first edition, addresses the conceptual and theoretical linkages between motivation, satisfaction, and management. These relationships lead to the concept of empowerment, which is also discussed in Chapter 2. Of course, it is very tempting simply to skip the theoretical link. This is actually all too common an occurrence in empirical research. Even though nearly every published journal article contains the obligatory first paragraph discussing theory, there is frequently no link between the theory and the measurements used. The link between theory and measurement is the whole rationale for this or any chapter addressing the conceptual framework of motivation and satisfaction. Measurement is supposed to come from theories and concepts; in fact, the conceptualization process should predict the measure. Anyone who does a library search for articles on nurse satisfaction is rather quickly impressed with the sheer quantity of studies. Close examination of these studies reveals much diversity—not just in measurements, but also in conceptualization. Diversity is not in and of itself a negative thing; however, confusion of conceptual terms is not a helpful process. Chapter 2 seeks to clarify some of these terms, while at the same time examining the relationship between concepts such as satisfaction and empowerment.

Chapter 3 focuses on the empirical research that has been done on nurse satisfaction in the last ten years. These published studies all have in common the attempt to measure satisfaction: about half of them use the IWS. In comparison to the empirical literature of the early 1980s, research on nurse satisfaction in the early 1990s focused more on the role of the organization in determining the satisfaction level of the nurses. Many of the studies described here operationalize the conceptual framework of empowerment, including restructuring patient care delivery systems and redesigning organizations to be more participative. A variety of specific examples are included here, such as team nursing, primary nursing, recognition and reward programs including clinical ladders, several types of case management, as well as quality programs, including total quality management (TQM) and continuous quality improvement (CQI). Satisfaction has become a more important outcome variable, one that is increasingly being used to evaluate management innovations within organizations. Chapter 3 ends with an analysis of the types of measurements used to quantify satisfaction, with a particular focus on the IWS.

An integral part of the scale-development process has been the contact with the many researchers who are using the IWS; their comments have encouraged continued revision of the IWS. We conducted a survey of investigators using the IWS prior to the first edition. Their comments helped us revise the scale, as presented in 1986. I conducted a second survey of users as part of the work for this revision, and the results are included in Chapter 4. This survey suggested a few revisions in the IWS, which are incorporated in the form of the IWS appearing in Appendix A. The last two sections of Appendix B present the rationale for these suggested revisions. Conducting this survey has provided an opportunity to meet one of the objectives that guided the original survey of users, described in Appendix B, which involved gathering comparative data. However, the 1983 survey revealed that the use of the IWS was not sufficiently standardized for such comparative studies to be useful. One of the effects of the 1986 book was to encourage a more standardized use and scoring of the IWS, and in this second survey (conducted in 1994–95), the ability to provide comparisons is much greater. This has led to the establishment of a comparative database that will be available to investigators using the IWS. At the moment, this is a generalized database; as more data are entered, more specific comparisons will become possible, which will be much more useful. This, of course, raises several controversial issues, including whether having a database will lead to the establishment of standards for level of satisfaction of nurses. Chapter 4 concludes with a discussion of several of these issues.

There are several other outcomes of the 1994–95 survey besides the sharing of data and feedback on the IWS as a measurement tool. One of the objectives was to formalize the network of people using the IWS, so that requests for information about what others are studying can be directed to the investigators themselves. Of the 50 different investigators who responded to this survey and contributed data to the beginning database, 40 agreed to have their names and addresses, and often telephone numbers, published in this book. These people are all willing to be contacted for more information about their studies or to talk about the process of studying nurse satisfaction.

Perhaps the most rewarding part of this second edition is the opportunity to increase the dissemination of information about using the IWS to measure level of satisfaction as well as about the various types of organizational redesign initiatives occurring in the nursing field. These examples have been labeled practice-based research; and they all share common perspectives, regardless of whether the research has been conducted by an academic or a practitioner. The organizations studied do not "hold still" for the research process. Each of these practice-based research examples helps to erase the line between research and practice.

Clearly the hardest part of writing this second edition is recognizing the space constraints involved in one volume. Not all of the contributions could be included in their entirety. The practice-based research contributions can be found in three places in this book. Chapter 5 contains five examples of using the IWS in an organizational setting, either as part of an ongoing monitoring system or to evaluate an innovation in nursing practice. Appendix E contains another 15 examples, some of which evaluate organizational redesign (such as shared governance) or a change in patient care (including case management). Other examples in Appendix E provide sophisticated models designed to address the issue of nurse retention. Some focus on nurses working in rural areas, others on specific specialties in nursing. All of these are presented as research briefs, a much shortened version of the original contribution. The final collection of 20 practice-based research examples can be found in Appendix F, where the presentation is in the form of abstracts. There is a tremendous variation in this collection, with several having an organizational or management emphasis, some investigating specialties of nurses or specific settings in which nurses work, and a few using regional or national samples to obtain more general perceptions of nurses about their profession. All of these contributions were shortened, many of them considerably. In some cases, data were not included. Interested readers are urged to contact the investigators to obtain the full report of their research.

Each of these contributions is clearly practice-based, but this does not mean they lack a research orientation or have disregarded the "rules" of research. Although many have not been previously published, several have been. One of the major contributions of this edition is the presentation of so many interesting research examples, many of which are unpublished. Taken together with the published studies using the IWS— as well as other measures of satisfaction—these contributions provide several significant insights into both research and practice in nursing.

The last chapter is an attempt to summarize what has now been 20 years of working to establish a statistically validated and useful measurement tool that can be used to assess level of nurse satisfaction as well as provide guidance to the redesign of jobs and organizations in order to provide more rewarding work environments for nurses. Even though the IWS has been well received in the field, it does not mean that the revision process should stop, nor does it mean that no other measures of nurse satisfaction should be developed. As noted throughout this book, it is important to continue the process of evaluating this measurement as well as developing new measures that may better reflect the variety of practice and organizational settings in which nurses work.

The IWS has obviously contributed to the acceptance of nurse satisfaction as an important variable to add to those used to evaluate organizational innovations. Part of the impetus is the increased focus on how to help people working in hierarchical organizations be more empowered, and able to participate more fully in the decision-making process. Another part of the impetus is the increased use of techniques used to improve quality. Many of these quality assurance activities involve more teamwork between clinical providers. Also inherent in several of the quality assurance programs is the idea of gathering a few indicators around which to monitor changes. All of these systems are termed "patient-oriented;" and, although it is true that medical care should be patient-oriented, there is ample evidence that organizations and care settings should also be "nurse-oriented." Level of satisfaction of nurses remains far too low in many settings. The IWS provides an easy way to monitor satisfaction level of nurses as one of several important effects of organizational change. Improving the level of satisfaction will not only improve the working conditions of nurses but will also improve the quality of patient care. It is my hope that this book will contribute to the increasing recognition of the importance of providing professionally satisfying work environments for nurses.

CONCEPTUAL FRAMEWORK: IDENTIFYING RELATIONSHIPS BETWEEN MOTIVATION, SATISFACTION, AND MANAGEMENT

This chapter is about theory: both the relationship between motivation and satisfaction, and the relationship between work redesign and empowerment. An additional topic is the appropriate role of management. It is tempting to ignore this material, since it is often difficult to relate a theoretical focus to the practical problems of low job satisfaction of nurses. It is far more gratifying to just plunge in and measure job satisfaction. However, without an appropriate theoretical framework, the measures developed for satisfaction are not adequate. As will be seen in Chapter 3, this urge has serious consequences for the credibility of findings from empirical studies.

This chapter focuses on an examination of the relationship between motivation, satisfaction, and management in organizations. The first two sections summarize major theories of motivation, as well as several different theories of satisfaction. Although the names of the researchers and the names of the models may be the same, there are stark differences in emphasis. Motivation is related to behavior and is actually what management can affect. Satisfaction is how people feel about their jobs. Some of these theories are built on the idea that motivation leads to satisfaction, while others are based on satisfaction increasing motivation. These two sections are, by necessity, historical, since much of the theoretical research on motivation and satisfaction took place in the 1930s and 1940s.

The third section describes three models that are more organizational in perspective. Two of these depend on a systems analysis perspective. One (Newman 1989) was specifically developed for nurses, while the other (Grant 1986) was developed for other professional groups as well. The third theoretical model is empowerment, which is both a process and an end result. These three models use different terms, but share a common theme: the structure and communication process within organizations are important factors and can be changed. These three models create a much more complex picture, but one that is undoubtedly more realistic.

When organizations make changes, outcomes result: something happens. Some outcomes are behavioral, such as turnover rate, absenteeism, and other withdrawal behaviors. Some outcomes relate to the perception of satisfaction. The last section explores the relationship between satisfaction and some of these behavioral outcomes.

The major effort of this chapter is to clarify and separate the several concepts that all too often are used interchangeably. The theories do not all agree with each other. In fact, there are some very significant differences. However, of greater concern than the variation is the confusion of concepts that is all too prevalent. Clarifying the difference between the concepts will allow for more precise measures to be developed as a result of operationalizing the concepts.

It is a common mistake to confuse motivation and satisfaction, since the terms are often used interchangeably, in spite of the significant differences between them. Motivation is mainly concerned with behavior, while satisfaction is primarily concerned with how people feel. Motivation is frequently defined as needs, wants, impulses, or drives that influence people to certain behaviors or actions. In other words, motives or needs provide an explanation of why people engage in certain behaviors. Successful motivation of employees is usually related to providing appropriate goals, whose achievement will provide satisfaction (Hersey and Blanchard 1982).

The ability to achieve a goal is one of the work-related activities that produces satisfaction. When the achievement is blocked for one reason or another, dissatisfaction may occur, and frequently some sort of coping behavior related to the inability to meet the need—or to accomplish the goal—occurs (Hersey and Blanchard 1982). Coping with such inability to achieve objectives may generate a range of behaviors including poor performance, low productivity, absenteeism, and perhaps even ultimately leaving the job. It is the appearance of these negative behaviors that usually produces concern about how satisfied—or dissatisfied—employees are. At this point in time, people may talk of a "management problem" or an "employee morale" problem. The role of management in an organization is actually not to produce satisfaction, but rather to increase motivation to perform activities to reach a goal and to ensure that resources are available for employees to be able to meet their work-related goals.

Theories of Motivation

There are several distinct theories of motivation and a variety of ways to organize or categorize them. The traditional way is to describe three general groupings of theories (Cherrington 1982). The first includes what are termed "needs" theories, emphasizing internal causes of behavior. These theories have in common an understanding that each individual has a set of needs, and that the goal of each person is to satisfy these needs. Perhaps the most commonly cited example of this arises from Maslow's work (Maslow 1954). The second category of motivation theories is based on what are termed reinforcement theories, concentrating on those external factors that influence behavior. This group of theories focuses on the relative advantages and disadvantages of positive reinforcement strategies or negative reinforcement strategies—rewards and punishments. The third category is usually termed expectancy theories; these place heavy emphasis on individual perceptions and expectations in a particular situation.

An alternative classification of motivation theories presented by Rakich, Longest, and Darr (1985) is more useful when the primary interest is in analyzing the relationship between motivation and satisfaction. They describe two categories of motivation theories: content theories and process theories. Content theories focus on what motivates behavior, regardless of whether the variables are within the individual or within the organization. Process theories concentrate more on how such behavior may be either initiated or sustained through organizational action or intervention.

Content Theories

The content theories are those that are viewed as the classical motivation paradigms, and one of the most well recognized is that of Taylor, who is usually referred to as the founder of so-called "scientific management." His 1911 work *The Principles of Scientific Management* was based on the assumption that individuals would be motivated to do their work well if rewards were directly related to their performance of carefully planned tasks (Taylor 1911). Taylor further believed that the primary motivator for people was economic, which led him to consider money as the only meaningful reward. Taylor's legacy still significantly affects the management field, despite the fact that several of his assumptions are explicitly questioned today.

The questioning of money as the primary motivator began formally in 1954 with Maslow, who suggested that behavior is governed by a hierarchy of needs, each of which becomes a motivator as lower-level needs are met (Maslow 1954). Maslow's needs hierarchy began with physiological needs, which he viewed as the lowest-level needs, and worked up a hierarchy to include safety and security, affection and social activity, esteem and status, and finally self-actualization, which is expressed as fulfillment. It was Maslow who first introduced the notion of the relationship of motivation and satisfaction by indicating that, once a lower-level need was "satisfied," a higher-level need then became dominant. Maslow also was the first to suggest that most people are both partially satisfied and dissatisfied in all these basic needs at the same time (Maslow 1964).

Maslow's work has been extremely influential in directing research in motivation and satisfaction. McClelland (1961) modified Maslow's basic work by suggesting that people are motivated by only three types of needs: achievement, power, and affiliation. The most significant modification of Maslow's work came from Herzberg, Mausner, and Snyderman (1959), who drew the two concepts of motivation and satisfaction closer together. They suggested that people have only two basic sets of needs, and that one set of needs produces satisfaction while the other set of needs produces dissatisfaction. Those factors that lead to dissatisfaction are termed hygiene (or more commonly today maintenance) factors, since they are viewed as being necessary to maintaining a reasonable level of satisfaction. Although managers view many of these factors (such as organizational policy, technical supervision, salary, and job security) as motivators, Herzberg, Mausner, and Snyderman view them as being more potent in providing dissatisfaction when absent. Those factors that are viewed as satisfiers or providing motivation include achievement, recognition, and responsibility. If these conditions are not present, they are not necessarily dissatisfiers.

Both Maslow's model and Herzberg's model emphasize the same set of relationships. They focus on the individual or situational factors motivating behavior. Maslow tends to emphasize individual needs while Herzberg focuses more on how job conditions affect a person's motivation, thus implying that motivation is derived from work itself. By focusing on what motivates people, both Maslow and Herzberg models are classified as content theories. An alternative perspective is to focus on how to initiate the desired behavior. Two process theories of motivation address this.

Process Theories

An alternative to theories that focus on individuals are those that emphasize the organizational process by which a person's motivation may be initiated or sustained. The first of these two process theories is often called the expectancy model, which postulates that people are motivated to perform well at work if they believe (or expect) they will be rewarded. In developing this model, Vroom (1964) described the two major parts of this motivation theory as preference and expectancy. A preference refers to an outcome that a person experiences as a result of a behavior. This outcome may be positive or negative. An expectancy is the individual's belief or expectation that a certain behavior will produce a desired outcome. A person with a preference for an outcome must feel that it can be achieved by doing certain activities. Vroom's model explains motivation as a function of an individual's perception of preference and expectations.

Porter and Lawler (1968) developed a more comprehensive view of preferences and expectations. They built their motivation model around the notion that people are motivated by future expectations that are based on previous experience and influenced by several variables, including personality and skills. This model explicitly includes the concept of satisfaction, by suggesting that performance in the job is what causes satisfaction. This view differs from others (including Maslow's) that postulate that high levels of satisfaction cause better job performance. This distinction is important since, in one theoretical model, satisfaction is a dependent variable, and in the other model, satisfaction is an independent variable.

Theories of Satisfaction

Job satisfaction is deceptively easy to describe, since the most common definition (even in textbooks) is simply the extent to which employees like their jobs (Rakich, Longest, and Darr 1985; Schmermerhorn 1984). Left unexplored in this definition are several significant issues including the notion that jobs have a variety of components that may be quite distinct and an individual may like one part more than another. Other important issues are whether absence of satisfaction means dissatisfaction, and whether satisfaction is related to performance or productivity. Of course, all of these questions are the ones that are of most interest to those trying to measure satisfaction. Before such measurement takes place, however, it is important to understand the theory of satisfaction. Although there are many theories, there are four that are most important: Maslow's, Herzberg's Dual-Factor Theory, two models within the need fulfillment theory, and the social reference group or equity theory. These are all also motivation theories, which were described in the previous section. This section will focus on the concept of satisfaction, rather than motivation.

Maslow (1964), whose hierarchy of needs is probably the best known of all motivation theories, views satisfaction as an important variable but only in the sense of motivation. For Maslow, when a need becomes satisfied it is no longer a motivator (i.e., people are motivated by what they are seeking, not by what they have). So, in Maslow's view, dissatisfaction is actually a more powerful motivator than satisfaction.

Herzberg's *Dual-Factor Theory of Job Satisfaction and Motivation* is much more specific about the relationship between satisfaction and motivation (House and Wigdor 1967). Herzberg suggested ten factors that act specifically as dissatisfiers or demotivators. These include: organizational policy and administration; technical supervision; interpersonal relations with supervisors, peers, and subordinates; salary; job security; personal life; work conditions; and status. He identified six factors as being satisfiers or motivators, including achievement, recognition, advancement, the nature of the work itself, the potential for growth, and responsibility. Herzberg's view is that these latter six factors contribute to job satisfaction; if they are not present, they are not strong dissatisfiers. However, the absence of the ten previous factors contribute significantly to job dissatisfaction (Rakich, Longest, and Darr 1985; Herzberg, Mausner, and Snyderman 1959; House and Wigdor 1967). Also, Herzberg suggested that a person may be both satisfied and dissatisfied with a work situation at the same time, although he theorized that dissatisfaction is more related to the characteristics of the job itself (Herzberg, Mausner, and Snyderman 1959).

Unlike Maslow, Herzberg views satisfaction and motivation as arising primarily from the work itself. Maslow views satisfaction as arising not just from work but also from other parts of one's life. Later theorists enlarged this thought, as will be seen in the next section. Herzberg's Dual-Factor Theory has been extensively criticized, perhaps because of the unique way in which he views satisfaction and dissatisfaction.

A major theory of job satisfaction may be categorized under the rubric of *need fulfillment*, which actually encompasses Vroom's theory of motivation, but also very nicely accommodates Maslow's ideas. This need-fulfillment theory of job satisfaction is a broad theoretical perspective that indicates that work satisfaction is a function of the degree to which a person's needs are met in the work situation (Korman 1971). The greater the need, the more satisfied the person when it is fulfilled; and if it is a great need, dissatisfaction will result from its being unfulfilled. There are two distinct subtypes within this need-fulfillment theory: the discrepancy or the subtractive model and the multiplicative model. The discrepancy or subtractive model modifies the ideas represented by need fulfillment by noting that work satisfaction represents the difference between what an individual needs and the extent to which the work environment fulfills those needs. This model views work satisfaction as the difference between the actual amount of outcome and the desired amount of outcome divided by the desired amount, with outcome being some aspect of work, such as pay or autonomy (Porter and Lawler 1968). The assumption here is that, the more workers want a particular outcome, the more dissatisfied they are with increasing discrepancy between desired and actual amounts of that outcome.

The discrepancy or subtractive model is unable to distinguish adequately between various nuances of work satisfaction. It does not consider the value placed on these expectations. Thus, although the discrepancy theory takes account of these expectations, it does not attempt to weight them differentially. Some further refinements pursue this point but are not frequently used.

An alternative to the discrepancy model is the multiplicative model, a variation on the theory developed by Vroom. The multiplicative model hypothesizes that an individual's work satisfaction is a product of the relative importance or weightings of various work-related and personal needs. Therefore, the degree to which the current job fulfills those needs is a measurement of satisfaction, and the sum of these products is a measure of the level of work satisfaction (Vroom 1964). This approach makes the important modification that work satisfaction cannot be taken as a totally separate factor from other, extra-work personal contributors to satisfaction. Although this model assigns weights for components of work satisfaction, it neglects the perceptions of satisfaction of other workers in similar situations. The importance of this comparison with peer groups is stressed in a separate theory of job satisfaction, the social reference group theory.

Sometimes known as the equity theory, social reference group theory arises from criticisms of the need-fulfillment theory. It holds that work satisfaction is a function of—or is at least positively related to—the characteristics of the job that meet the desires of those groups to which a worker looks for guidance in evaluating his or her own reality (Korman 1971). Social reference group theory significantly departs from the need-fulfillment theory because it stresses the importance of what other people feel in shaping the individual's stated needs. Philosophically, the theory means that persons can only measure their satisfaction when compared to their peer group.

Adams (1973) maintains work satisfaction is "determined by the perceived ratio of what a person receives from his job relative to what a person puts into his job." He notes that this ratio, computed internally, is dependent on how a person judges the satisfaction that others in the same or similar work situations are receiving. Thus, this theory sees satisfaction as a function of the magnitude of the discrepancy between the real and expected outcomes—like the previous theory—but adds two notions of how this process works: (1) the expected outcomes are determined by comparing one's work and rewards to others doing a similar job, and (2) it recognizes that dissatisfaction may be caused both by overrewarding and underrewarding. Overrewarding may bring out feelings of guilt; underrewarding may lead to feelings of unfair treatment. This theory makes a step forward in trying to state how a worker evaluates his or her situation as satisfying or dissatisfying, and also reveals some of the complexity of the notion of work satisfaction.

Organizational Theories and Empowerment

Most of the traditional theoretical views of motivation and job satisfaction focus on the work itself, usually on the specific job, rather than on the person. Those that include individual differences do so in terms of accomplishing a job. The role of a manager is to control or change a job to increase performance or productivity. Although this makes for a narrower and simpler theoretical understanding, it clearly does not fit the personal experience of all of us as workers. Satisfaction with work and even motivation to work may lie outside the work environment and may involve factors over which managers have no control. Coupled with the view that satisfaction may be significantly affected by factors external to the work setting is the view that satisfaction of an individual may also be influenced by organizational factors that may not have a direct relationship to the specific job itself. Including both organizational factors and factors external to the work setting creates a much more complex—but also more realistic—model. Two such models are especially appropriate to the health field.

Newman's Systems Model

The first model uses a systems perspective. This views the organization as one system with resources as inputs, and achievement of objectives as the outputs. This perspective is generally used with organizations as the model of analysis and is frequently used to evaluate organizations. Newman (1989; Chesnis 1990) describes a systems model that is specific to nursing personnel. The model centers on the nurse, identifying a variety of factors as being part of what he or she terms the core structure, including physical aspects (health, physical stamina), psychological aspects (ego strength, role perceptions, individual attitudes), sociocultural aspects (ethnicity, cultural background, age, sex), developmental aspects (specialty, board certification, length of professional experience), and spiritual aspects.

The second component is the client system, which is an open system interacting with both the environment and the nurse. This client system is conceptualized as lines of defenses, all of which protect the integrity of the nurse and all of which are dependent on job satisfaction. The utmost level is a "flexible line of defense" that expands and contracts depending on the job satisfaction of the nurse. It expands as job satisfaction increases; as satisfaction increases, the nurse has less need for protection from the client system as it interacts with the nurse core system. This level can be equated with the highest of Maslow's needs, self-actualization. A protective line of defense is related to a moderate level of job satisfaction, similar to the middle level of Maslow's hierarchy. The innermost line of defense is activated by extreme dissatisfaction. Behaviors related to this include increased physical symptomatology that may cause absenteeism, leaving the job, or some decreased quality of care, a syndrome generally labeled as burnout.

The environment of the system includes internal and external stresses that affect the nurse. These stresses may arise from the clients, from the job (internal stress), or from outside the work setting (environmental or external). Three ways of mediating these stresses are conceptualized as three levels of prevention, all of which involve some type of management intervention. The point of this model is to consider the nurse as the center of a system with many pressures brought to bear. The pressures frequently are from patients, with subsequent "lines of defense" that are directly related to job satisfaction. Other pressures are related to the work environment, some of which can be mediated by management and some of which cannot be very successfully mediated by management. The key to this model, based on an open systems theory, is that equilibrium of the nurse needs to be maintained. In this model, job satisfaction is critical and may be significantly affected by the patient or by the organization.

Exchange Flow System

Grant (1986) has developed a second alternative framework, one that involves yet another variation of a systems perspective, a flow process model specifically designed for management of employees for the purpose of improving job performance. The core concept on which this model is based is that employment is an exchange process, with both the employee and the organization having needs and providing contributions. The model is deceptively simple. It starts with designing both the work system and the reward structure and training or developing appropriate staff. The model uses several important and unusual control feedback mechanisms based on performance. These control mechanisms recognize the importance of managing rewards as well as individuals. One of the unusual features of this approach is where motivation and satisfaction fit in. It is postulated that the several factors which affect performance (the working conditions, the nature of the organization, the person's life outside of the organization, the degree of organizational decentralization) affect performance *through* employee satisfaction. This is termed an Effort–Net Return (ENR) model of motivation and satisfaction.

One very important part of the ENR model is the understanding that motivation and satisfaction of employees are not just functions of the job goal system, but that systems that are completely outside of the work environment frequently play an important role. Since an individual is viewed as one who strives to maximize total aggregate satisfaction, the satisfaction gained from outside the work environment must also be included in the analysis. Because of consideration of aggregate satisfaction from all sources, this model assumes that individuals have multiple goals to which they devote effort and energy and that some of these goals lie outside the organization and thus outside the domain of work. Therefore, this model indicates that how satisfied people are with their jobs has nothing to do with motivation, except in terms of their motive to achieve all the goals in their life, both work and nonwork goals. In this model, satisfaction (or dissatisfaction) becomes a variable to manipulate, since it is recognized to cause certain negative behaviors including employee turnover, absenteeism, and alcoholism.

This particular model reevaluates motivation, satisfaction, and the role of managers in ways that are particularly appropriate to the health field. Grant (1986) points out the existence of several "myths" about motivation that permeate academic literature, including management, the first of which is that high levels of motivation lead to increased productivity. This is one of those statements that intuitively seems to be true, but which cannot be empirically documented. Related to this is the notion that managers should always strive to maximize motivation. In fact, there can be too highly motivated a worker, whose efforts may or may not be in line with the needs and goals of the organization. High levels of motivation will produce higher levels of effort, but the result may be increased frustration rather than increased productivity. Maximizing motivation frequently involves a trade-off with satisfaction: a highly motivated, hard-working person may have very low satisfaction. In fact, this is often the situation that leads to burnout: high levels of effort that do not always produce the organizational response the worker desires.

Another accepted notion is that a "happy" worker is more motivated, and the corollary to this is that motivation is inherent within a person. This confuses satisfaction and motivation. Motivation produces high effort on a job. If the effort is rewarded and thus viewed by the organization as appropriate, satisfaction may result. However, satisfaction also arises from many factors outside the job. Satisfaction produces a different set of behaviors than does motivation. Satisfied workers are absent less often, submit grievances less often, and leave their jobs less often.

Managers are not trained to believe that motivation is something that is inherent: to believe this is to question a central role of management, which is to provide motivation through rewards. But the topic of rewards is problematic, since a whole set of expectations exist with respect to rewards, some of which are conflicting. One myth is that greater rewards cause greater motivation. Although it is clear that rewards do motivate, the ability of a reward to motivate is actually highly dependent on the necessary effort. The economic principle of declining marginal utility operates here. For many professionals, the trade-off of money and leisure time is such that increased rewards do not induce more time at work. The common assumption is that the most obvious reward is money. Although money obviously matters, it is not the best motivator. Other factors that affect motivation more include job security, interesting and challenging work, and status, as well as good relationships with supervisors and coworkers. The value of money as a motivator is partially dependent on the workers' view of the adequacy of their income and the negative trade-offs in their personal lives that more income from work may cause.

This line of thinking encourages reflection about the nature of work and whether it is inherently distasteful or undesirable, which is a common view of both workers and managers in U.S. society. There is really nothing to indicate that work is inherently undesirable and much to indicate the opposite. Grant (1986) feels that it is the design of the work system that makes work unsatisfying, as do those who do research in empowerment. In fact, people can and do derive satisfaction from their jobs. Several factors affect this degree of satisfaction, one of which is the way in which the work itself is designed. Other factors include the physical conditions in which the work is carried out, and the social conditions within the organization. The social system of an organization seems to be a strong determinant of employee satisfaction. An important facet of this social system is organizational communication, both within similar levels of employees and between the hierarchies within organizations. As will be seen in the next section, increasing communication is a central value in the empowerment model.

Empowerment

Many of the same themes evident in the conceptual framework of these two systems theories are found in the empowerment literature. The term "empowerment" has many definitions. Webster's dictionary definition includes "to give official authority to." Steiner uses the phrase "earned autonomy based on consistent contributions as a situational leader, for the good of the employee, the customer, and the organization" (McGraw 1992). Although delegation of authority is clearly implied in these definitions, empowerment is conceptualized as more than delegation. Tebbitt (1993) articulates five conceptual components of empowerment, most of which focus on the organization, including the necessity of a cultural change process involving the mission and basic values of the organization.

The concept of empowerment addresses the balance of power in organizations. Unlike more traditional ways of viewing power, this concept as described by Kanter (1977) views power in organizations as being derived from the structure of organizations, both formally and informally. The formal sources of power include jobs that are visible and central to the major purpose of the organization. Informal power arises from the alliances made by people within the organization. These informal alliances are instrumental in enabling individuals to get the cooperation they need to get things done, which further enhances their power (Laschinger 1996).

Empowerment is often described as enabling. The process of enabling is directed at gaining more access to power. This implies that individuals and groups are enabled to participate in decision making within an organizational context that will support a more equitable distribution of power. This concept is consistent with current feminist theory and is especially relevant to the nursing profession (Mason, Backer, and Georges 1991).

Although there is much literature today on empowerment, it is important to note that this is not a new theory. Much of the theory as used today arises from Kanter's 1977 book entitled *Men and Women of the Corporation*. Her development of this theory owes much to Freire, whose 1970 work is also used as the basis of community development work. Even though the theory of empowerment is a critique of prevalent management practices, there are many references to the ideas of empowerment sprinkled throughout management literature. For example, in 1968 Tannenbaum did an analysis of power and control in organizations that concluded with the observation that organizational effectiveness and productivity increased as supervisors shared power with others within the organization (Conger and Kanungo 1988). Research in leadership and team building in the 1960s includes many references to what is termed empowerment today (Conger and Kanungo 1988). Most of the work in the 1960s was derived from Maslow's hierarchy of needs, first developed in 1954 (Maslow 1970). Maslow's highest need is self-actualization or "becoming what one is capable of becoming." This is analogous to being empowered. Maslow's lower-level needs are analogous to the necessary organizational support required for the empowerment process to be realized (McGraw 1992).

This is not to diminish this current line of research. If anything, the consistent expression of the concept strengthens the importance of continuing to address the question of why employees in organizations feel so "un-empowered." This question is particularly appropriate to the nursing profession, especially those nurses that work within the hospital setting. Hospitals are among the most hierarchical of all organizations. Nurses are skilled professionals whose knowledge base is absolutely critical to the ability of the hospital to provide care for patients. Yet, the absence of nurses being involved in the running of hospitals has been well documented by the Institute of Medicine (1983), the National Commission on Nursing (1983), the American Academy of Nursing's study of magnet hospitals (1983), and the report of the Secretary's Commission on Nursing (U.S. Department of Health and Human Services 1988). Not only are nurses noticeably absent from the power structure of the hospital, very frequently the organizational structure dictates the way nursing care is delivered. Stillwaggon's (1989) brief but pointed historical analysis of nursing patterns concluded that a specific nursing care delivery system was related more to the prevalent management theories of a given era than any other variable. Despite the many changes in nursing care practices throughout the century, the bureaucratic structure of the hospital has remained basically unchanged (Stillwaggon 1989).

Empowerment is clearly related to management, management style, and especially communication patterns within organizations. The theory of empowerment provides strong reinforcement of the notion of the leader rather than the manager being effective in motivating people to work at their highest level. Although this is not a new idea by any means, the more recent nursing management books provide strong emphasis for the importance of nursing managers being leaders rather than managers (Tappen 1995). Of course, having the nurse supervisor be an effective leader does not necessarily affect the rest of the organization. Much of the current research emphasizes the necessity of including the whole organization in an empowerment process (Conger and Kanungo 1988; Laschinger 1996; McGraw 1992; Schmieding 1993; Tebbitt 1993). Since the process is about equitable distribution of power within the whole organization, the entire hospital structure must be involved.

This process requires some way to operationalize the concept of empowerment. Since the concept of empowerment is itself fuzzy, it should not be surprising that some of the initiatives may seem to fall short of the conceptual expectations. After all, most of the efforts are occurring in hospitals, an overwhelmingly hierarchical organizational setting. Almost all of the efforts involve delegation of authority, which has led many people to equate delegation of authority to the empowerment process. Among the many who note that delegation is not empowerment, Tebbitt (1993) is most direct, as she talks about the need for change to be included in all levels of the organization.

One of the most common ways to operationalize empowerment is the concept of participative management. Although there are many ways to institute participative management, shared governance is a very common approach. This involves nurses becoming involved in the management structure of the hospital, including policy development and decision making (Jenkins 1991; Mason, Backer, and Georges 1991; Schmieding 1993). Shared governance is concerned with effective communication, and especially with the need for communication patterns to be established between the higher levels of the organization and the middle and lower levels. Communication is recognized as a primary way of maintaining power within organizations (Heinzelman 1994; Schmieding 1993). This is an example of an innovation that has strong historical roots in theory, but only recently have there been many serious attempts actually to implement shared decision making (Allen, Calkin, and Peterson 1988).

Another common way to operationalize empowerment is to restructure patient care delivery systems. Some of the more popular methods include team nursing, primary nursing, and case management. Team nursing originally developed as a way to cope with nursing shortages, but it also seemed to increase the perception of autonomy of nurses. Primary nursing is a more common way of achieving this autonomy in the current environment. Case management is another way in which hospitals attempt to operationalize empowerment. Primary nursing and case management are complementary; there are many examples of these innovations being combined (Coulter et al. 1995).

Recognition and reward programs are strategies traditionally used to improve both performance and productivity. These involve many different types of rewards, including pay. However, in order to be considered a method of empowerment, such programs must also involve some other recognition. A very typical one is the use of clinical ladders, a way in which nurses may advance within the organization, either in management or in clinical practice. Clinical ladders are an example of a method that is arguable in terms of achieving empowerment. The effect of the recognition process is generally on only a few nurses, and they are frequently those who have indicated interest. There is little effect on the whole organization, and there is generally little or no effect on distribution of power in an organization.

Another innovation that is more frequently being used in an attempt to operationalize empowerment is that of TQM. This model has been successful in other industries, and is increasingly being applied to the health field. TQM is an organized and integrated system of continuous quality improvement that is aimed at meeting the needs of the consumers. Although the system is clearly oriented toward consumer satisfaction and increased productivity, implementation of a TQM model involves a transformation of the whole organization. This model relies on teamwork that also involves shared decision making. Inherent in the process is the increased communication throughout all levels of an organization. Like Tebbitt (1993), who refers to the necessity of a "cultural change" within an organization, TQM requires a "cultural transformation of the entire organization with changing beliefs, attitudes, and behaviors" (Zonsius and Murphy 1995). Instituting TQM programs requires a commitment of higher-level administrators and managers to sharing decision making and power within an organization (Johnson 1993; Matherly and Lasater 1992; Zonsius and Murphy 1995). Because of this, TQM is conceptually closer to the empowerment principle than are either clinical ladder programs or any other programs that emphasize redesigning the job without also addressing the distribution of power in the organization.

Sometimes language, which is meant to clarify, instead confuses important issues. Some of the conceptual research in this area uses the term job or work "redesign" in conjunction with the word empowerment, and often indicates that one way to achieve empowerment is through the redesign of work. Work redesign itself has a long history that draws on theories from several academic disciplines, including management, engineering, psychology, sociology, and economics. One of the most helpful ways of incorporating these various perspectives is by using the systems analysis model detailed in the previous section and work redesign efforts often do this. By using this analytic approach, both of two important levels of implementation inherent in work redesign can be addressed.

The first redesign level is a macro orientation, which involves restructuring the entire organization to improve productivity and quality. Using this perspective, redesigning the nursing care delivery system may take place in the context of addressing the necessary organizational changes. Dienemann and Gessner (1992) describe a model that includes all management and professional groups in an effort to create an environment in which professionals can make autonomous decisions within some explicit parameters. Dienemann and Gessner also include TQM as another way of restructuring the whole system or working at this macro level. Several other models of system redesign are evident in the literature. Often, some form of case management will be used, with the most common examples being in the New England Medical Center, Sharp Medical Center, Tucson Medical Center, and the Robert Wood Johnson University Hospital (Redman and Ketefian 1995). The common theme in all of these specific examples is the necessity of involving the whole organization. Even when the emphasis is on individuals, restructuring efforts will only be successful when all levels of the organization are involved. When the whole organization is included, this meets the conceptual definition of empowerment.

A micro approach involves a focus that is specific to a particular job or one unit. This is more likely to be a bottom-up approach, where one particular job is redesigned to increase productivity. Sometimes, this is termed job enrichment, especially if the person is given the opportunity to use additional skills in their job. Although the micro level recognizes the importance of the commitment of the larger organization to any particular redesign effort, the major emphasis is on making a particular job more interesting. Clinical ladders are an especially good example of this approach to job redesign, but primary nursing and even shared governance (Davis 1992) may fall under this approach if the orientation is on one particular job or one particular unit within a hospital rather than the whole hospital. Unit-based approaches are the most common of the empowerment innovations within hospital nursing (Havens and Mills 1992). Unit-based innovations that do not also involve the redistribution of power within the organization do not meet the conceptual definition of empowerment.

There are several different models of work redesign or work reengineering, as it is sometimes called. Some of these models emphasize the work that needs to be done, others emphasize the structure of a specific job, while others focus on the structure of either a unit or an organization in which the job is located. It is beyond the scope of this chapter to describe all the variations, although there are many good analyses available, including identification of factors that are common to work redesign projects that have succeeded as well as those that have failed (Brown 1995; Kelly 1995). One important insight to remember is that each of the different concepts will suggest different strategies for work redesign.

Some of these strategies will encourage the empowerment process, while some will not have much influence on the distribution of power within an organization. It is important to look behind the language and analyze the actual implementation of a specific strategy. For example, many of these strategies delegate responsibility, but not all also delegate authority or decision-making power.

Regardless of the concept or the particular implementation of a re-design strategy, one theme is common. Empowerment, or work redesign, is supposed to have an effect on the nursing staff. By far the single most common effect either mentioned or measured is level of satisfaction. There are a variety of other effects noted, including increased retention, decreased absenteeism, increased productivity, and improved patient out-comes. All of these seem to be related to increased satisfaction. In fact, within this empowerment literature, there is considerable confusion of terms and concepts. Frequently, an empowered worker is referred to as a satisfied worker. In fact, this may or may not be true: not all workers want power within an organization. As shown in the previous sections, it is important to differentiate carefully between the relevant concepts, including motivation, satisfaction, and empowerment.

The collection of articles that might be labeled the "empowerment literature" demonstrates the same conclusion as Grant (1986) and New-man (1989): organizations can manage the work environment in such a way as to produce certain outcomes or effects. Some of these effects are a perception of being more satisfied with a particular job. For some people, this will be due to feeling empowered; for others, it may be due to having a very clearly defined job responsibility or having enough scheduling freedom to attend to personal matters. How this level of satisfaction then translates into behavior is complicated. This is the subject of the next section.

Satisfaction and Behavioral Outcomes

Definitive theories of work satisfaction have been elusive because of the complexity of determining what makes workers happy or unhappy. As discussed in the first section of this chapter, the earliest studies con-centrated on individuals' psychological needs, and behavioral outcomes were given insufficient attention, except for those studies that focused on productivity. Most of the empirical attempts to link work satisfaction with productivity are neither consistent nor conclusive. A stronger rela-tionship seems to exist between dissatisfaction and absenteeism, turnover rate, and accidents, all of which are more likely to be included in studies as behavioral outcomes instead of productivity. Both absenteeism and turnover rate reduce organizational effectiveness and, although both are related to satisfaction, the direction and nature of the relationship is not always clear. As will be seen in the next chapter, a lot of empirical research has focused on the relationship between these distancing behaviors and satisfaction.

The link between productivity or performance and job satisfaction (or motivation) remains strongly felt, but also without consistent empirical documentation. Both productivity and performance are obviously of central concern for the health field. An especially catchy management concept is the notion of managing for productivity, or managing for job performance, which can easily be seen in several management textbooks (Schmermerhorn 1984; Grant 1986).

One of the central problems, of course, is understanding satisfaction. By some theoretical models, including Maslow's (1954), high levels of satisfaction are likely to result in high levels of performance. Other theoretical models, including Porter and Lawler's (1968), indicate that it is job performance that is a significant cause of satisfaction. And, of course, other theoreticians (Taylor in 1911 and Vroom in 1964) argue that appropriate rewards can improve both job performance and job satisfaction (Cherrington 1982). Grant (1986) notes that these notions are all far too simplistic, when arguing that his exchange model is more appropriate by recognizing that an individual strives to maximize aggregate satisfaction arising from within the job and outside the job in exchange for a certain amount of effort. For Grant, satisfaction has little to do with motivation and thus, not much to do with performance. Satisfaction has a big effect on employee behaviors such as turnover, absenteeism, and grievances, however.

The supposed relationship between satisfaction and performance has always been suggested, even in the face of conflicting results from empirical studies. A review of the theoretical and applied literature from both a sociological and management perspective suggests three conclusions are evident. The first conclusion is that one major problem is a failure to be attentive to the appropriate theoretical framework. It is important to separate motivation and satisfaction. Motivation seems to produce what are interpreted as more positive job-related behaviors, including performance and productivity. It seems that motivation can be improved with appropriately designed rewards. Much of managerial activity can be seen to lie in this arena.

Job satisfaction, however, is a separate phenomenon. At one level, it may be viewed as an outcome of being able to be successful in acting in accordance with one's motivation. In this sense, satisfaction arises not from performance of the job as such, but from the ability to have a need or motive satisfied. Satisfaction is not independent of job performance, but it is not primarily dependent on performance. At another level, satisfaction could be viewed as Grant (1986) views it: this feeling is complicated and arises from many sources in our lives, some of which are job related and some of which are not. In this view, any individual tries to maximize all possible sources of satisfaction, both those arising from within the job and those arising from outside the job. In some situations, and these are probably more frequent than any manager wants to admit, employees maximize their total satisfaction by lessening their time at work, a behavior that may well decrease performance and productivity.

The second conclusion is that it is far easier to see and recognize the behaviors related to low levels of satisfaction than those related to high levels. This strongly supports the conceptualization of satisfaction put forward by Herzberg, Mausner, and Snyderman (1959), which indicates that satisfaction and dissatisfaction are two distinct factors. Herzberg's analysis even noted that some job-related factors produce satisfaction while others produce dissatisfaction. Those factors that produce satisfaction include motivation; achievement, recognition, and opportunities for advancement; the work itself; and level of responsibility. Those factors that he described as dissatisfying are more closely related to what we recognize as part of management or administration of the job. These include organizational policy and administration; supervision; personal relationships with supervisors, peers, and subordinates; salary, security, work conditions, and status. Herzberg even included in this group the "personal life," an inclusion that was far before his time, in light of the fact that most contemporary theoreticians failed to recognize any factors outside of the work environment.

It is true that, when conceptualizing satisfaction, we think mostly of behaviors associated with dissatisfaction, and much of the research in this area supports this notion. Low levels of satisfaction seem to produce behaviors that are costly for organizations to cope with, both in personal terms and in economic terms. As only one example, high rates of absenteeism and turnover are considered to be strongly related to low levels of satisfaction.

This chapter has focused on clarifying the theoretical understanding of motivation and satisfaction as well as differentiating between empowerment and work redesign. The role of management has also been addressed from a theoretical level. However, satisfaction levels of workers in organizations, including health and human services organizations, is a practical problem as well as a theoretical problem, which requires making a transition from theory to practice. So, the third conclusion that arises from this review of the management, sociological, and psychological literature is that everybody wants to measure either satisfaction or dissatisfaction. It doesn't matter whether one is working within the conceptual model of empowerment or motivation, or Newman's (1989) systems approach. The primary variable of interest is level of satisfaction. As a variable, satisfaction may be conceptualized as being independent or dependent. In some of these theoretical models it has everything to do with performance, and in others it has nothing to do with performance. However, regardless of how it is conceptualized, some type of measurement is needed. The measurement should be rooted in the appropriate theoretical framework and should be accurate and valid, but also must be simple enough to use in organizations. The next chapter makes this transition from theory to practice by considering results from those studies that have measured satisfaction, as well as addressing several problems in trying to measure satisfaction.

References

Adams, J. S. 1973. "Toward an Understanding of Inequity." In *Motivation in Work Organizations*, edited by E. E. Lawler, 127. Los Angeles, CA: Brooks/Cole.

Allen, D., J. Calkin, and M. Peterson. 1988. "Making Shared Governance Work: A Conceptual Model." *Journal of Nursing Administration* 18: 37–41.

American Academy of Nursing. 1983. *Magnet Hospitals: Attraction and Retention of Professional Nurses*. Kansas City, MO: American Nurses Association.

Brown, C. L. 1995. "Successful and 'Failed' Work Redesign Projects: Illuminating the Creative Tension." In *Health Care Work Redesign*, edited by K. Kelly. Series on Nursing Administration. Thousand Oaks, CA: Sage.

Cherrington, D. J. 1982. *Personal Management: The Management of Human Resources*. Dubuque, IA: W. M. L. Brown.

Chesnis, R. M. R. 1990. "How Does Leadership Behavior Affect Job Satisfaction of Subordinates?" Master's thesis, Anna Maria College, Paxton, MA.

Conger, J. A., and R. N. Kanungo. 1988. "The Empowerment Process: Integrating Theory and Practice." *Academy of Management Review* 13: 471–82.

Coulter, S. J., C. A. Wind, C. Miller, and L. J. Lewicki. 1995. "Nursing Case Management to Achieve Integrated Clinical Expertise and Improved Resource Utilization." In *Health Care Work Redesign*, edited by K. Kelly. Series on Nursing Administration. Thousand Oaks, CA: Sage.

Davis, P. A. 1992. "Unit-Based Shared Governance: Nurturing the Vision." *Journal of Nursing Administration* 22: 46–50.

Dienemann, J., and T. Gessner. 1992. "Restructuring Nursing Care Delivery Systems." *Nursing Economic$* 10: 253–58.

Freire, P. 1970. *Pedagogy of the Oppressed*. New York: Continuum.

Grant, P. 1986. *The Performance Management Process: An Integrative Approach to Human Resource Management*. Dubuque, IA: Kendall/Hunt.

Havens, D. S., and M. E. Mills. 1992. "Staff Nurse Empowerment: Current Status and Future Projections." *Nursing Administration Quarterly* 16: 65–71.

Heinzelman, S. 1994. "Collaborative Management: Revitalizing an OR." *Nursing Management* 25: 48F–48H.

Hersey, P., and K. H. Blanchard. 1982. *Management of Organizational Behavior: Utilizing Human Resources*, 4th ed. Englewood Cliffs, NJ: Prentice-Hall.

Herzberg, F., B. Mausner, and B. Snyderman. 1959. *The Motivation to Work*, 2nd ed. New York: John Wiley and Sons.

House, R. J., and L. A. Wigdor. 1967. "Herzberg's Dual-Factor Theory of Job Satisfaction and Motivation: A Review of the Evidence and a Criticism." *Personnel Psychology* 20: 13, 20.

Institute of Medicine. 1983. *Nursing and Nursing Education: Public Policies and Private Actions*. Washington, DC: National Academy Press.

Jenkins, J. E. 1991. "Professional Governance: The Missing Link." *Nursing Management* 22: 26–30.

Johnson, R. S. 1993. "TQM: Leadership for the Quality Transformation (Part 4)." *Quality Progress* 25: 47–49.

Kanter, R. 1977. *Men and Women of the Corporation*. New York: Basic Books.

Kelly, K. 1995. *Health Care Work Redesign*. Series on Nursing Administration. Thousands Oaks, CA: Sage.

Korman, A. 1971. *Industrial and Organizational Psychology*. Englewood Cliffs, NJ: Prentice-Hall.

Laschinger, H. K. S. 1996. "A Theoretical Approach to Studying Work Empowerment in Nursing: A Review of Studies Testing Kanter's Theory of Structural Power in Organizations." *Nursing Administration Quarterly* 20: 25–41.

Maslow, A. 1954. *Motivation and Personality*. New York: Harper & Row.

———. 1964. "A Theory of Human Motivation." In *Readings in Managerial Psychology*, edited by H. J. Leavett and L. R. Pondy. Chicago: University of Chicago Press.

———. 1970. *Motivation and Personality*, 2nd ed. New York: Harper & Row.

Mason, D. J., B. A. Backer, and C. A. Georges. 1996. "Toward a Feminist Model for the Political Empowerment of Nurses." *Image* 23: 72–77.

Matherly, L. L., and A. H. Lasater. 1992. "Implementing TQM in a Hospital." *Quality Progress* 25: 81–84.

McClelland, D. C. 1961. *The Achieving Society*. Princeton, NJ: Von Nostrand Reinhold.

McGraw, J. P. 1992. "The Road to Empowerment." *Nursing Administration Quarterly* 16: 16–19.

National Commission on Nursing. 1983. *Summary Report and Recommendations*. Chicago: Hospital Research and Educational Trust.

Newman, B. 1989. *The Newman Systems Model*, 2nd ed. Norwalk, CT: Appleton and Lange.

Porter, L. W., and E. E. Lawler. 1968. *Managerial Attitudes and Performance*. Homewood, IL: Dorsey Press.

Rakich, J. S., B. B. Longest, and K. Darr. 1985. *Managing Health Services Organizations*, 2nd ed. Philadelphia, PA: W. B. Saunders Co.

Redman, R., and S. Ketefian. 1995. "Defining and Measuring Work Redesign: A Field Study." In *Health Care Work Redesign*, edited by K. Kelly. Series on Nursing Administration. Thousand Oaks, CA: Sage.

Schmermerhorn, J. R. 1984. *Management for Productivity*. New York: John Wiley and Sons.

Schmieding, N. J. 1993. "Nurse Empowerment Through Context, Structure, and Process." *Journal of Professional Nursing* 9: 239–45.

Stillwaggon, C. A. 1989. "The Impact of Nurse Managed Care on the Cost of Nurse Practice and Nurse Satisfaction." *Journal of Nursing Administration* 19: 21–27.

Tappen, R. M. 1995. *Nursing Leadership and Management: Concepts and Practice*, 3rd ed. Philadelphia, PA: F. A. Davis.

Taylor, F. 1911. *The Principles of Scientific Management*. New York: Harper.

Tebbitt, B. V. 1993. "Demystifying Organizational Empowerment." *Journal of Nursing Administration* 23: 18–23.

U. S. Department of Health and Human Services, Public Health Service. 1988. *Secretary's Commission on Nursing, Final Report*. Washington, DC: U.S. Government Printing Office.

Vroom, U. H. 1964. *Work and Motivation*. New York: John Wiley.

Zonsius, M. K., and M. Murphy. 1995. "Use of Total Quality Management Sparks Staff Nurse Participation in Continuous Quality Improvement." *Nursing Clinics of North America* 30: 1–12.

MEASURING RELATIONSHIPS:
SATISFACTION IN ORGANIZATIONS

Nearly every empirical study on satisfaction begins with some type of theoretical framework; however, in many cases, it seems that this is primarily a historical review, one that establishes that the investigator has read the literature. A review of theoretical literature has a purpose, which is to delineate the conceptual framework being used by the investigator. This is important because the type of measure selected is at least partially dependent on this framework. In some cases, the theoretical framework is quite different. For example, Porter and Lawler (1968) viewed satisfaction as a dependent variable, which is affected by job performance. Maslow (1954), on the other hand, viewed satisfaction as an independent variable, in that high levels of satisfaction were likely to cause better job performance.

Although a great many studies mention Maslow's work, few actually use his theory as the orienting device for their particular study. It is far more common for a study to use Herzberg's Dual-Factor Theory as the orienting framework. This framework (Herzberg, Mausner, and Snyderman 1959) considers satisfaction to be dependent on the nature of a specific job. Although controversial when it was developed, over time this theory has been used more than any other in the nursing research literature. This is probably because of the fact that Herzberg conceptualized satisfaction not as a continuum, but rather as two separate sets of factors, some of which cause satisfaction while others cause dissatisfaction. The terms he originally used have been changed, but the theory of identifying some factors that provide satisfaction and others that provide dissatisfaction has made measurement of satisfaction easier. Recent examples of studies that use Herzberg's theory include efforts to describe what is satisfying and not satisfying to nurse practitioners (Koelbel, Fuller, and Misener 1991), critical care and medical-surgical nurses (Williams 1990), and intensive care unit and coronary care unit nurses (Malik 1991). Increasingly, research is emphasizing the link between satisfaction levels and organizational intervention. Factors identified as satisfiers are viewed as those that hospital administration should in some way support in an effort to decrease nurse turnover (Blegen et al. 1992; Butler and Parsons 1989; Johnston 1991).

However, when one reviews all this literature, a consistent picture does not emerge. Not only are the findings contradictory, the ways in which job satisfaction is conceptualized and measured are diverse. In her meta-analysis of published empirical research on job satisfaction, Blegen (1993) quantified some of these relationships. One of her observations is instructive here. Autonomy, one of the most common variables to be included in satisfaction studies, had six different labels in the literature she surveyed. Although the descriptions for all of these labels were quite similar, each was associated with different measures.

In the published literature, job satisfaction is conceptualized in one of three ways. Some studies measure job satisfaction as if it were an independent variable, although they do not always explicitly so define it. The focus of these studies tends to be the relationship between satisfaction and personal characteristics of nurses, including psychological and personality traits as well as demographic characteristics.

A second category of studies conceptualizes job satisfaction as a dependent variable, something that occurs as a result of something else. Some of these studies treat job satisfaction as arising as a result of the specific job that nurses do. A third, related category conceptualizes job satisfaction as a response to the structure of the organization itself, using as an orienting framework the concept of empowerment.

Although this conceptual variation produces sometimes conflicting and confusing research, it is neither unexpected nor negative. In fact, as Chapter 2 showed, job satisfaction has been conceptualized in different ways for a long time. This diversity will contribute to a better understanding of the complex concept of satisfaction. Two problems should be noted, however. First, it is very important that the focus of the study be consistent with the theory. For example, if Maslow's theoretical framework is used, then the research should treat satisfaction as an independent variable. If the theoretical framework is that organizational factors affect satisfaction, then there must be a measure of some organizational variable, such as organizational climate, not a job-specific measure. The second issue of concern is that, as more knowledge about satisfaction is disseminated within the field, the results from a variety of research studies are contrasted and compared. In some cases, this is not appropriate, since different measures are being used. Not only are the measures assessing different things, sometimes they represent a completely different way of thinking about satisfaction.

There has been extensive research in the area of nurse satisfaction. Because of the increasing knowledge base, there has been a gradual shift from descriptive studies to more analytic ones. Based on this knowledge, the nursing profession is moving beyond simply describing the problem to attempting to resolve it. One such example is the 1994 Joint Commission Accreditation Manual for Hospitals (JCAHO 1993), which requires each hospital to show evidence of developing, implementing, and evaluating programs to promote recruitment and retention of nurses, as well as evidence of providing opportunities for development and continuing education for nurses in an effort to improve satisfaction levels. Other examples include the increasing research that attempts to link satisfaction levels not only to performance and productivity, but also to quality of care and patient outcomes.

This is an appropriate time to move from descriptive studies to evaluative and analytic ones that may be more likely to present suggestions for resolution of the low levels of nurse satisfaction. However, it is important to remain sensitive to the relationship between theory and measurement. This chapter will focus on measurement, to provide a complement to Chapter 2, which focused on theory. The purpose of this chapter is to summarize the body of literature categorized as "nurse satisfaction," while focusing on how satisfaction is conceptualized and measured. The first part of the chapter presents studies that use satisfaction as an independent variable, emphasizing the relationship between satisfaction and personal characteristics of the nurse. Next are studies that focus on analyzing job satisfaction as an outcome of a specific job, followed by a section in which studies consider satisfaction to be an outcome of an organizational structure. The next section describes studies that attempt to demonstrate a link between satisfaction and several negative behaviors, including turnover. This chapter concludes with analysis of the types of measures that are currently being used for job satisfaction.

Demographic and Personal Factors

Nearly every study collects some type of demographic information. In most cases, this information is gathered out of curiosity or because "everyone else does." Sometimes a demographic characteristic may help explain a finding or set it in a more understandable context. In some situations, a study is specifically designed to explore the effect of some demographic variable on satisfaction levels. The most common ones used are education, gender, age, and personality factors.

Education

This is perhaps the single most frequently included of the demographic variables, primarily because the educational preparation in nursing is diverse and there are large differences in the various educational pathways. Intuitively, researchers feel that there should be a relationship between educational preparation and satisfaction. However, demonstrating this empirically has not been very successful, despite several different approaches. Most often, educational preparation is simply included in the data-gathering process, and the relationship is analyzed by correlating the findings. In some cases, a specific study is done, with the express purpose of investigating the relationship between educational preparation and satisfaction. One example is a survey of graduates of three different schools of nursing—an associate degree program, a diploma program, and a baccalaureate program (Stewart-Dedmon 1988). This study analyzed how well each program prepared its graduates as well as how satisfied they were. Of 23 different job characteristics, there were significant differences by education for 7 characteristics. In terms of satisfaction, baccalaureate and diploma nurses were significantly less satisfied than their associate degree peers, although there was a lot of variation in the responses to specific areas of satisfaction and dissatisfaction. Because of the variation, the author concludes that although educational preparation is an important factor in influencing job satisfaction, it cannot be identified as the predominant factor.

Another example is a study by Schutzenhofer and Musser (1994), who also surveyed graduates of different types of educational programs. They categorized educational preparation in two levels—a basic nursing program and a "highest degree" level. Instead of directly assessing the relationship of education and satisfaction, they measured the association between education and autonomy, since autonomy is thought to be positively related to satisfaction. They were able to show a positive relationship between highest level of nursing education and autonomy.

Johnson (1988) used a different approach in a meta-analysis of 139 studies published between 1958 and 1985 that examined the effects of education on a range of nursing behaviors. This often-cited study found mixed evidence for the effect of educational preparation. A meta-analysis by Blegen (1993) on the satisfaction literature examined how often variables were included in studies assessing levels of nurse satisfaction. Education was frequently included, but only small relationships were noted between education and satisfaction.

Undoubtedly, the relationship between education and satisfaction is complicated. Hinshaw, Smeltzer, and Atwood (1987) demonstrated some of these complexities when they created a model to explain turnover: education was one of the variables that helped explain the choice to stay. In their model, a higher educational degree was associated with a tendency to leave.

Gender

Another variable that is frequently mentioned in satisfaction studies is gender, and, like education, the results are mixed. Gender is of interest because of the nature of the nursing profession, which is predominantly composed of women. Although nursing can be accurately categorized as a female-dominated profession, this only means that women hold the highest number of positions, not necessarily the most powerful ones. For nursing, the picture is even more complicated because of the traditional male-dominated medical profession and hospital hierarchy in which most nurses work. In a national survey of nurses, Seymour and Buscherhof (1991) found that gender roles and women's socialization issues were the third most frequently mentioned concern by the respondents.

Studying the effect of gender is actually not easy, even though it is obviously easy to delineate whether a respondent is male or female. The consequences of this variable are hard to assess. Some investigators use the concept of sex-role orientation (Schutzenhofer and Musser 1994; Krausz et al. 1992), while others are more likely to use feminist theory, which explores the nature of power. Koeckeritz (Appendix E, Selection 15) does an excellent job of reviewing the literature on the consequences of gender analysis in the health field, with a special emphasis on nurses.

Age

Age is another demographic variable that is frequently included in studies. This is sometimes operationalized as age, while other times it is operationalized as length of time in a specific job or sometimes, length of overall professional experience. Blegen (1993) found age was included in the same number of studies as education. Like education, it had only a small effect on satisfaction levels. When examining level of satisfaction in relation to participative management initiatives, Lucas (1991) also found little relationship between age and satisfaction; however, there was a relationship between satisfaction and length of time in a specific job. Both Agho (1993) and Baggs and Ryan (1990) found a relationship between age and level of satisfaction. For both of these studies, younger nurses and less experienced nurses were more satisfied. Others have noted that satisfaction increases with age (Malik 1991; Williams 1990; Blegen 1993; deSavorgnani, Haring, and Galloway 1993; Wade 1993).

Personality Factors

Some studies also look at personality when examining factors that might be related to satisfaction. Agho's (1993) study is an example of this, suggesting that the Price-Mueller model be modified to include personality, specifically negative or positive affect. McCrea (Appendix E, Selection 7) summarizes the latest research within the stress and satisfaction area, which includes an emphasis on factors that affect an individual's perception of and response to stress, sometimes called personality hardiness. The results of her study suggest that recruitment efforts should include consideration of "hardiness" as part of the selection process, especially for nurses in critical care areas.

It is interesting to note that, although demographic variables seem very straightforward, demonstrating an empirical relationship with satisfaction level is difficult. This may be because the relative power of a demographic characteristic is probably a smaller influence on satisfaction than is either a specific job or the managerial climate within an organization. Certainly, it is more common for satisfaction to be conceptualized as a dependent variable, and as an outcome of a job or a more generalized organizational climate.

Satisfaction as a Function of a Specific Job

Most of the studies on nurse satisfaction conceptualize job satisfaction as being an outcome, or a dependent variable, although there is not agreement on what independent variable determines satisfaction levels. In general, there seem to be two distinct schools of thought. The first is that job satisfaction is an outcome of a particular type of job, or a specific unit in a hospital or even in a specific type of hospital. Many, but not all of the studies that fall under this conceptualization, are descriptive in nature. The ones that are not descriptive usually evaluate some type of innovation, one that changes the specific job rather than the organization itself. The second school of thought is that job satisfaction arises not primarily from the specific job, but rather from organizational characteristics and management style. In the 1980s, the most common type of research conducted was analyzing job satisfaction as a dependent variable arising from a specific type of job. In the 1990s, there has been a trend toward conceptualizing satisfaction as arising from larger organizational issues. This section will summarize the research that treats job satisfaction as primarily arising from a specific job, while the next section will address job satisfaction as an outcome of larger, organizational issues.

Not surprisingly, a large majority of the studies are located in hospitals. This is reflective of where nurses work, since two-thirds of all nurses work in a hospital setting. In the 1980s, the major purpose of most of the research done in hospitals was to describe the level of satisfaction of nurses. Although this descriptive focus has been less common in the 1990s, it is still a predominant theme in the literature. Most studies limit themselves to registered nurses (RNs), although some studies do include the entire nursing staff. One study that assessed role strain of hospital employees included all hospital staff members, although most of the sample were in fact nurses (Steffy and Jones 1990). Johnston (1991) did an interesting descriptive study that focused on RNs. She used the IWS with a sample of 385 RNs and identified two clusters, the first of which included pay, professional status, and autonomy, the scores of which were so close together that satisfaction in one is predictive of satisfaction in another. Her view is that these may represent the cultural values of the nursing profession. The second cluster included interaction, task requirements, and organizational policies representing the values of the organizational culture. The differences in scores for these components are slightly larger, indicating that these are more independent.

Studies that focus on specific types of nursing jobs are able to contribute to the depth of understanding about one particular aspect of nursing. By far the most conventional emphasis is to study nurses in critical care, and especially to compare satisfaction levels of critical care and other nurses, although the results are not consistent (Williams 1990). Studies frequently have a more narrow focus, such as examining increased control of work shifts (Houston 1990) or the amount of collaboration between physicians and nurses in the ICU setting (Baggs and Ryan 1990).

Increasingly, researchers are analyzing interventions that are designed to improve a specific job. Some of these analyze the effect of types of recognition programs (Blegen et al. 1992; Goode and Blegen 1992; Goode, Ibarra, and Blegen 1993) while others focus on a specific type of recognition program, such as clinical ladders (Joy and Malay 1992; Malik 1991). Changes in nursing care delivery systems are thought to have an effect on nurse satisfaction, and this is a particular focus of several of the examples of practice-based research included in Chapter 5 and Appendix E. Often, such research will have a pre- and posttest design to allow more careful evaluation of the innovation (Blenkarn, D'Amico, and Virtue 1988). A particularly interesting—and somewhat unusual—initiative is that of assisting nurses in information management. This large study occurred in an 800-bed teaching hospital and evaluates the effect of a computerized, decision-support system that provides assistance not only with patient care but also with discharge planning. Although the nurses in this study found the computer system valuable, it did not increase their level of satisfaction, and the authors offer several observations to explain this (Thompson, Ryan, and Baggs 1991).

Most research on nurse satisfaction in the 1980s took place in single-hospital settings. In the 1990s there has been an increasing amount of research taking place in multiple-hospital settings, or in surveys of nurses outside of their specific job setting. Sometimes, the multiple-hospital setting is especially appropriate because of the type of nurse studied. For example, Tumulty (1992) used 10 hospitals to get a sample of 110 head nurses. She found that satisfaction was significantly related to job characteristics, and also to unit outcomes. Research that focuses on rural nurses also frequently utilizes multiple hospitals, primarily for reasons of sample size. Bushy and Banik (1991) surveyed nurses working in eight South Dakota hospitals. One of their unexpected findings was that the more satisfied workers were those that worked the evening and night shifts. This is consistent with Schmidt and Martin's observation (Appendix E, Selection 1) that nurses working night and evening shifts may have increased decision-making authority. Bushy and Banik (1991) note that this needs to be investigated more, since it is a common practice to offer new nurse employees a day shift as a retention strategy. Coward et al. (1995) investigated the level of satisfaction of nurses working in long-term care facilities. Included in the sample were urban and rural nurses drawn from nursing homes within a ten-county area in north Florida. The researchers measured satisfaction by using a shortened version of the IWS. They found no differences in level of satisfaction between urban and rural nurses. One of the largest of the multiple-hospital studies used 65 hospitals and included 8,500 hospital employees, most of whom were nurses (Steffy and Jones 1990). This study, which was conducted by an insurance company, was trying to determine whether satisfaction levels of part-time employees are any different than satisfaction levels of full-time employees. Satisfaction in this study was conceptualized as being related to role strain. Although part-time employees did experience more role strain than full-time employees, there was no effect on satisfaction levels, which was an unexpected finding.

Two studies used multiple hospitals to collect data in order to investigate a more specific issue. Kovner et al. (1994) collected data in 37 acute care hospitals in New Jersey in an effort to evaluate one of the five different innovations being introduced in the hospitals. The innovations included a variety of programs, all aimed at changing the specific job or unit on which the nurse worked. Kovner's findings were similar to Johnston's (1991) in that the same two clusters were identified. Also, Kovner noted that the two components most affected by the changes were task requirements and interaction. In general, nurses were more satisfied in the new work environments. Blegen et al. (1992) evaluated recognition programs in 16 Iowa hospitals. They identified several important recognition programs that positively affected nurse satisfaction. Although pay was obviously an important one, there were a range of other ways in which supervising nurses were able to provide recognition in such a way as to improve levels of satisfaction.

Other investigators choose to describe level of satisfaction of nurses by collecting data from nurses in settings other than the hospital. Schutzenhofer and Musser (1994) surveyed 2,000 RNs from four different states—Idaho, Missouri, Florida, and Maryland. This descriptive study explored the relationship of several personal and job characteristics and autonomy, using autonomy as a measure for satisfaction. Seymour and Buscherhof (1991) summarized the findings of a national survey of employed nurses conducted for the Center for Nursing Research. This study included quantitative and qualitative findings. Some of the strongest dissatisfiers included structural problems in controlling work schedules, and issues related to pay and other forms of recognition. National and regional studies such as these are very helpful in identifying issues important to nurses; the results often help to guide other, more specialized research efforts.

As shown above, the investigations into nurse satisfaction are so varied in nature that it is difficult to provide a summary of results; it is far easier to summarize the studies by examining some aspect of methodology. Although clearly not the only measure used, the IWS is the single most commonly used measure for nurse satisfaction. Several of the other measures used have clearly been developed based on the IWS. Thus, as might be expected, much of the descriptive literature focuses on components included as part of the IWS that are satisfying or dissatisfying to nurses. By far the two most frequently mentioned of these components are autonomy and pay.

Autonomy

It is not surprising that autonomy is frequently included as a variable. Increased autonomy for the staff nurse is a well-recognized goal in the nursing profession. In Blegen's (1993) meta-analysis, autonomy was one of the most commonly included variables, but its effect on satisfaction was only moderate. The two variables with a stronger relationship to satisfaction were stress and organizational commitment. This is especially interesting, since the relationship between autonomy and satisfaction is thought to be so strong and direct that some investigators use autonomy as a pseudo-measure for satisfaction. Schutzenhofer and Musser (1994) have a "professional activities" scale that measures perception of autonomy; they and others use it to measure level of satisfaction. McCloskey (1990) used the autonomy subscale of the Job Characteristics Inventory, a scale developed in 1976 by Sims, Szilaggi, and Keller, to investigate the relationship between social integration and autonomy in nurse retention. Her results indicate that both are important, although social integration seems to be able to buffer the negative effect of low autonomy.

Other investigators often measure both satisfaction and autonomy. Tumulty (1992) identified autonomy as one of the three role components that best predict both satisfaction and performance of nurses. Her study included a measure for both satisfaction and autonomy. All research that includes autonomy, however it is measured, finds autonomy to have some effect on nurse satisfaction, but the empirical studies do not generally find it to be the most important determinant of satisfaction. Although there are many explanations for this, one likely possibility is that the studies that investigate job-specific or unit-specific interventions or that provide descriptive analyses of satisfaction levels of nurses have respondents that are accustomed to the limited autonomy that is so common in the traditional nursing position so their expectations are limited. As will be shown in the next section, when the analytic focus is switched to the organization, findings related to the relationship between satisfaction and autonomy are more consistent.

Pay

One of the most important methods of recognition is pay, and it is intuitively important to level of satisfaction. In Seymour and Buscherhof's (1991) national survey of what nurses find satisfying and dissatisfying in their work, level of pay was the second most important source of dissatisfaction. Of all possible recognition behaviors identified in the 1992 study by Blegen et al., pay was most important in terms of increasing satisfaction.

Despite this, not every study is able to support the importance of pay as a satisfier. One interesting example is among home care nurses, where level of satisfaction is high despite lower pay levels (deSavorgnani,

Haring, and Galloway 1993). And Blegen's (1993) meta-analysis did not even include pay because it did not appear often enough in the literature she surveyed.

Of course, part of the problem here is that autonomy and pay are not completely distinct from each other, since the more autonomous professions usually have a higher salary (Kovner et al. 1994). Home care nurses may be the exception to this rule, since they perceive more professional autonomy but seem to be more satisfied with lower levels of pay (deSavorgnani, Haring, and Galloway 1993). Another part of the problem is that staff nurses are perhaps more aware of what researchers have only recently acknowledged: increased autonomy cannot be realized through changes in a specific job without the involvement of the whole organization.

Satisfaction as a Function of the Organization

The published literature may be taken both as a reflection of current interests and as direction for new areas that need to be investigated. The published literature that focuses on nurse satisfaction represents this dual function nicely. In the 1980s the primary focus of researchers was descriptive. They were concerned mainly with identifying what satisfaction is related to, and examining how satisfaction can be measured. Job satisfaction was sometimes viewed as an independent variable, one that managers cannot control (Agho 1993), but it was more commonly viewed as a dependent variable.

What satisfaction depends on, however, has been an interesting question for both empirical and conceptual researchers. In the 1980s, the primary answer to this question was that job satisfaction depended primarily on something related to a specific job, a particular role definition, or perhaps a particular unit in a hospital. The results of this literature were mixed, to say the least. No clear patterns emerged. Perhaps because of this, many articles ended with an acknowledgment that satisfaction is more complex than first realized. Some of the complexity obviously involves measurement problems, which is where this chapter will end up. But some of this research also acknowledged the conceptual complexity, with particular recognition that specific jobs and particular units exist within an organizational structure. The role of management was frequently included as a possible factor, the influence of which could not be determined.

The literature of the late 1980s and the 1990s, with increasing frequency, directly addresses this complex relationship, both by examining empirical data and by reexamining conceptual relationships. Increasingly, satisfaction of the nursing staff is thought to be the result of an organizational structure as well as an organizational climate or culture. This larger climate is viewed as affecting specific jobs and particular units within a hospital. The role of management is more frequently included in the research, and satisfaction is increasingly used as a criterion to evaluate the effectiveness of some type of management intervention. The development of such empirical efforts has coincided with the emergence of some of the newer, organizationally based theories discussed in Chapter 2.

This section will describe and summarize some of the predominant themes in this literature. Some specific types of organizational interventions, such as control of work hours, and changing the nursing care delivery system will be described first. Empirical research focusing on the relationship of management style to nurse satisfaction will be addressed next, including research on participative management innovations. If there is one single variable that is more likely to be included in this literature, it is something related to organizational climate: the next section will describe some of this literature. This section will conclude with a brief description of the efforts to quantify the concept that is the basis of this research, which is empowerment.

Making distinctions between research efforts in this category—those with an emphasis on organizational aspects—rather than the previous category, which emphasized the specific job, is not always easy. If the research is mostly concerned with the effect of a specific job or the effect of one unit, with little or no attention paid to the larger organizational issues, it is considered to belong to the previous category. There are several examples of the ambiguity of such delineations. For example, recognition programs, including clinical ladders, are included in the previous section, because, although many studies that investigate recognition programs use empowerment as a theoretical framework, they do not measure any organizational variables. Even though the concept of autonomy is an important part of thinking about the effect of the organization on the individual, most of the research currently focusing on autonomy is included in the previous section, not this one. This is because most of the empirical research addresses the question of how a particular job can be changed to increase the decision-making authority of the nurse, rather than how nurses can have greater autonomy within the organization itself. In order for a study to be included in this section, the unit of analysis must be the organization, not the nurse, the job, or the unit. There also must be some measure of these organizational variables. The question addressed must not be limited to autonomy within a certain job description, but rather include control over the nature of the job itself. The first two examples—control of work hours and changing the nursing care delivery system—are not as clear examples as are later parts of this section, but they are included here because each of the studies acknowledges the importance of the whole organization in the analysis of job satisfaction of nurses.

Control of Work Hours

Research on the effect of the shift or hours worked on satisfaction of nurses is not new. Blenkarn, D'Amico, and Virtue's (1988) study is supportive of the general assumption that nurses are more satisfied with 8-hour shifts than 12-hour shifts, although Houston's (1990) study showed that 12-hour shifts had a positive effect on satisfaction levels. However, Houston's study, although anecdotal, involved nurses themselves choosing whether to work 12-hour shifts. It is a truism worth repeating that the important issue may be how much control—or choice—nurses feel they have in controlling the nature of their work responsibilities, rather than the amount of autonomy they may be allowed to exercise within parameters of a job they are not able to define. When nurses are allowed choice in defining the nature of their work conditions, the results are sometimes surprising. For example, Bushy and Banik (1991) noted the somewhat surprising finding that, in their rural setting, nurses working the evening and night shifts had higher levels of satisfaction. The nursing administrators in these rural hospitals had a tradition of offering day shifts to new nurses in order to increase retention, based on the assumption that this shift is associated with increased satisfaction. The important point is not whether satisfaction is higher for nurses on day or evening or night shifts: the salient point is nurses will be more satisfied the more they are able to choose their working hours for themselves. Obviously, this choice cannot be entirely free, since there are organizational constraints, but how the constraints are presented may be more relevant than the existence of the constraints.

The appropriate way in which to view issues related to shifts, hours worked, and other scheduling issues is as part of the work environment or work climate; a part that is controlled by the larger organization. The extent that the organization allows nurses to choose—that is, to exercise their autonomy—is important to satisfaction levels. Schaefer and Moos (1996) examined the importance of this relationship in a study involving 405 nurses in 14 long-term care facilities, where morale was measured rather than satisfaction. In this study, workload and scheduling stressors had the strongest negative effect on both morale and the level of physical functioning at work.

Changing Nursing Care Delivery Systems

This is another area in which there has been research for a long time, but the emphasis is changing from the concept of teams or even primary nursing to an increased emphasis on "reengineering," which involves more patient-focused care, and a "debureaucratized" organization (Schweikhart and Smith-Daniels 1996). It seems clear that changes in nursing care delivery systems that involve primary nursing increase work satisfaction, but in those studies that also measure amount of control over work, there is often no effect (Blenkarn, D'Amica, and Virtue 1988; Lancero and Gerber 1995). This may be because satisfaction has in fact increased, but without an increase in organizational autonomy. Some investigators have conceptualized redefining the role of nursing care delivery systems as a way to improve the work environment, as did Mularz et al. (1995), who used Theory "M" to integrate the redesigned roles into the organization. Kramer and Schmalenberg (1993) describe primary nursing as a method of empowerment—or organizational change—but only if the whole organizational "culture of excellence" is established. Their work with what are termed magnet hospitals is an example of attempting to change the organizational climate so it will be more satisfying to nurses.

Instituting these changes takes time, as several of the selections in Chapter 5 and Appendix E note; instituting the whole program is also important, as Ingersoll et al. (Chapter 5, Selection 1) observe. When changes are introduced, the effect on satisfaction is usually positive. Kovner et al. (1994) analyzed the effect of five different innovations—including case management, shared governance, and various reorganizations of nursing delivery—in 37 hospitals. All of the innovations gave nurses more decision-making authority, and all of them increased the level of satisfaction, which was measured using the IWS. Kovner et al. noted that sometimes the effect of programs cannot be immediately seen, since incorporating changes into the organizational climate requires time. This is an acute problem for evaluating innovations that involve such organizational changes: the rate of change is sometimes slow enough that the research timeline is not able to capture it.

Management Style

There are several assumptions about management inherent in this research. The first is that management style can—and does—affect level of nurse satisfaction. Another assumption is that management can change the organizational environment. In fact, some of these studies assume that the nurse manager is the gatekeeper for the nurse's access to the organization. For the hospital nurse, this person is usually a head nurse, and it is not surprising that some very interesting research centers on the head nurse position. The head nurse has long been recognized as a supervisor; more and more, this position is being associated with leadership responsibilities. An increasing amount of empirical research is devoted to demonstrating the relationship between leadership and level of satisfaction among head nurses (Hansen et al. 1995; Garrett 1991; Irvine and Evans 1995). Tumulty (1992) examined the role characteristics of head nurses and found that the level of satisfaction of the head nurses themselves was higher (as measured by the IWS) when the hospital provided more autonomy to this position.

Some of this research does not limit itself to head nurses specifically, but rather focuses on management style, thus trying to capture the climate of the entire organization. Most of this research supports the positive relationship between satisfaction or morale, as it is sometimes termed, and either confidence in management (MacRobert, Schmele, and Henson 1993) or communication behavior in managers (Kennedy, Camden, and Timmesman 1990). In a large-scale research project, Weisman et al. (1993) examined level of satisfaction of nurses involved in a unit self-management innovation. The self-management model included gain sharing and salaried compensation in a 900-bed teaching hospital. In comparing traditional units and these self-managed units, the self-managed units had higher levels of satisfaction and higher retention rates. Nurses in these units also worked longer hours, but they earned more money. Interestingly enough, the measures of control over work schedule and participation in decision making did not show a relationship to level of satisfaction, which may reveal the difficulty of measuring the level of organizational involvement.

One recurring theme throughout this research is the idea that level of satisfaction is related to management styles that are more participative. Drews and Fisher (1996) used the IWS to demonstrate that, as supervising nurses' management style became increasingly participative, there were higher levels of satisfaction among the staff nurses. Lucas (1991) studied 505 nurses in four different hospitals and, using Likert's Management Systems Theory to measure management style and Munson and Heda's satisfaction measure, showed that a more participative management style has a strong relationship to satisfaction.

A particular innovation that is designed to increase participative management style is shared governance, and several selections in Chapter 5 and Appendix E show how satisfaction levels can be used to measure the effect of this management model. Jones et al. (1993) collected data annually for three years in a 611-bed hospital that had instituted a shared-governance program. Using Hinshaw's adaptation of the IWS, they showed a significant improvement in satisfaction, especially with organizational policies and professional job satisfaction.

Organizational Structure and Organizational Climate

The assumption underlying participative management models of various types, including shared-governance models, is the recognition that the organization itself is different if there is a real commitment to participative management. Of course, there are many examples of failed efforts in increasing participation in the decision-making process of the organization. The common theme among the success stories seems to be the extent to which the larger organization itself "buys in" to what is a power-sharing process. Kramer and Schmalenberg (1993) also describe this process as "debureaucratizing" or empowering. In their study of 1,800 nurses, those who worked in magnet hospitals had higher morale, because of the different kind of organizational climate found there.

Recent research has concentrated on both measurement and better conceptualization of the relationship between organizational climate and satisfaction. The most common conceptualization is to recognize organizational climate as an intervening variable. For example, Peter (1994) conceptualized organizational structure as an independent variable, organizational commitment and satisfaction as intervening variables, and intent to leave as the dependent variable. Gillies, Franklin, and Child (1990) analyzed the difference between those who stayed and those who left a hospital. They found that 80 percent of those who left as well as 60 percent of those who stayed viewed lack of support from hospital administrators as an unfavorable aspect of their job. Certain organizational climate factors were strongly related to satisfaction levels: responsibility, warmth, and support were among the most important factors in level of satisfaction.

Not all research that includes organizational climate is able to document a positive relationship between organizational factors and level of satisfaction. Begley and Czajka (1993) were not able to demonstrate a relationship between organizational climate and satisfaction, but they were able to show that organizational factors provided a moderating effect on dissatisfaction. Wells (1990) looked at decentralized management as a structural feature of an organization. Her study involved 137 nurse managers from eight hospitals, some of which had a more centralized administrative structure and some that had a more decentralized administrative structure. She found no differences in level of satisfaction (measured by a shortened version of the IWS) for nurse managers working in a more decentralized hospital setting, although the time allowed for the study may not have been sufficient for an effect on level of satisfaction to be noticed.

Empowerment

The literature characterized by the word "empowerment" is concerned with the ideas of power and communication within organizations. Although the term empowerment is often used in the theoretical framework of studies, it is not often operationalized to permit measurement and data collection. A few investigators have attempted to measure empowerment, and their work has helped to clarify the important conceptual issues in trying to identify the complex relationships between organizational structure, organizational climate, and feelings of satisfaction. Chandler (1991) has developed a measure that assesses how empowered a nurse feels in a particular organization. In a study involving 268 nurses, she defined an empowering environment as one that included support, information, and opportunity. She developed a measurement tool, the Work Effectiveness Questionnaire (WEQ), to assess the perception of nurses. This questionnaire was used in a study in conjunction with the IWS to determine if these two tools were measuring the same constructs. In general, nurses who scored higher on the WEQ (indicating higher levels of feeling empowered) were also more likely to report higher levels of satisfaction, as measured by the IWS. Some specific components were more strongly correlated than others, with organizational policies and task requirements showing the strongest relationship. The conclusion of this study is that, although empowerment and satisfaction share some constructs, they are also different and should be measured specifically (Scherr 1995). Chandler (1992) has also addressed the problem of how empowerment and delegation of authority can exist in the hospital structure, by asking a smaller sample of nurses (56) to describe carefully when they felt empowered in a hospital working environment.

Building on these ideas, Wilson and Laschinger (1994) collected information from 92 staff nurses to help identify how work environments could be structured to allow nurses to experience more organizational power. In a very small study involving only 20 nurses, Radice (1994) explored the relationship between empowerment and satisfaction. She used a Hospital Nurse Experience Questionnaire to measure organizational constraint and the IWS to measure satisfaction. She found a positive relationship between low constraints in the organization and higher levels of satisfaction.

This is obviously just the beginning in trying to address some complex relationships that involve not only individuals' perception of satisfaction with their job, but also their perception of satisfaction with an organizational climate, which involves a perception of access to power. There are, of course, important measurement problems here: measuring perception of power and organizational climate is very complex, as is the measurement of the perception of satisfaction. However, these studies also raise another issue, one that further complicates the development of measurements, and that is the conceptualization of power within an organization. In a study concerned with the structural power of women's occupations, Jenkins (1994) observed that structural power involves task-role power and hierarchical-role power. This study identified a paradox for women, which is that supervisory power roles usually involve more structural power as well as more autonomy within an organization; but less relational power with individuals. In analyzing female occupations, Jenkins observed that women viewed relational power as being more significant than hierarchical power. Although this study was not focused on nurses, this observation obviously raises many interesting issues, especially when considering the role of the head nurse, the staff nurse, and the larger hospital organizational structure.

Satisfaction and Negative Employee Behaviors

Creating working conditions and designing specific jobs to ensure a high level of nurse satisfaction is an end in and of itself since satisfaction with one's job has obvious inherent value. However true this may be, it is not the most common rationale for investigating level of satisfaction. The single most common reason is the belief of the link between level of satisfaction and nursing turnover, with high levels of turnover described as "plaguing the profession" for years (Blegen 1993). So universal is the concern about nursing turnover that nearly every article on satisfaction begins with a statement about either turnover, retention, or shortage. This is still true in the 1990s, even in the presence of organizational downsizing and mergers, which often result in decrease of nursing staff. Estimates of the overall turnover problem range from 10 percent to 70 percent of a given nursing staff yearly (Peter 1994), a range so large that it is almost not helpful.

It is important to be more clear about what is meant by turnover and also how to measure it. One way is to compare the turnover rate of nursing with that of other female-dominated professions. For example, nurses have 3 times the turnover rate of teachers and 1½ times the turnover rate of social workers (Kennedy, Camden, and Timmesman 1990). Although this is a useful comparison, it still leaves turnover undefined.

One definition is that of nurses who voluntarily leave their jobs. However, in some cases, this involves nurses leaving the profession itself. Kennedy, Camden, and Timmesman (1990) noted that between 35 percent and 67 percent of nurses leave the profession yearly, with 75 percent of these being voluntary.

Others use turnover to indicate the percentage of vacant nursing positions within a hospital or a unit. Vacancy rates vary by care setting. Estimates for vacancy rates in hospitals range from 12 percent to 14 percent. Vacancy rates are usually higher in nursing home and long-term care settings, often around 20 percent (Coward et al. 1995; Johnston 1991; Gillies, Franklin, and Child 1990; Schaefer and Moos 1996). High vacancy rates seem to exist in inner-city public hospitals, where the estimate is also around 20 percent (Gillies, Franklin, and Child 1990). Vacancy rates are sometimes used synonomously with shortage rates (Baggs and Ryan 1990; Gillies, Franklin, and Child 1990; deSavorgnani, Haring, and Galloway 1993; Corcoran, Meyer, and Magliaro 1990).

Turnover is more than nurses leaving either their job or the profession, however. It also includes nurses transferring to other units or jobs within the same hospital. This may be substantial; in one University hospital, this accounted for 33 percent of the turnover (Peter 1994). Although in some ways, this internal transferring is less disruptive to the hospital, there are still important effects and significant costs associated with such internal moves. As technology and specialization of units continue to increase within the hospital setting, nurses are not interchangeable with one another, but require more and more specific training. Higher costs for replacing nurses in intensive care units and coronary care units reflect this (Hinshaw, Smeltzer, and Atwood 1987; Fernandez et al. 1990).

Regardless of whether the vacancies result from nurses leaving the job or the profession, or from moving within the hospital to another job, the cost to the hospital is significant. Hospitals are labor-intensive organizations, and personnel account for 75 percent of most hospital budgets (Johnston 1991). The amount of money spent by a given hospital in one year to replace nursing staff will obviously vary, but it is not unusual for a hospital to spend 10 percent to 15 percent of its total nursing budget replacing nurses (Peter 1994; Garrett 1991; Butler and Parsons 1989). The cost to replace one nurse ranges from $1,300 to $8,000, depending on the specialty (Garrett 1991; Kennedy, Camden, and Timmesman 1990; Robinson et al. 1991; MacRobert, Schmele, and Henson 1993). Others give estimates that are much higher, including Kennedy, Camden, and Timmesman (1990) who quote a figure of $19,000, which includes all costs. Increasingly, investigators designate all costs related to recruitment, including advertising and interviewing candidates; orienting new employees; paying new nurses while they are being oriented, and paying existing nurses to provide "double coverage." Peter (1994) notes several stages involved in replacing a nurse, besides the obvious recruiting and selecting tasks. These include the need to socialize new staff to both unit and organizational expectations, the need to provide time for a social balance to develop between new staff and existing staff, and the need to maintain either old or extra temporary staff while new staff members are being trained.

Other costs can also be incurred as a result of dealing with turnover. For example, at Albany Medical Center, the use of supplemental agency nurses increased from 30 percent to 45 percent in two years. A 20 percent turnover rate caused beds to be closed, which resulted in a $500,000 monthly loss of revenue for the hospital (Fernandez et al. 1990).

A high rate of nursing turnover is almost universally viewed as a sign of high levels of dissatisfaction. The high turnover rates in nursing homes, for example, are often used as prima facie evidence of a care setting that provides less satisfaction than other settings. So ingrained is this relationship between dissatisfaction and turnover rates that many investigators view it as an assumption, although several are continuing to attempt to document the relationship empirically. Irvine and Evans (1995) did a meta-analysis of literature examining turnover. Most studies described a multistage process beginning with an attitude, usually described as dissatisfaction; proceeding through a decisional phase, during which the intent to leave is formed; and then ending with a behavioral outcome, which is the act of leaving a job. In their review of literature, they looked for evidence of a number of factors affecting turnover. A consistent finding is that, as satisfaction decreases, turnover behavior increases. Some research has focused on specific specialties of nurses. Perhaps because of the high costs associated with their replacement, intensive care unit nurses are frequently studied. The link between satisfaction and turnover is just as well documented for these nurses, with a special emphasis on the satisfaction with nurse-physician collaboration (Baggs and Ryan 1990).

During the last ten years, the relationship between dissatisfaction and turnover has been increasingly conceptualized as being related to head nurse—or leadership—behavior as well as larger organizational issues. For example, Blegen et al. (1992) concentrated on head nurse recognition behaviors and how these can be augmented to increase staff nurse satisfaction and thus reduce turnover of staff nurses.

Leader behavior is linked to a larger organizational climate. In their study of 1,600 nurses in 15 hospitals, Hinshaw, Smeltzer, and Atwood

(1987) discovered that retention strategies, particularly for critical care nurses, need to focus on organizational job satisfiers, especially administrative style. This finding was later reinforced by Gillies, Franklin, and Child (1990) for all nursing staff; in their study, organizational climate was strongly related to satisfaction, which was in turn negatively associated with turnover. A vast majority of those who left cited the need for more administrative support within the organization. A Swedish study also demonstrated that factors related to lack of administrative support as well as interaction with coworkers were significantly related to dissatisfaction, which was one of the prime reasons for turnover (Bjorvell and Brodin 1992).

For many, the main conclusion here is to figure out a way to prevent turnover, even in the current economic climate of organizational downsizing, hospital closures, and mergers, which often produce a smaller nursing staff. The evidence is overwhelming that turnover is costly, both in monetary terms and in quality of the product. Johnston (1991) notes that in the hospital, care is the core product, a product that is primarily organized and delivered by nurses. Improving the quality of this core product is dependent on improving the professional satisfaction of nurses. Retention programs are mentioned more and more often in the literature (Johnston 1991; Baggs and Ryan 1990; Fernandez et al. 1990). Corcoran, Meyer, and Magliaro (1990) cite the need for developing a retention plan as part of a strategic plan. This approach has produced in their hospital a 5 percent nurse vacancy rate, despite an increase in RN positions because of new services being offered. The turnover rate is only 8 percent, and more than 40 percent of the nurses have been on staff for at least ten years. Both of these indicators are much better than similar ones across the nation (Corcoran, Meyer, and Magliaro 1990).

As people investigate the relationship between satisfaction and turnover, the terms stress and burnout are also introduced with increasing frequency. The relationship between satisfaction, stress, and turnover has been investigated for many years (Hinshaw and Atwood 1983; Blegen 1993). A growing body of research suggests that work stressors and a negative work climate affect staff negatively, especially in terms of job satisfaction, but also in terms of physical ability to perform the job (Schaefer and Moos 1996). For some people, high levels of dissatisfaction automatically cause stress, although this is not always true. Schaefer and Moos (1996) have an especially helpful discussion in which they identify the various stresses in clinical roles. There is a fine line between stressors related to poor outcomes (including turnover), and stressors related to challenging or rewarding job tasks. These latter stressors are related to positive outcomes, including higher levels of satisfaction. Schaefer and

Moos's research supports earlier work that describes at least two distinct categories of stressors. The first are those related to patient care. These stressors are associated with challenging patient care, which is associated with higher levels of satisfaction for all direct care professionals (Stamps and Cruz 1994; Shaefer and Moos 1996; Chappell and Novak 1992; Marshall et al. 1991). Those stressors associated with dissatisfaction—the second category—are consistently related to heavy workloads leading to overwork, as well as chronic interpersonal strain. In Schaefer and Moos's (1996) study, workload and scheduling stressors had the greatest negative effect on mental and physical functioning, as well as on intent to stay.

The various measures used to quantify stress are diverse and, for the most part, not standardized. Two scales are used most frequently. One scale is by Schaefer and Moos (1996), a Work Stressors Inventory that measures several stressors, including relationship, task, and system. Using this measure, Schaefer and Moos found the presence of sicker patients in a nursing home did not increase dissatisfaction, since patient care tasks are stressors that are linked to satisfaction rather than dissatisfaction. Jones et al. (1993) used the Bailey and Claus 1987 Job Stress Scale to evaluate changes in stress levels after two years experience with a shared-governance model. Begley and Czajka (1993) measured stress by asking only one question: "How stressed do changes make you feel?" This was used in a study that evaluated the level of stress in an organization undergoing downsizing. Stress was viewed as an independent variable, as was intent to quit; while satisfaction and somatic complaints, as well as leaving the job, were all viewed as dependent variables.

One of the behavioral consequences of stress is burnout, "a syndrome of physical and emotional exhaustion involving the development of a negative self-concept, negative job attitude and a loss of concern and feeling for client" (Butler and Parsons 1989). One of the most common measures of burnout is the Maslach Burnout Inventory, developed in 1986. Robinson et al. (1991) used this with a sample of 354 nurses to investigate the consequences of burnout, which included turnover. They discovered that excessive work pressure and limited participation caused nurses to withdraw. Appropriate managerial control and support were important factors in mediating such withdrawal behavior, especially with nurses working on day shifts. These same results were obtained in England, in a study that also used Maslach's Inventory (Matrunola 1996). Both of these studies also noted a significant level of involvement with physical and somatic complaints, a major feature of the burnout syndrome.

Regardless of whether it is satisfaction or stress or burnout, the assumption in these studies is that dissatisfaction is related to turnover.

A few studies attempt to document this relationship empirically. Even though turnover seems a straightforward variable to measure, there are in fact three different measurement possibilities found in the published literature. It is important to assess these, since the type of measurement reflects the way turnover is conceptualized.

Measurement of Turnover

Turnover is operationalized in one of three different ways. One of the ways is to count the number of people who actually leave their job, either for another job within the same institution or for a job in another institution, or because they leave the profession itself. This is a behavioral measure, and in some ways is the easiest measure. However, this does not provide much insight into the process involved in turnover, nor does it allow intervention or prevention of the turnover. Increasingly, investigators are using intentions so that retention programs may be developed on the basis of research conducted on turnover. Studies that use intentions may use either intent to leave or intent to stay.

Since turnover is a frequently investigated topic, there are many interesting examples of each of these types of measures. Investigators using either intent to leave or intent to stay must also establish the link between intentions and actual behavior. Hinshaw, Smeltzer, and Atwood (1987) used the term "anticipated turnover," which is really intent to leave, since a turnover is a leaving of the job. In their study, which they used to create a theoretical model that has functioned as a guide to much of the later research, they determined that actual turnover was weakly predicted by intent to leave: 72 percent of those who stayed in 15 different hospitals could be predicted by a combination of self-reported anticipated turnover scores and educational level and clinical service. Jones et al. (1993) used the Anticipated Turnover Scale developed by Hinshaw and Atwood (1983) to evaluate the effect of a shared-governance model by measuring management style, group cohesion, job stress, satisfaction, and intent to leave. They found that the staff were less likely to leave after the implementation of a shared-governance model, which reinforces the link between satisfaction and intent to leave, since satisfaction levels do seem to improve with the implementation of participative management, including shared governance.

Research that assesses the effect of organizational climate and participative management styles on levels of satisfaction stresses the importance of organizational factors on satisfaction, as discussed previously. Begley and Czajka (1993) extended this research by investigating what happens in an organization that is downsizing. They measured intent to quit, health status, and level of satisfaction after an organization had consolidated and was in the process of downsizing. They measured intent to leave by a two-item scale: "As soon as I can find a better job, I'll quit," and "I often think about quitting my job." They discovered a much higher "intent to leave" after the organization had downsized.

Not all research documents the link between low satisfaction and intent to leave. In a study done in Sweden, investigators found that, in spite of relatively high levels of satisfaction, about half the staff wanted to leave anyway (Bjorvell and Brodin 1992). As a result of these findings, they view the link between satisfaction and intent to leave as being more tenuous.

Since the goal is to keep staff, not lose them, it makes sense to try to measure intent to stay, rather than intent to leave. If more knowledge can be gained about what makes people want to stay in their jobs, then it may be easier to develop retention programs. Increasingly, researchers are more likely to use intent to stay rather than intent to leave, and to view intent to stay as a better predictor of turnover (Drews and Fisher 1996; Peter 1994). In their meta-analysis, Irvine and Evans (1995) found a strong correlation between behavioral intentions and turnover. Schulz (1993) measured actual turnover and intent to stay and found a positive correlation. Yoder (1995) measured intent to stay by using seven questions, including those addressing staying in the current job, staying in the nursing profession, and staying in the army. She evaluated the effect of what she termed "career development relationships" on intent to stay, which did not seem to have much effect.

Because of the tenuous relationship between intentions—regardless of whether these are intentions to stay or to leave—and behavior, some investigators still prefer to measure actual behavior. Several investigators use both. For example, Jones et al. (1993) who used intent to leave, also measured actual turnover, which decreased from 22 percent to 16 percent after two years of a shared-governance program. Peter (1994) also used both intent to remain as well as actual turnover in her study, which examined the effect of educational workshops for nurse managers. The units associated with the nurse managers who had experienced the workshops had turnover rates of 16 percent, while the units with the nurse managers who had not experienced the workshops had a turnover rate of 46 percent.

Schultz's 1993 study made clear the complexity of the relationships between satisfaction and negative employee behaviors, including turnover. A hospital established a clinical advancement system to improve nurse retention rates. Schultz evaluated the first eight years of this system, using both satisfaction rates and actual turnover rates. The clinically advanced nurses did have lower turnover rates and higher satisfaction levels each year that the system operated. The differences for turnover rates were quite pronounced: the turnover rate experienced for Level I nurses was between 18 percent and 21 percent, while the turnover rate experienced by the advanced (Level II) nurses was between 4 percent and 8 percent. Schultz also did a cost-benefit analysis, which demonstrated that this clinical advancement system actually cost the hospital more than the turnover rates would have, although, as Schultz points out, placing a cost on all the benefits of such a system is very difficult.

Measuring Satisfaction

The focus of this chapter has been on studies that have quantified level of satisfaction. Not surprisingly, there are many different ways to measure satisfaction, each of which also represent a different way to conceptualize this variable. Blegen's (1993) meta-analysis on studies measuring satisfaction noted 21 different measures used to operationalize satisfaction. This section will present an analysis that will focus not on the findings, as Blegen did, but rather on the measurements themselves. Although the research described in this chapter includes measurement of many other variables besides satisfaction, the focus here will be limited. For a similar analysis of how other variables (including organizational culture and climate, personality, and social support networks) are measured, see Stamps (1997).

In doing any type of meta-analysis, it is necessary to set some criteria. In this case, in order for a study to be included, it must have been done after 1986, the year in which the final, revised version of the IWS became widely available. If the IWS is the measure used, it must be this version. This effectively limits the time period to research conducted within the past ten years.

The research must actually measure satisfaction. Some articles have satisfaction as a prominent variable but do not actually measure it. One example of this is the 1992 article by Blegen et al., which assesses the effect of recognition programs on satisfaction but includes no measure of satisfaction. Another example is the study by Butler and Parsons (1989), which surveyed 152 decision makers and 212 nurses to determine which environmental factors would cause satisfaction but left the respondents to use their own perception of increased level of satisfaction. A third example includes those studies that mention satisfaction, but measure stress (Matrunola 1996). Stress and satisfaction are not the same thing: more research is clearly needed to clarify the relationship between stress, dissatisfaction, and satisfaction among direct care providers. Some studies used the term "morale," but if their measures were clearly within the general conceptualization of satisfaction, they are included here. For example, MacRobert, Schmele, and Henson (1993) used the Science Research Associates morale inventory to measure employees' attitudes toward the work environment in order to determine "specific areas of satisfaction and dissatisfaction among employees."

In the 36 studies that met these criteria, by far the most common measure used for satisfaction was the IWS. Table 3.1 presents the 18 studies that used this tool as a measure for satisfaction. Most of these studies used only Part B, the attitude scale measuring the current level of satisfaction, and most of them view satisfaction as a dependent variable, with the specific job characteristics being the most important of the variables affecting satisfaction. The last four studies included in this table either modified the IWS significantly or used it to measure a different construct than satisfaction. In all cases they identified their instrument as coming from the IWS, although each used a slightly shorter version of the IWS. Additionally, as can be seen in Table 3.1, Coward et al. (1995) modified the scale for use with long-term care nurses, and Lancero and Gerber (1995) modified the tool for specific use with a case management model.

The remaining 18 studies used a variety of other tools to measure satisfaction. Three of these studies used all or part of the satisfaction scale developed in 1951 by Brayfield and Rothe (Agho 1993; Hinshaw, Smeltzer, and Atwood 1987; Koelbel, Fuller, and Misener 1991). Two studies used all or a part of the Job Description Index, originally developed by Smith, Kendall, and Hulin in 1969; and modified by Hackman and Oldham in 1975 (Roedel and Nystrom 1988; Garrett 1991). Two studies used the 20-item Minnesota Satisfaction Questionnaire, developed by Weiss in 1967 (Begley and Czajka 1993; Koelbel, Fuller, and Misener 1991).

A few of these studies created measures of satisfaction by selecting items from more than one tool. For example, Hinshaw, Smeltzer, and Atwood (1987) used the old version of the IWS to measure "organizational satisfaction" and adapted the Brayfield and Rothe scale to measure "professional and occupational satisfaction." Jones et al. (1993) later used the Hinshaw adaptation of the IWS to measure organizational satisfaction. Koebel, Fuller, and Misener (1991) used the Brayfield and Rothe Index of Job Satisfaction and the Minnesota Satisfaction Questionnaire to create a new global satisfaction measure. Begley and Czajka (1993) used the Minnesota Satisfaction Questionnaire and a single item meant to measure global satisfaction.

The use of either a single or a very small number of items to measure what is termed global satisfaction is easier to analyze than a scale with

Table 3.1 Summary of Published Studies Using the IWS as a Measure of Satisfaction

Author, Date	Purpose of Study/Setting of Study	Form of IWS Used in Study
Blenkarn et al. 1988	Evaluation of institution of primary nursing in psychiatric units in a hospital in Canada; Pre- and post-test design	IWS, Part B
Houston, 1990	Evaluation of an innovation involving 8-hour versus 12-hour work shifts; ICU unit; multiple data collection points	IWS, Part B
Baggs and Ryan, 1990	Descriptive study of relationship between nurse-physician collaboration and satisfaction in ICU settings	IWS, Part B
Williams, 1990	Descriptive study comparing satisfaction of critical care and med/surg nurses	IWS, Parts A and B
Johnston, 1991	Descriptive study showing relationship between turnover and satisfaction; a 300-bed hospital	IWS, Parts A and B
Bushy and Banik, 1991	Descriptive study of the relationship between satisfaction and a variety of job and personal factors among rural nurses	IWS, Parts A and B
Thompson et al. 1991	Evaluating the introduction of a computer-based decision-support system in an 800-bed teaching hospital; experimental and control units	IWS, Part B
Malik, 1991	Descriptive study comparing the satisfaction of ICU/CCU nurses in a career ladder setting and those not in a career ladder setting	IWS, Parts A and B
Joy and Malay, 1992	Evaluate professional practice model; includes clinical ladder	IWS, Part B
Tumulty, 1992	Descriptive study to determine relationship between satisfaction and job characteristics of head nurses; collected data on 110 nurses in 10 hospitals	IWS, Parts A and B
Kovner et al. 1994	Evaluation of impact of five different changes in nursing care delivery models in 37 different hospitals in New Jersey	IWS, Parts A and B

Continued

Table 3.1 Continued

Author, Date	Purpose of Study/Setting of Study	Form of IWS Used in Study
Mularz et al. 1995	Evaluating changes in the nursing care delivery system; control and experimental units	IWS, Part B
Drews and Fisher, 1996	Descriptive study on the relationship between perception of management style and satisfaction; in an acute-care public-university children's hospital	IWS, Part B
Hinshaw et al. 1987	Testing a theoretical model predicting turnover; data collected from 1,597 nurses working in seven urban and eight rural hospitals	IWS, Part B, used to measure 'organizational satisfaction'
Wells, 1990	Descriptive study on the influence of the facility organizational structure on the level of satisfaction of nurse managers; data collected from 137 nurse managers in eight hospitals	A 'Staff Satisfaction Scale' was used to measure satisfaction; this was a 38-item modification of the IWS by Hall and VonEndt
Gillies and Child, 1990	Descriptive study of the relationship between organizational climate and satisfaction; sample was 34 nurses from four different units in an urban teaching hospital	IWS, Part B; Pay Component excluded; also Nurse-Physician interaction
Coward et al. 1995	Descriptive study on the satisfaction of nurses in rural and urban nursing homes	IWS, shortened and modified for a nursing home setting
Lancero and Gerber, 1995	Descriptive analysis of the impact of case management on level of satisfaction; compared satisfaction levels in two different models of case management	Used a 29-item modification of the IWS, with wording changes to make it appropriate to a case management model; deleted the pay component

several components. Recognizing the possible disadvantage of creating too general a measure, some investigators use this approach in combination with other items or another scale (Begley and Czajka 1993). Others use an existing scale and reduce it to a small number of items that seem to assess general satisfaction. Weisman et al. (1993) used a four-item global satisfaction measure based on the 1977 Quality of Employment Survey. Both McCloskey (1990) and Schaefer and Moos (1996) modified work done by Hackman and Oldham in 1975; with McCloskey using three items and Schaefer and Moos six.

Many researchers use scales that have been developed by others. Some choose scales that are well recognized, but older, such as Munson and Heda's 1974 adaptation of Porter and Lawler's scale (Lucas 1991) or Bullough's Job Satisfaction Scale, developed in 1974 (Parsons and Felton 1992). Others use scales that are newer, but not designed specifically for nurses. MacRobert, Schmele, and Henson (1993) used the Science Research Associates morale inventory; and Steffy and Jones (1990) used the Human Factors Inventory. Peter (1994) modified Prestholdt's questionnaire, which originally measured intent to stay, and created a 90-item questionnaire that included measures of satisfaction, intent to stay, and perception of a variety of organizational characteristics.

Some investigators noted they wanted to use a scale designed for nurses, but did not wish to use the IWS, either because they viewed the scoring as too cumbersome or because the way the scale operationalizes satisfaction was inconsistent with their research objectives. Pranulis et al. (1995) measured satisfaction by using the Personal Satisfaction Inventory, developed by Dyer especially for nurses in a Veterans Administration setting. Yoder (1995) used the Nursing Work Index developed by Kramer and Hafner in 1989, based on their work with magnet hospitals. In 1990, Mueller and McCloskey developed a new measure for nurse satisfaction, aimed partly at reducing the complexity of scoring required by the IWS. Their article presents the testing of the factor structure of this scale.

When the measurements used to quantify level of nurse satisfaction are examined closely, it is no wonder that no clear pattern seems to emerge when one analyzes this body of literature. Although the IWS is the most frequently used measuring tool, that frequency of use does not mean that the IWS is the only tool that should be used. If the purpose of the research is comparative, or to evaluate a particular innovation, the IWS may well be the best choice. But if the purpose is to ensure that satisfaction has been appropriately conceptualized, it is important that investigations continue on the development of new measures for nurse satisfaction.

It is clear that quantifying the level of nurse satisfaction is increasingly well accepted, not only among staff nurses, but also among managers and administrators. Evidence for this can be found in the 1994 Accreditation Standards, which require some assessment of level of nurse satisfaction (JCAHO 1993). It may be that the IWS is the tool of choice for this increasingly application-oriented use. However, again, new research needs to continue on the development of other measures of satisfaction. One obvious approach is to assess multiple measures of satisfaction against each other. For example, administering the IWS, the Mueller and

McCloskey Scale, and a global scale to the same group of respondents would be helpful in evaluating the relative strengths of each of these measures.

This is basic research, not applied; but the benefits will clearly be worth the time spent. The one single conclusion that can be drawn from the published literature is that satisfaction is an important variable, one that nearly every study wishes to assess. Nursing care delivery systems are increasingly patient-focused, especially in organizations that are instituting quality control systems. However, the research indicates that there is a direct and positive relationship between satisfaction levels of nurses, and their productivity and performance, as well as patient outcomes. This means that if nursing delivery systems are made nursing-oriented, the same positive patient outcomes can be achieved. One of the barriers to this is the need for several possible measures for nurse satisfaction levels.

Having the IWS available has certainly increased researchers' ability to compare results and, despite what some view as complicated scoring techniques, the IWS has enabled organizations to use satisfaction levels more easily as one way to evaluate managerial and organizational innovations. This chapter has focused on what can be found in the published literature, but the IWS is used widely in practice. The rest of this book will focus on such practice-based uses of the IWS, in an effort to increase the dissemination of information about levels of nurse satisfaction. Chapter 4 focuses on the systematic collection of information from many of the people who have used the IWS over the last ten years, and Chapter 5 and Appendixes E and F contain many examples of practice-based research using the IWS as the measure of satisfaction.

References

Agho, A. 1993. "The Moderating Effects of Dispositional Affectivity on Relationships Between Job Characteristics and Nurses' Job Satisfaction." *Research in Nursing and Health* 16: 451–58.

Baggs, J. G., and S. A. Ryan. 1990. "ICU Nurse-Physician Collaboration & Nursing Satisfaction." *Nursing Economic$* 8: 386–92.

Begley, T. M., and J. M. Czajka. 1993. "Panel Analysis of the Moderating Effects of Commitment on Job Satisfaction, Intent to Quit, and Health Following Organizational Change." *Journal of Applied Psychology* 78: 552–56.

Bjorvell, H., and B. Brodin. 1992. "Hospital Staff Members Are Satisfied with Their Jobs." *Scandinavian Journal of Caring Science* 6: 9–16.

Blegen, M. A. 1993. "Nurses' Job Satisfaction: A Meta-Analysis of Related Variables." *Nursing Research* 42: 36–41.

Blegen, M. A., C. J. Goode, M. Johnson, M. L. Maas, J. C. McCloskey, and S. A. Moorhead.

1992. "Recognizing Staff Nurse Job Performance and Achievements." *Research in Nursing and Health* 15: 57–66.

Blenkarn, H., M. D'Amico, and E. Virtue. 1988. "Primary Nursing and Job Satisfaction." *Nursing Management* 19 (April): 41–42.

Bushy, A., and D. Banik. 1991. "Nurse Satisfaction with Work in Rural Hospitals." *Journal of Nursing Administration* 21: 35–38.

Butler, J., and R. J. Parsons. 1989. "Hospital Perceptions of Job Satisfaction." *Nursing Management* 20: 45–48.

Chandler, G. E. 1991. "Creating an Environment to Empower Nurses." *Nursing Management* 22: 20–23.

———. 1992. "The Source and Process of Empowerment." *Nursing Administration Quarterly* 16: 65–71.

Chappell, N. C., and M. Novak. 1992. "The Role of Support in Alleviating Stress among Nursing Assistants." *The Gerontologist* 32: 351–59.

Corcoran, N. M., L. A. Meyer, and B. L. Magliaro. 1990. "Retention: The Key to the 21st Century for Health Care Institutions." *Nursing Administration Quarterly* 14: 23–31.

Coward, R. T., T. L. Hogan, R. P. Duncan, C. H. Horne, M. A. Hilker, and L. M. Felsen. 1995. "Job Satisfaction of Nurses Employed in Rural and Urban Long-Term Care Facilities." *Research in Nursing and Health* 18: 271–84.

deSavorgnani, A. A., R. C. Haring, and S. Galloway. 1993. "Recruiting and Retaining Registered Nurses in Home HealthCare." *Journal of Nursing Administration* 23: 42–46.

Drews, T. T., and M. C. Fisher. 1996. "Job Satisfaction and Intent to Stay: RNs' Perceptions." *Nursing Management* 27: 58.

Fernandez, R., M. L. Brennan, A. R. Alvarez, and M. R. Duff. 1990. "Theory-Based Practice: A Model for Nurse Retention." *Nursing Administration Quarterly* 14: 47–53.

Garrett, B. H. 1991. "The Relationship among Leadership Preferences, Head Nurse Leader Style and Job Satisfaction of Staff Nurses." *Journal of New York State Nurses Association* 22: 11–14.

Gillies, D. A., M. Franklin, and D. A. Child. 1990. "Relationship Between Organizational Climate and Job Satisfaction of Nursing Personnel." *Nursing Administration Quarterly* 14: 15–22.

Goode, C. J., and M. A. Blegen. 1992. "Development and Evaluation of a Research-Based Management Intervention." *Journal of Nursing Administration* 23: 61–66.

Goode, L. J., U. Ibarra, M. A. Blegen, J. Anderson-Bruner, T. Boshart-Yoder, E. Cram, L. Finn, R. Mills, and C. Winty. 1993. "What Kind of Recognition Do Staff Nurses Want?" *American Journal of Nursing* 7: 64–68.

Hansen, H. E., C. Q. Woods, D. K. Boyle, M. J. Bott, and R. L. Taunton. 1995. "Nurse Manager Personal Traits and Leadership Characteristics." *Nursing Administration Quarterly* 19: 23–35.

Herzberg, F., B. Mausner, and B. Snyderman. 1959. *The Motivation to Work*, 2nd ed. New York: John Wiley and Sons.

Hinshaw, A. S., and J. R. Atwood. 1983. "Nursing Staff Turnover, Stress and Satisfaction: Models, Measures and Management." In *Annual Review of Nursing Research*, edited by H. H. Werley and J. J. Fitzpatrick, 133–53. New York: Springer.

Hinshaw, A. S., C. H. Smeltzer, and J. R. Atwood. 1987. "Innovative Retention Strategies for Nursing Staff." *Journal of Nursing Administration* 17: 8–16.

Houston, R. 1990. "Twelve-Hour Shifts: Answer to Job Satisfaction." *Nursing Management* 21: 88F–88H.

Irvine, D., and M. G. Evans. 1995. "Job Satisfaction and Turnover among Nurses: Integrating Research Findings Across Studies." *Nursing Research* 44: 246–51.

Jenkins, S. R. 1994. "Structural Power and Experienced Job Satisfactions: The Empowerment Paradox for Women." *Sex Roles* 30: 347–67.

Johnson, J. H. 1988. "Differences in the Performance of Baccaulareate, Associate Degree and Diploma Nurses: A Meta-Analysis." *Research in Nursing and Health* 11: 183–97.

Johnston, C. L. 1991. "Sources of Work Satisfaction/Dissatisfaction for Hospital Registered Nurses." *Western Journal of Nursing Research* 13: 503–13.

Joint Commission on Accreditation of Healthcare Organizations. 1993. *1994 Accreditation Manual for Hospitals. Volume 1, Standards*. Oakbrook Terrace, IL: The Commission.

Jones, C. B., S. Stasiowski, B. J. Simons, N. J. Boyd, and M. D. Lucas. 1993. "Shared Governance and Nursing Practice." *Nursing Economics* 11: 208–14.

Joy, L., and M. Malay. 1992. "Evaluation Instruments to Measure Professional Nursing Practice." *Nursing Management* 23: 73–77.

Kennedy, C. W., C. T. Camden, and G. M. Timmesman. 1990. "Relationships among Perceived Supervisor Communication, Nurse Morale and Sociocultural Variables." *Nursing Administration Quarterly* 14: 38–46.

Koelbel, P., S. G. Fuller, and T. R. Misener. 1991. "An Explanatory Model of Nurse Practitioner Job Satisfaction." *Journal of the American Academy of Nurse Practitioners* 3: 17–24.

Kovner, C. T., G. Hendrickson, J. R. Knickman, and S. A. Finkler. 1994. "Nursing Care Delivery Models and Nurse Satisfaction." *Nursing Administration Quarterly* 19: 74–85.

Kramer, M., and C. Schmalenberg. 1993. "Learning from Success: Autonomy and Empowerment." *Nursing Management* 24: 58–64.

Krausz, M., P. Kedem, Z. Tal, and Y. Amir. 1992. "Sex-Role Orientation and Work Adaptation of Male Nurses." *Research in Nursing and Health* 15: 391–98.

Lancero, A. W., and R. M. Gerber. 1995. "Comparing Work Satisfaction in Two Case Management Models." *Nursing Management* 26: 45–48.

Lucas, M. D. 1991. "Management Style and Staff Nurse Job Satisfaction." *Journal of Professional Nursing* 7: 119–25.

MacRobert, M., J. A. Schmele, and R. Henson. 1993. "An Analysis of Job Morale Factors of Community Health Nurses Who Report a Low Turnover Rate." *Journal of Nursing Administration* 23: 22–28.

Malik, D. M. 1991. "Career Ladders: Position Enrichment vis-a-vis Tenure." *Nursing Management* 22: 120A–120F.

Marshall, N. C., R. C. Barnett, G. K. Baruch, and J. Pleck. 1991. "More Than a Job: Women and Stress in Care-Giving Occupations." In *Current Research on Occupations and Professions*, edited by H. Lapata and J. A. Levy, VI: 61–81. Greenwich, CT: JAL Press.

Maslow, A. 1954. *Motivation and Personality*. New York: Harper & Row.

Matrunola, P. 1996. "Is There a Relationship Between Job Satisfaction and Absenteeism?" *Journal of Advanced Nursing* 23: 827–34.

McCloskey, J. C. 1990. "Two Requirements for Job Contentment: Autonomy and Social Integration." *Image: Journal of Nursing Scholarship* 22: 140–43.

Mueller, C. W., and J. C. McCloskey. 1990. "Nurses' Job Satisfaction: A Proposed Measure." *Nursing Research* 39: 113–17.

Mularz, L. A., M. Maher, A. P. Johnson, B. Rolston-Blenman, and M. A. Anderson. 1995. "Theory M: A Restructuring Process." *Nursing Management* 26: 49–51.

Parsons, M. A., and G. M. Felton. 1992. "Role Performance and Job Satisfaction of School Nurses." *Western Journal of Nursing Research* 14: 498–511.

Peter, M. A. 1994. "Making the Hidden Obvious: Management Education Through Survey Feedback." *Journal of Nursing Administration* 24: 13–19.

Porter, L. W., and E. E. Lawler. 1968. *Managerial Attitudes and Performance*. Homewood, IL: Dorsey Press.

Pranulis, M. F., A. Renwanz-Boyle, A. S. Kontas, and W. L. Hodson. 1995. "Identifying Nurses Vulnerable to Role Conflict." *International Nursing Review* 42: 45–50.

Radice, B. 1994. "The Relationship Between Nurse Empowerment in the Hospital Work Environment and Job Satisfaction: A Pilot Study." *Journal of New York State Nurses Association* 25: 14–17.

Robinson, S. E., S. L. Roth, J. Keim, M. Levenson, J. R. Flentje, and K. Bashor. 1991. "Nurse Burnout: Work Related and Demographic Factors as Culprits." *Research in Nursing Health* 14: 223–28.

Roedel, R. R., and P. C. Nystrom. 1988. "Nursing Jobs and Satisfaction." *Nursing Management* 19: 34–38.

Schaefer, J. A., and R. A. Moos. 1996. "Effects of Work Stressors and Work Climate on Long-Term Care Staff's Job Morale and Functioning." *Research in Nursing and Health* 19: 63–73.

Scherr, D. D. 1995. "Nurses' Work Satisfaction and Empowerment: A Construct Validation Study." Master's thesis: University of Massachusetts.

Schultz, A. W. 1993. "Evaluation of a Clinical Advancement System." *Journal of Nursing Administration* 25: 13–19.

Schutzenhofer, K. K., and D. B. Musser. 1994. "Nurse Characteristics and Professional Autonomy." *Image: Journal of Nursing Scholarship* 26: 201–5.

Schweikhart, S. B., and V. Smith-Daniels. 1996. "Reengineering the Work of Caregivers: Role Redefinition, Team Structures, and Organizational Design." *Hospital & Health Services Administration* 41 (1): 1–27.

Seymour, E., and J. R. Buscherhof. 1991. "Sources and Consequences of Satisfaction and Dissatisfaction in Nursing: Findings from a National Sample." *International Journal of Nursing Studies* 28: 109–24.

Sims, H. P., A. D. Szilaggi, and R. T. Keller. 1976. "The Measurement of Job Characteristics." *Academy of Management Journal* 19: 195–212.

Stamps, P. L. 1997. "Relationship of Theory and Measurement." Under review.

Stamps, P. L., and N. T. B. Cruz. 1994. *Issues in Physician Satisfaction: New Perspectives*. Chicago: Health Administration Press.

Steffy, B. D., and J. W. Jones. 1990. "Differences Between Full-Time and Part-Time

Employees in Perceived Role Strain and Work Satisfaction." *Journal of Organizational Behavior* 11: 321–29.

Stewart-Dedmon, M. 1988. "Job Satisfaction of New Graduates." *Western Journal of Nursing Research* 10: 66–72.

Thompson, C., S. A. Ryan, and J. Baggs. 1991. "Testing of a Computer-Based Decisions Support System in an Acute Care Hospital." In *Nursing Informatics '91*, Proceedings of the Fourth International Conference on Nursing Use of Computers and Information Science, Melbourne, Australia, April 1991.

Tumulty, G. 1992. "Head Nurse Role Redesign: Improving Satisfaction and Performance." *Journal of Nursing Administration* 22: 41–48.

Wade, B. E. 1993. "The Job Satisfaction of Health Visitors, District Nurses and Practice Nurses Working in Areas Served by Four Trusts: Year 1." *Journal of Advanced Nursing* 18: 992–1004.

Weisman, C. S., D. L. Gordon, S. D. Cassard, M. Bergner, and R. Wong. 1993. "The Effects of Unit Self-Management on Hospital Nurses' Work Process, Work Satisfaction, and Retention." *Medical Care* 31: 381–93.

Wells, G. T. 1990. "Influence of Organizational Structure on Nurse Manager Job Satisfaction." *Nursing Administration Quarterly* 14: 1–8.

Williams, C. 1990. "Job Satisfaction: Comparing CC and Med/Surg. Nurses." *Nursing Management* 21: 104A–104H.

Wilson, B., and H. K. S. Laschinger. 1994. "Staff Nurse Perception of Job Empowerment and Organizational Commitment." *Journal of Nursing Administration* 24: 39–47.

Yoder, L. H. 1995. "Staff Nurses' Career Development Relationships and Self-Reports of Professionalism, Job Satisfaction, and Intent to Stay." *Nursing Research* 44: 290–99.

USING THE IWS IN THE FIELD:
A SURVEY OF RESEARCHERS

nvestigators who use the IWS in their research have played a major role in the development of this measurement tool. Their comments on the scale itself, as well as the scoring procedures, have provided valuable guidance in its design, leading to several revisions that have allowed the IWS to continue measuring important aspects of professional satisfaction. These investigators have also provided the impetus for making the transition from measuring satisfaction to creating more satisfying work environments for nurses. Input from those who use the IWS has been obtained both formally and informally. The first formal survey of researchers using the IWS was conducted in 1983 and was the basis for the final revision of the scale. The 1986 book included the results of this survey, the final validated questionnaire, and scoring procedures and suggestions.

The publication of the first edition greatly increased the informal contact with researchers, so that an extensive network of those using the IWS in their research developed. A wide variety of studies have used the IWS over the past ten years. Many of these practice-based research studies were not published, for a variety of reasons. Some, of course, do not meet the methodological standards required for publication. However, two other factors have an effect. First of all, research-oriented journals are often less interested in reporting uses of a well-established measurement instrument than in reporting research on the development of new measures. Second, managers who use the IWS in a monitoring context to evaluate some type of nursing practice innovation are frequently not interested in publishing their experiences: their emphasis is on implementing the findings. Among these practice-based research studies, the IWS was frequently used to evaluate the effect of some type of innovation in nursing practice.

The IWS was also showing up in the published literature, of course, as shown in Chapter 3. The research studies published in the past ten years have been diverse, although the evaluative use of the IWS has increased. Also increasing is the use of the IWS to assess some innovation instituted as a part of an effort to increase empowerment in an organization.

In both the published literature and the many personal and informal contacts, one persistent theme has emerged. It is captured by this question: "Has anybody else studied the group I am studying?" Inherent in this question is first a desire to compare the results of one study with others, and second a desire to talk with others about the results of their research. The desire for comparative results is not new: this was one of the objectives in the first survey conducted in 1983. As discussed in Appendix B, it was not possible to do any comparisons among the many studies using the IWS at that time because of the extreme variability in the use of the IWS, in terms of both the questionnaire itself and the scoring procedures. The 1986 book strongly encouraged more standardized use of the IWS to facilitate comparability.

The continued desire of IWS users for access to comparative results was one of the reasons for the second formal survey of people using the IWS. An additional motivation was to stimulate the dissemination of the results of some of the important research being done in the field. A lot of interesting research was not well represented in the published literature. As a result, the field was not sufficiently aware of the innovations in nursing practice being tried in different settings.

There were five objectives for the 1994–95 survey of investigators. The first was to determine what researchers using the IWS perceive as its strengths and weaknesses. After all, the IWS was originally developed in 1972, although it has been modified several times since then. It was important to know if the measurement tool was still useful to investigators. A second objective was to determine whether IWS use in the field is standardized enough to merit the development of any comparative data. Although there are obvious advantages to having comparisons, one significant disadvantage is the need for more standardized use, which decreases flexibility for researchers. The third objective depended on the first two: if the IWS seems to be measuring satisfaction of nurses, and if its use seems standardized enough, then a comparative database could be constructed. The fourth objective was to provide a way in which the many examples of practice-based research could be shared with other researchers and practitioners in the nursing field. The last objective arose from these four, which is to formalize the network of investigators using the IWS in an effort to promote dissemination of knowledge.

Achieving these objectives required solving several problems. The first was identifying investigators who use the IWS and obtaining responses from them that include their numerical data. Because of previous experience in surveying users of the IWS, this was not a difficult problem to solve. However, this second survey required additional feedback from those using the IWS, that is, more extensive reports of their research to share with others. Also, creating a network of users requires a willingness to be contacted by others. Last, but definitely not least, this survey required some type of computer system in order to create and maintain a data base, without restricting the free and available use of the IWS.

As will be seen in the rest of this book, the process of conducting the second survey was an extremely positive experience and resulted in an extremely positive outcome. Many investigators responded, sharing data as well as the results of their research. Of course, not all the problems were successfully resolved. The construction of a database, which always seemed like such a good idea, carries with it a range of technical and philosophical issues. Not all are resolved with this book. Also, although the IWS is clearly the most frequently used and most well-accepted measure of satisfaction in the field, this book does not mean to imply that the measure is perfect or that there should be no more research devoted to developing a new measure for nurse satisfaction. Neither of those statements is true. However, this second survey made possible significant progress in the ability of the IWS to measure level of satisfaction of nurses and to change the working environments of nurses to make them more satisfying. Further, this survey produced a significant amount of information both on satisfaction and on innovations in the nursing profession. The rest of this book is devoted to presenting the results of this survey and to integrating the results of the practice-based research with the published research in this area.

This chapter focuses on the survey and the construction of the comparative database. The first two sections describe the survey process and the types of studies using the IWS to measure level of satisfaction. The third section focuses on investigators' comments about the IWS, their view of its adequacy as a measure, and their suggestions for modification. The next section describes the type of numerical responses and presents them as the first description of what might be termed a comprehensive database.

The next section in this chapter focuses on the several issues that arise from the use of such a database. Some of these issues are technical, including the use of the component weighting coefficient (from the paired-comparisons part of the IWS) as well as advantages and disadvantages in greater standardization of the IWS. Other issues are conceptual, including what use may be made of a comparative database. Of all the problems identified earlier, these conceptual issues remain and need to be addressed so that the use of this database will not exceed our ability to measure and interpret level of satisfaction of nurses. This chapter ends with a concluding section addressing a few final thoughts and observations about using the IWS to assess the level of nurse satisfaction.

This chapter is supported by three appendixes, particularly Appendixes B and C, which describe the scale-development process and guidelines for using the IWS in a study, respectively. Also important to this chapter is Appendix D, which describes the technical support necessary for the more specific comparative database described at the end of the chapter.

The Survey Process

The data-gathering process sought three different types of information. The first was the range of purposes for studies using the IWS. The second was how people "like" the IWS, both in terms of what it is able to measure and in terms of practicality, including feedback on scoring methods. The third was the numerical scores, which would contribute to the effort to make comparative information available to other researchers.

This section will describe the questionnaire, as well as the process of deciding on the sample. Because of the obvious difficulty of contacting users of the IWS, there was no goal of representativeness or randomness; rather the effort focused on gathering as much information as possible.

Developing the Questionnaire

A questionnaire was developed that would provide information in the three areas noted above. The first part of the questionnaire gathers information about the study in which the IWS is being used, including the major purpose of the study, such as whether the emphasis is on research or management; the setting of the study; and the type and size of the sample. The second part ascertains what the investigators think of the IWS as a measurement tool, including any modifications made; how useful they found the results; whether the scale administration, scoring, and interpretation presented any problems; and any suggestions for revisions to the IWS. The last part of the questionnaire asks the investigators to share as much of their numerical data as possible.

Identifying the Sample

A process for using the IWS was developed in 1986. Investigators wanting to use this tool in their research were supposed to gain permission by writing to the author of the scale (Paula Stamps) and to Health Administration Press, which held the copyright to the scale itself in 1986. (Appendix D describes the new process for obtaining permission to use the scale.) The 465 requests to use the 1986 scale obviously do not represent the complete population of users, as not all who used the IWS sought permission. Also, there are people who wrote to seek permission but who may not actually have used the scale. However, this group of 465 letters does provide a way to identify one specific group of people who have used the IWS. Because of the difficulty of even determining a population, it is not appropriate to attempt to achieve either a representative or a random sample. The major goal of identifying the sample is to collect as much usable information as possible in order to document the use of the IWS in the field.

Four criteria were identified to produce a sample that would be appropriate for a mailed survey:

- **Sample size.** Only those studies that had an initial planned sample size of at least 50 were included. This is mainly because of the response rate problem: if a study started with a planned sample size of 50, even a 50 percent response rate would produce only 25 responses. Even though the IWS is used and is appropriate for small institutions, the objectives of constructing a comparative database are best met through studies with planned samples of more than 50.
- **Recent contact.** The survey included only those studies conducted since 1990. This was primarily to increase the likelihood of contacting a respondent. This also meant that the studies were more homogenous with respect to the larger healthcare environment.
- **Use of revised IWS.** Since several articles appeared before the publication of the revised scale in the first edition of *Nurses and Work Satisfaction*, some people writing to seek permission still planned to use the previous version of the IWS. Since one of the primary objectives of the survey was to gain a sense of the comparability of results, it was important to have similar numbers contributed. So, in order for a study to be included, the investigator had to use the scale as published in 1986. The investigator also had to have plans to use the whole scale, with only minor modifications. Some requests were for one particular subscale, or for major modification

of the scale for use with other groups of healthcare professionals. Researchers seeking permission to use the IWS with healthcare groups other than nurses, or planning to make major changes to the questionnaire, were excluded from the sample.

- **United States or Canadian use.** Eighteen studies in these files used the IWS in a setting other than the United States or Canada, including two in Japan. These were excluded primarily because the summary numbers obtained from an international setting might well have different meanings than those obtained in the United States or Canada. Even if the IWS is appropriate for use internationally, it is probably not appropriate to include those numbers in a database intended for U.S. use.

Applying these four criteria resulted in 248 individuals being selected to receive the questionnaire. No follow-up phase was planned, since the objectives of the survey did not include representative use of the IWS.

Description of Studies Using the IWS

Response Rate to the Questionnaire

Questionnaires were sent to the 248 individuals whose letters met the four criteria. Of these, 28 were returned with no forwarding address. Another 15 investigators responded by indicating they had not used the IWS. Most of these noted that their study had not been funded or approved by the hospital in which they were working. A total of 65 people responded, representing 50 different studies and 88 separate administrations of the IWS. As might be expected, several studies had more than one investigator: the original mailing list often had individual listings for each investigator, especially if both investigators had written, which was often the case.

In this situation, calculating a response rate to the survey may not have much meaning. This is especially true since the original 465 studies did not represent a whole population. In this data-gathering effort, the whole population was unknown, since people frequently used the IWS without asking permission. Even so, the 65 people who responded to the survey represent 44 percent of the questionnaires that were mailed out. It was gratifying to receive as many responses as this, since they were clearly sufficient to begin the process of constructing a meaningful database. Also, the group was large and diverse enough to provide significant feedback in terms of what people feel about the IWS.

The studies came from all parts of the United States, with 18 from the eastern states and 21 from the Midwest. There were six studies from Ohio; five each from Massachusetts, New York, and Illinois; four each from Michigan and New Jersey; and three each from Arizona and Texas. States with one study included Colorado, Nebraska, North Carolina, Wisconsin, Pennsylvania, Florida, Missouri, California, Indiana, Hawaii, and Connecticut. One study was nationwide and one study was from Canada.

Year of Study

As might be expected, the year in which the study was conducted was constrained by wide availability of the final version of the IWS and the time it takes to complete a study of nurse satisfaction. The earliest that people had access to the final version of the IWS was 1986. A small number of studies (6 percent) took place in 1988, with 12 percent taking place in each of 1989 and 1990. Only 5 percent occurred in 1991. Fourteen percent of the studies took place in 1992; 21 percent in 1993; and 25 percent in 1994. Not surprisingly, only a small number (5 percent) took place in 1995, since that was the year in which the survey was conducted.

Person Doing the Study

In many of the studies, more than one person was involved. Forty percent of the studies involved students, mostly graduate nursing students, although one or two were undergraduate students. Twenty-seven percent of the studies involved a nurse administrator or manager, and 16 percent involved a staff nurse. Only 3 percent involved a hospital administrator or manager. Academic researchers conducted 13 percent of the studies.

Purpose of the Study

Personal communications with investigators over the years suggested that studies involving the IWS had one or the other of two major objectives: research or management. Interestingly, in the 50 sample studies, there was no such clear delineation. Twenty-nine studies (58 percent) did identify their primary purpose as research, and another 21 (42 percent) identified their major purpose as management. However, investigators also classified 20 of the 50 studies as a mixture of research and management. There seemed to be few uses of the IWS that were clearly either management or research; rather, there seemed to be real overlapping and integration of functions. Twenty-nine studies (58 percent) were used as part of an academic training program, with the vast majority of these involving a master's program. Many of these were classified by the respondent as serving a primarily management purpose. Also, although these were being used as part of a graduate degree program, more than one respondent indicated that the major purpose of the study was to maintain a level of scholarship as a nurse administrator.

Studies that were mostly related to research arose from a personal interest, including problem identification, or simply an interest in documenting the level of nurse satisfaction. Of the studies with a strong management purpose, the most common specific use was to evaluate programs aimed at either restructuring patient care delivery systems or establishing a shared-governance model of management. Studies using the IWS for mainly managerial purposes focused on improving nurse retention programs, improving communication within the organization, or suggesting additional criteria for selection of the nursing staff.

Of the studies whose purpose included both management and research, the respondent was most likely to write additional comments about the management orientation. Some studies began as part of an evaluation of some type of managerial intervention. Several then noted the evolution of using the IWS as a monitoring tool to keep track of the progress of the intervention. In many of the larger hospitals, the research team and the managers worked together to design studies and to make organizational decisions based on the results of the research.

Eighty percent of the studies that identified some management focus found the information gathered by the IWS to be useful. About one-third of these indicated that redesign initiatives were part of the administration of the IWS, and 20 percent noted that other administrative programs were developed as a result of the study.

One indication of the use of the IWS as part of a redesign program is how often it is given. In only about one-third of all the studies is the IWS administered more than once, with most of these involving a pretest and posttest around some type of specific management intervention. A few used the IWS in a monitoring situation, especially those trying to create a TQM/CQI program. Some of the selections in Chapter 5 are good examples of this. The next section will provide more information on the types of redesign programs.

Setting of the Study and Type of Nursing Staff

The majority of these studies took place in one or more hospital settings. Two were conducted in nursing homes and six involved regional surveys of nurses. Of those in hospitals, the vast majority were in acute care, community hospitals (33 or 66 percent). Two were in children's hospitals; five in tertiary, teaching centers, and two in psychiatric hospitals.

As Table 4.1 shows, the studies using the IWS involved hospitals of all sizes, with a fairly equal distribution. As shown in Table 4.2, half of all studies involved sample sizes of less than 100, and one-third had sample sizes of more than 300. However, four studies each involved over 700 nursing staff, demonstrating that the IWS was also being used in larger hospital and multihospital settings. Response rates varied; slightly over half of all the studies had a response rate of less than 50 percent.

Most studies included all specialties of nurses, but a significant number focused on more specialized groups of nurses. For example, three studies concentrated on pediatric nurses. Other specialties included: neonatal or intensive care nurses (two studies); medical/surgical nurses (two studies); critical care nurses (one study); psychiatric nurses (one study); operating room nurses (one study); long-term care or nursing home nurses (three studies); and oncology nurses (two studies). Two studies looked not at specialty but at where the nurse respondents were in their careers: these two studies examined entry-level nurses in comparison to advanced, more experienced nurses.

Table 4.1 IWS Use, by Hospital Size

Number of Beds	Number and Percentage of Studies	
Less than 100	6	12%
101–199	7	13%
200–299	5	9%
300–399	7	13%
400–499	6	12%
500–599	4	8%
600–699	4	8%
700–799	6	12%
Over 800	7	13%

Note: Some studies involved more than one hospital.

Table 4.2 Sample Size in 88 Adminstrations of the IWS

Number of Nurses in Sample	Number and Percentage of Studies	
Less than 100	40	45%
101–199	11	13%
200–299	8	9%
300–399	14	16%
400–499	8	9%
Over 500	7	8%

Response Rate

An important aspect of administering the IWS—regardless of whether it is primarily for research or for management concerns—is the response rate. Obviously, a higher response rate gives more confidence in a management intervention or the credibility of a research result. Not surprisingly, the response rate in the sample studies seemed to be somewhat related to the method of administration. Thirty-four percent of the studies distributed the questionnaire in a group setting and retrieved it at that time, while 37 percent distributed it individually and retrieved it individually. Both of these methods of distribution and retrieval took place within the organizational setting. Slightly over one-quarter of the studies used a mail survey outside the organizational setting.

Even though the intraorganizational distribution and retrieval of questionnaires should lead to higher response rates, the reported rates were variable. Investigators with higher response rates were more likely to have distributed and retrieved the questionnaire from within the organization, although whether they distributed the questionnaire in a group or in an individual setting had little effect on response rate. Studies using a mail survey technique outside the organizational setting had the lowest response rates. As noted above, slightly over half of all the studies involved response rates of less than 50 percent, which limits the ability of a project to suggest meaningful conclusions or to identify the management interventions that might work most effectively.

Comments and Suggestions about the IWS

What people thought of the IWS in a general way depended to some extent on the purpose of their study. The most frequent comments about the IWS were contributed by those respondents whose study had some management orientation, which is about three-fourths of all the respondents. Of this group, 80 percent indicated that the IWS gathered information that was very useful to their organization. Perhaps the largest single category of information involved identifying the relationship of nurse satisfaction to programs established within the organization. These included clinical advancement systems, personality issues that might be used to better screen nurses in the hiring process, and several managerial interventions, especially participative management systems such as shared governance. In some cases, the IWS was used in combination with the management intervention. In other cases, the results from an administration of the IWS were used to validate initiatives already begun. Several cases viewed the IWS as providing information to supplement other routine management data.

A few studies used the IWS in planning, with positive comments focusing on its usefulness in assigning priorities to needs. A few studies pointed out the importance of having several administrative levels involved in the process of administering the IWS and interpreting the results. More than one study specifically noted the value of the IWS in terms of gathering feedback from the nursing staff, in order "to let them know how they were perceiving changes. This was also useful to me to distinguish 'noise' from valid concerns."

About one-third of the respondents indicated that redesign initiatives were part of the administration of the IWS, and another 20 percent noted that the IWS process led to additional administrative programs. Among these respondents, by far the most frequent comment was that the IWS was useful as one of several measurement tools used to guide, evaluate, or monitor the redesign process. Specific examples of programs included shared governance, primary nursing, and clinical advancement systems. In one case, after the administration of the IWS, a comprehensive salary survey and compensation program were undertaken. A different hospital used the IWS as one of the mechanisms to redesign and improve communication with the staff. Another hospital formed joint research-management teams to pursue issues identified in the IWS survey process.

The survey of researchers asked respondents specifically to indicate whether they had made any changes in the IWS, either in the wording of the scale or in the scoring process. Of course, because of the sampling process, most of these respondents had made only minor modifications to the IWS. And, in fact, the vast majority of investigators used the IWS scale without any modifications. Those who modified the wording did so to meet their specific needs, such as substituting "nursing staff" for "nurse" to include a variety of nursing levels. One study in particular compared the level of satisfaction of current and previous employees, changing the wording to represent the past experience of previous employees. A few respondents did not use all the subscales. The most common omission was the pay component. When investigators deleted this component, it was primarily because they felt they "could not do anything about pay, anyway."

By far the largest category of negative comments concerns the issue of incorporating the component-weighting coefficient (the values computed from the paired comparisons, Part A of the IWS) into a final weighted score, which is actually the Index itself. These critical comments take several forms, with some people referring to the component-weighting coefficient itself and others referring to "scoring problems." Some investigators resolved the problem by not using the paired comparisons; they used only Part B, which measures current level of satisfaction.

They either did not construct the weighted Index or used the values reported in the 1986 edition of this book, a practice that edition supported. Others struggled through the scoring process, but made several—all negative—comments about it, such as, "I found it necessary to hire a statistics graduate student to write the program to assist in data analysis. SAS was utilized for data analysis. I would like to utilize the IWS for my dissertation and look forward to simplification of the scoring procedure."

A few of the respondents also commented on the difficulty of understanding the need for reversing the scoring of some items in Part B. Some indicated they had reversed the scoring on other items besides the suggested ones or had not reversed the scoring on the designated items. The reversal of items is inherent in a Likert attitude scale, but is somewhat confusing. Appendix B, Sections IV and V present a slightly different way to think about these required reversals. This appendix also presents more technical information related to the structure of the scale itself.

The impression received from the many comments about the IWS is that people were very satisfied with the type of information the tool provided. They were also very pleased with the way in which the management system of the organization was able to use the information gained from the IWS. The only major source of unhappiness concerned the scoring process, which really relates to the issue of creating a weighted score, one that includes information about expectations as well as current level of satisfaction. This is, in fact, a critical issue and will be discussed later in this chapter.

The comments and the first level of analysis of the responses to the survey made it obvious that the use of the IWS in the field was far more standardized after the publication of the first edition of this book than before that version of the IWS became available. A higher proportion of investigators used the scale without modification, and a higher proportion used both parts of the scale, although some investigators struggled with the scoring procedures. This finding led to the next step in the analysis: comparison of the numerical results of the responding investigators' studies.

Comparison of Numerical Results

The first edition described the ten different types of numerical analyses suggested for the IWS. Some arise from the first part of the questionnaire (the paired comparisons), others arise from the second part (the Likert scale measuring the current level of satisfaction), and a final set of calculations involves numbers from both parts. The types of numerical analyses are briefly described here, with a complete description included in Appendix B. The questionnaire itself, which has been slightly revised as a result of this survey process, appears in Appendix A.

Numerical Analyses

From Paired Comparisons

The first part of the questionnaire presents each of the 6 components of the IWS with each of the other 5, to give 15 possible comparisons. Respondents are asked to choose which one of each pair is most important to them. The numerical value generated from this is called the Component Weighting Coefficient, and is used to calculate the actual Index value, which is described below. From this Component Weighting Coefficient can also be determined the ranking of each of the components in terms of level of importance. This can be used to understand what is important to the nursing staff, especially if the IWS is being used in conjunction with a management intervention, as has become increasingly common.

From the Likert Scale

The second part of the questionnaire is a 44-item Likert scale, which measures respondents' current level of satisfaction with each of the components ranked in Part A. The numerical values that arise from this part of the scale include a total score for each component and a mean score for each component. These are used to create a ranking of which components currently provide more satisfaction and which provide less satisfaction. It is very useful to compare the rankings of what is viewed as being most important with what currently provides most satisfaction. Also calculable are a total scale score and a total mean score, using all six components together, providing a total summary score for level of satisfaction.

Combinations of Values

The adjusted component score is created by multiplying the mean component score (from Part B) by the Component Weighting Coefficient (from Part A). The scores, which are given for each component separately, provide a numerical value that combines ranking of importance with current level of satisfaction. When these six adjusted scores are summed and divided by six (the number of components), one number is created, which is termed the Index of Work Satisfaction. This single weighted number represents both ranking of importance and level of satisfaction.

Numerical Values

The respondents to the survey were asked to share their data for each of these numerical values in a common format. Each of the returned data sets was examined to make sure the returned data fell within the established parameters of the numerical ranges for each calculation. If a contributed number fell outside this established range, the whole data set was excluded. Also, the numerical values were all examined carefully for "face validity." This was done to decrease the possibility of introducing into the database any numbers that might be inaccurate because of computation errors.

Sixty-five respondents contributed data from 50 different studies, and some of these studies involved multiple administrations of the IWS. Some of the multiple administrations involved separate hospitals; some involved different administrations over time in the same hospital. The database includes 88 different administrations of the IWS.

All of the information meeting the criteria was combined to create this database. The database now includes responses to the IWS from over 10,000 nurses. This section of this chapter will describe the basic numerical values for the IWS, using all responses combined together. In all cases, the unit of analysis employed here will be studies, rather than respondents. The last section of this chapter will address some of the methodological and philosophical issues that arise from such a combination of responses.

Component Weighting Coefficient

This value is calculated from Part A of the IWS questionnaire, a forced-choice paired comparisons technique. (This and all other technical details about the structure of the IWS appear in Appendix B.) The Component Weighting Coefficient is calculated using a proportion matrix based on the frequency distribution of how often one member of a pair is chosen over the other. The actual value is produced by use of a Z-table, which incorporates a distribution of all possible scores. The values of the Component Weighting Coefficient range from 0.9 to 5.3. The higher the Component Weighting Coefficient, the more important that particular component is to a respondent.

Figure 4.1 comprises six bar graphs. Each bar graph gives the frequency distribution for the Component Weighting Coefficient for one component—pay, autonomy, task requirements, organizational policies, professional status, or interaction—calculated from the 50 studies included in the survey. For this and the other figures in this section, the results are shown in terms of the number of studies in which a particular numerical value was obtained. The definition of a study is not exact, because some studies involved multiple administrations, as noted above. In the figures in this section, a study denotes one administration of the

IWS questionnaire. In cases where the IWS was used over time, only the first administration is counted as a "study."

Each bar graph of Figure 4.1 shows the number of studies that obtained a numerical value for the Component Weighting Coefficient of a particular component. Not all studies calculated the Component Weighting Coefficient: in fact, only about half of the studies did their own calculations. Several noted they used the values for the Component Weighting Coefficient that were reported in 1986. This is consistent with the feedback from the users of the IWS that scoring this part of the questionnaire was somewhat confusing.

As may be seen in Table 4.3, the order of ranking of importance of these components remained stable from 1986 to 1996. When all the values obtained from the 50 studies contributed to the database are averaged together, the numbers calculated as the Component Weighting Coefficient are within 4 percentage points of the values calculated in the final validation study of 1986.

Figure 4.1 shows the distributions of values for the Component Weighting Coefficients for the studies that calculated this value. These distributions are fairly compact and symmetrical, with small standard deviations. The least variation exists for the organizational policies and autonomy components, which have a range of scores of about 0.5, not counting the one outlier in the organizational policies component, where respondents in one study ranked this component as being very important. The most variation exists for pay and professional status, although the variation for interaction and task requirements is not much less. The largest range is 1.1, which is the range for the pay component.

When this method of analysis was suggested in 1986, it was not known how much variation would exist in terms of these expectations. The first edition of this book suggested that ranking of importance would be more consistent than current level of satisfaction, and Figure 4.1 does seem to support this observation. Even though the variation is small, the effect of such a range in calculating an adjusted score cannot be ignored. The 1986 guideline that expectations are consistent and thus need not be calculated for each study should be reexamined in light of these studies. This issue will be addressed in the last section of this chapter.

Current Level of Satisfaction Values

There are four separate numbers that may be calculated from the responses to the attitude items on Part B of the questionnaire, which measures current level of satisfaction. Two of these are related to the total scale: the total scale score (the sum of responses to all 44 items) and the total mean score (the mean of the scores for the total scale). The

Figure 4.1 Frequency Distribution of Component Weighting Coefficients

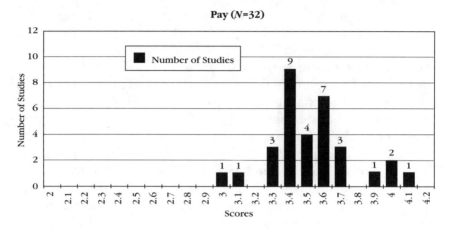

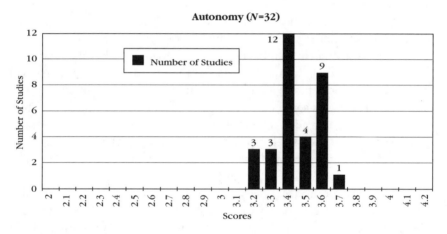

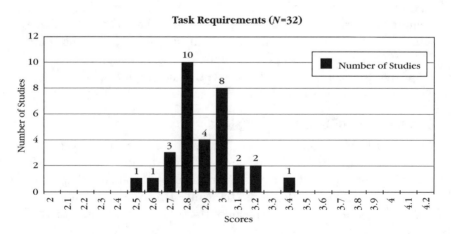

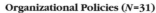

Organizational Policies (*N*=31)

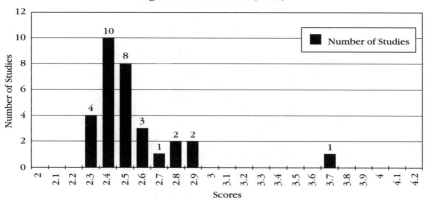

Professional Status (*N*=32)

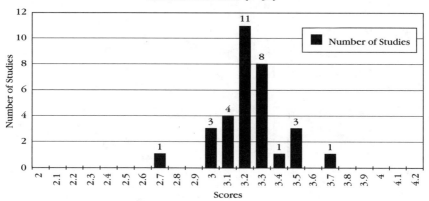

Interaction (*N*=30)

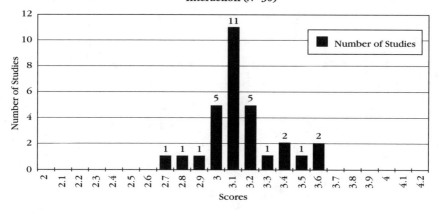

Table 4.3 Comparison of Ranking of Importance with Level of Satisfaction, 1986 and 1996 Studies

1986 Studies		1996 Studies	
Ranking of Importance	Level of Satisfaction	Ranking of Importance	Level of Satisfaction
1/2 Autonomy	1. Professional Status	1/2 Autonomy	1. Professional Status
1/2 Pay	2. Interaction	1/2 Pay	2. Interaction
3. Professional Status	3. Autonomy	3. Professional Status	3. Autonomy
4. Interaction	4. Task Requirements	4/5 Interaction	4. Task Requirements
5. Task Requirements	5. Organizational Policies	4/5 Task Requirements	5. Organizational Policies
6. Organizational Policies	6. Pay	6. Organizational Policies	6. Pay

other two numbers are based on each of the components: a total score for each separate component and a mean score for each component. Most studies calculated these two scores for each of the components separately, rather than using the total scale score for the entire questionnaire. Figure 4.2 compares the total scores for each component for 1986 and 1996; Figure 4.3 shows the frequency distributions for the total scores for each component in the 1996 survey; and Table 4.3 compares the rankings from both parts of the IWS questionnaire.

As Table 4.3 shows, there seems to be no change in the ranking of components from 1986 to 1996, either in level of importance or in level of satisfaction. Autonomy and pay continue to be the most important components to the nurse respondents; pay continues to be the component with which there is the highest level of dissatisfaction. Pay continues to be identified as an area in which change needs to occur, since it exhibits the largest dissonance between level of importance and level of satisfaction. However, it is not just components that rank high in terms of level of importance that deserve attention. As will be repeatedly demonstrated in Chapter 5 and Appendixes E and F, nurses have historically low expectations of organizational policies, in particular, and also of task requirements. However, these low expectations do not mean that either component is unimportant; rather they probably reflect nurses' professional and personal experience. In some of the selections in Chapter 5 and Appendix E, for example, the largest changes after

Figure 4.2 Total Scores for the Six Components, 1986 and 1996

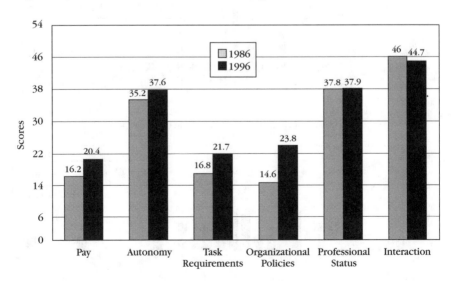

Figure 4.3 Frequency Distribution of Total Scores for Each Component

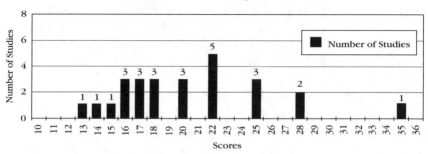

Pay (Theoretical Range 6–42, *N*=26)

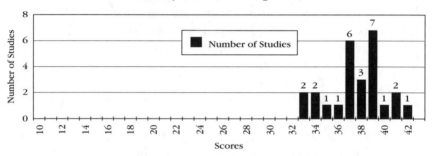

Autonomy (Theoretical Range 8–56, *N*=26)

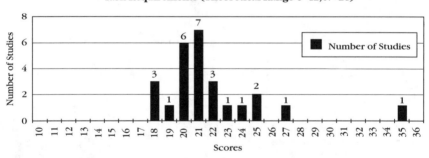

Task Requirements (Theoretical Range 6–42, *N*=26)

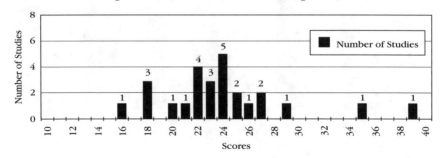

Organizational Policies (Theoretical Range 7–49, *N*=26)

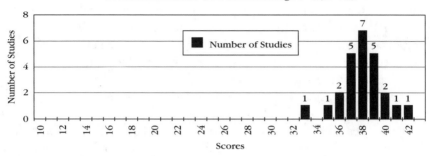

Professional Status (Theoretical Range 7–49, *N*=25)

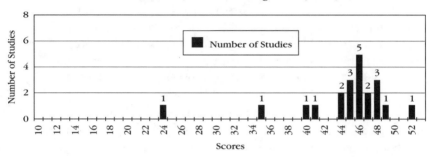

Interaction (Theoretical Range 10–70, *N*=21)

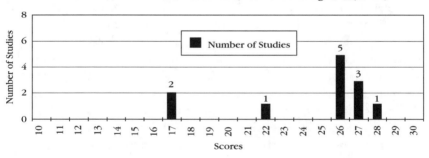

Nurse-Nurse Interaction Subscale (Theoretical Range 5–35, *N*=12)

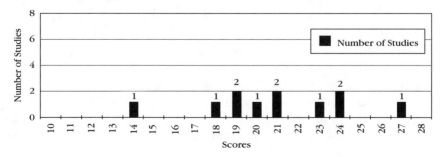

Nurse-Physician Interaction Subscale (Theoretical Range 5–35, *N*=11)

managerial interventions are often in the component of organizational policies.

The comparison of level of importance (or expectations) and level of current satisfaction is helpful in interpreting what the numbers generated by the IWS mean, as the above discussion shows. However, it is also important to consider the findings related to current level of satisfaction. In interpreting these scores, it is helpful to compare them with the total theoretical score for each component. To make comparisons easier, the theoretical score is divided into percentiles, or quartiles. This is especially important because each component has a different range, so comparing actual scores of the components is not very helpful. In this method of interpretation, a score in the first quartile would be at or below 25 percent of the theoretically possible score. A score in the second quartile would be between 26 percent and 50 percent of the theoretical maximum; a score in the third quartile would be between 51 percent and 75 percent, and a score in the fourth or highest quartile would be above 75 percent of the maximum possible. Interpreting what these scores mean is more problematic: nearly everyone would agree that a score in the first quartile is too low, but the limits of "acceptable" or "high" are arguable. This issue is addressed further in the last section of this chapter.

Figure 4.2 shows the total scores for level of satisfaction for each of the components. A comparison is shown here between the data reported in 1986 and the average of all the scores for the studies contributing to the 1996 database. Appendix B contains more information, including the actual numerical values for each quartile for each component.

The first observation, of course, is how low all the scores are, in comparison to the theoretical possible. The component with the highest level of satisfaction is professional status, with scores at the very bottom of the fourth quartile (77 percent of the total possible score). Interaction and autonomy each have scale scores that are about 65 percent of the total possible, placing them in the middle of the third quartile. When the interaction component is broken into its respective parts, the satisfaction with the interaction between nurses and physicians is lower, being closer to the bottom of the third quartile. Task requirements and organizational policies both have scores that are slightly under the 50 percent mark, placing them at the top of the second quartile. Pay, with the lowest score, is in the middle of the second quartile.

It is of obvious interest to determine whether there seem to have been any changes over time in these scores. Four of the six components do seem to show a positive change over time. The biggest of these seems to be in the pay component, which mirrors positive changes in income over time, especially for hospital nurses. The other three showing positive improvement are autonomy, task requirements, and organizational policies. The scores of the professional status component seem to have remained the same over time. Only the interaction component seems to show a decline in level of satisfaction over time. This decrease is more pronounced with the physician-nurse interaction, but is also present with nurse-nurse interaction. These changes are small and relative, and statistical tests of significance are not appropriate. Later, as more information is contributed to this database, it will be possible to examine differences more closely, including through statistical analysis of the significance of those differences.

The distributions of the scores for each of the components are interesting. Figure 4.3 shows total scores, and Figure 4.4 shows mean scores. Two of the components—autonomy and professional status—have a near-normal distribution of total scores (Figure 4.3). Both pay and organizational policies show a flatter-than-expected distribution, while task requirements shows a somewhat skewed distribution. Each of these components has one or two outliers that are highly satisfied with that particular component. The interaction component shows a fragmented distribution with several outliers, most of whom are dissatisfied. Figure 4.3 also shows the results of the interaction component broken down into its two subcomponents, based on the 12 studies that made this breakdown. The distribution of study averages for the nurse-physician subcomponent is very flat, indicating diverse perceptions about this important interaction. The distribution of study averages for the nurse-nurse interaction subcomponent is not as flat, but it is noteworthy that the outliers are all at the low end of the scores, indicating high levels of dissatisfaction perceived by respondents in some of the studies.

Figure 4.4 shows the frequency distributions of the mean scores for each component reported by the studies. Understandably, more studies (43) reported using the mean scores rather than the total scores (26), primarily because of the ease of comparing the various components. Figure 4.5 shows the comparison of mean scores for each component for the 1986 final validation study and the studies that responded to the 1996 survey. The changes over time shown here are consistent—as they should be—with the total scores shown in Figure 4.2, although it is probably easier to see the level of change over time when looking at mean scores. One additional piece of information shown in Figure 4.5 concerns the interaction component. When looking at either the mean or total scores over time, there seems to be little or no change. However, when the interaction component is broken into its two parts, there are some dramatic differences, actually the largest single difference noted in this type of meta-analysis. The level of satisfaction of the nurse respondents

Figure 4.4 Frequency Distribution of Mean Scores for Each Component

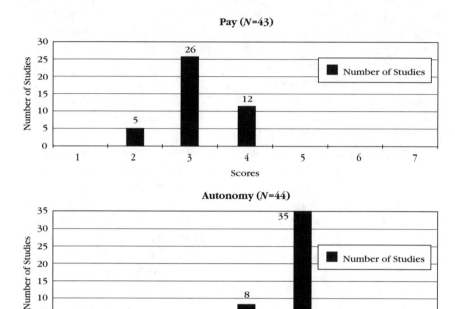

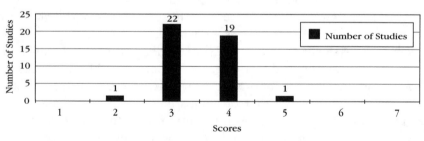

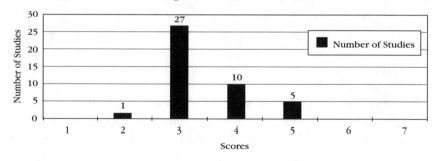

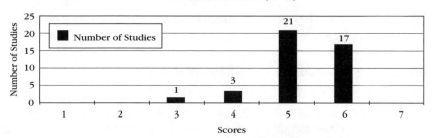

Professional Status (*N*=42)

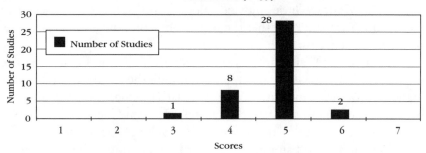

Interaction (*N*=39)

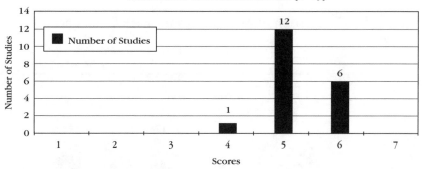

Nurse-Nurse Interaction Subscale (*N*=19)

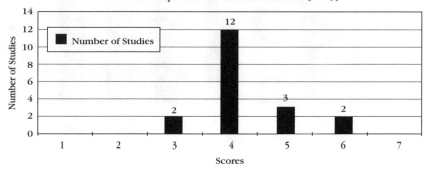

Nurse-Physician Interaction Subscale (*N*=19)

with nurse-physician interaction has significantly eroded over time. This may be due to the higher professional training and expectations of nurses who still encounter basically the same type of physician control over their professional decisions.

Calculating the Index of Work Satisfaction

The Index of Work Satisfaction is calculated by multiplying the mean score for each component, obtained from measuring current level of satisfaction, by the weighting coefficient of that component, producing adjusted scores, and then dividing by 6 (the number of components) to produce the Index. These adjusted values do not seem to be as sensitive to variation over time as either the total scale score, the total mean score, or the mean score for each component.

The Index of Work Satisfaction scores are shown in Figure 4.6. The most common value is around 13, even though the theoretical value is as high as 39.7, which indicates a low cumulative value. Over the ten-year period included in this survey, the average IWS score increased from 12.0 to 12.5. Although this may not seem like much of an increase, the Index itself is a complicated summary number that should not be expected to

Figure 4.5 Comparison of Mean Scores for Each Component, 1986 and 1996

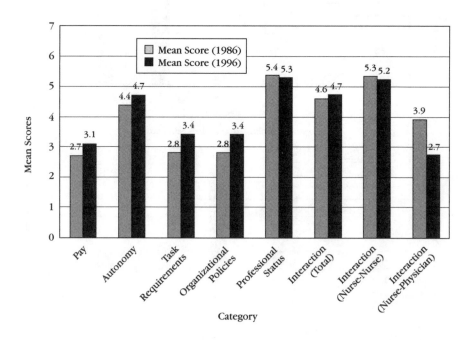

vary much. Based on these studies, it seems that the adjusted scores and the Index itself are not as sensitive to the changes that are observed in the component scores, both total and mean scores.

The analysis of the numerical results of these 50 studies representing 88 different administrations of the IWS provides a valuable context to any individual study of satisfaction using the IWS. Given the increased standardization of use of the questionnaire itself as well as the scoring procedures, these comparisons provide a high level of confidence in what the IWS is actually measuring. Having such comparisons available will increase investigators' ability to interpret findings from any individual study. This ability is not without some disadvantages, however, as the next section will demonstrate.

Issues in Creating a Comparative Database

Once comparisons of similar studies are available, a new level of research is possible. Many of the questions posed by this research concern a database. This section will begin by addressing the philosophical and conceptual issues related to establishing a database, and then move to a consideration of methodological and practical issues. Although the establishment of such a database adds a significant amount of information, it is far from answering all the relevant questions. In fact, the observation will be made throughout this section that more research is needed, often because new questions can be asked.

Philosophical and Conceptual Issues

There is a phenomenon in social sciences research known as reification, where the measurement used for the variable becomes the focus of attention, in place of the concept itself. Perhaps the most classic example of this phenomenon is the use of grades in schools. Nearly everyone— teachers, parents, and students—talks about the measurement as the outcome itself. When asked what they learned in a particular course, students commonly respond, "I got an A." Only upon reflection is it clear that receiving an A is not necessarily the same as achieving mastery of a subject.

Perhaps the greatest cause for hesitation in developing a comparative database is the fear that the numbers generated by the IWS will become the focus, rather than what the numbers represent. It is extremely important always to acknowledge that satisfaction is perceptual and also individualistic. Not every person responds the same way to organizational situations, or to stressful situations. Some of the practice-based investigations contained in Appendix E (especially Selections 6, 7,

Figure 4.6   IWS Scores, 1996 (Theoretical Range .5–39.7, (*N*=30)

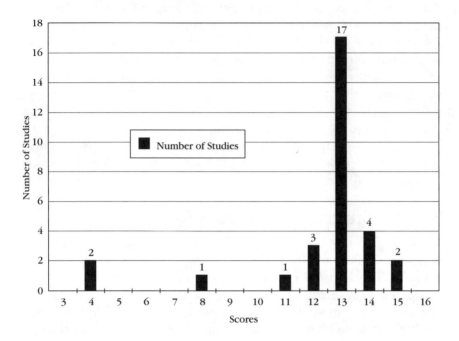

and 8) for example, describe research on what are commonly viewed as particularly stressful situations for nurses, but these studies demonstrate that not everyone views such settings as stressful. The published literature also reinforces this (Blegen 1993; Schaefer and Moos 1996; Chappell and Novak 1992).

There is much still unknown about satisfaction, and its relation to other variables, including level of stress and burnout as well as other outcomes, such as productivity and patient outcomes. Even the theoretical foundations of satisfaction are not consistent with one another. One view is that satisfaction is a continuum, with high levels of dissatisfaction leading to high levels of stress, and with both leading to burnout. One alternative view is that satisfaction is in a completely different category from dissatisfaction and that a person may be both satisfied and dissatisfied, depending on the circumstances, as shown in Chapter 2.

Small wonder that studies linking satisfaction to other variables such as productivity, other performance measures, or patient outcomes are so contradictory. All of these things are hard to quantify; and as measures are developed, if the process of reification occurs, the conclusions made—and actions taken—may be based on the measurement itself rather than the concept. The actions taken are often in the area of management interventions and job redesign. Evaluation of these actions is one of the primary ways in which level of satisfaction is measured. It is important that the appropriate conclusions are drawn about the effect of these actions on the level of nurse satisfaction. This is ensured by keeping in mind the limitations of any summary numerical score and by remembering what the number is meant to represent.

One of the most likely outcomes of the use of a database is the development of norms or standards for satisfaction. This is something that users of the IWS have been requesting since 1986. The desire for such standards is certainly understandable, since they would add context and a broader understanding of one's own results. This is appropriate and useful as long as users remember the meaning of the numbers, rather than making the numbers themselves the standards.

The 1994–95 survey of investigators using the IWS has added significantly to setting such a context, by beginning the comparison phase of this research. The satisfaction scores generated by the IWS seem low, particularly the Index itself. Nurses indicate the highest level of satisfaction with the professional satisfaction component; it has scores that are just barely in the top quartile, which is 75 percent of the total maximum possible. The lowest is satisfaction with pay, which has scores in the top of the second quartile, which means that they are only about half of the total possible. Using quartiles to interpret satisfaction is one way to recognize the ambiguity involved in trying to represent the individual perception of satisfaction by one summary number. However, as confidence in the numbers themselves improves, it will be tempting for some minimal standards to be set. One possibility that may be effective is for each institution to set its own goals for each individual component. For example, one hospital may try specifically to improve the sense of professional satisfaction, while another may wish to improve the feeling of autonomy that nurses perceive. Another possibility is to set an arbitrary general standard that would be applicable to all nurses at all hospitals. If this approach were taken, it would seem reasonable to aim for scores in at least the third quartile, which would mean that the scale scores on each component should be between 50 percent and 75 percent of the maximum possible. Clearly, research is needed here, especially to identify better what effect organizational innovations have on satisfaction to determine the specific innovations that have the greatest effect on satisfaction.

As the evidence for the link between organizational innovations and satisfaction increases, there will be increased interest in seeing the level of satisfaction change over time. As has been shown in this section, there do not seem to be dramatic differences in the scores generated by the IWS between 1986 and the studies reported here as 1996 data.

Three important caveats are relevant here. First of all, as noted earlier, the studies contributed to this research process took place over the ten-year period of time between 1986 and 1996, 60 percent of them between 1992 and 1994. Second, the comparisons presented here are between one study conducted in 1986 and many studies, the results of which are aggregated. It is perhaps unfair to expect large-scale changes in general levels of satisfaction, especially given the rapidly developing knowledge base about the effect of specific organizational and managerial innovations on level of satisfaction. As will be seen from some of the selections in Chapter 5 and Appendixes E and F, when specific comparisons are made the change noted is significant, especially when evaluating the effect of participative management models. The third caveat is to recognize that, in general, levels of nurse satisfaction are low, and although they are hard to modify over time, they are not impossible to modify. Change in level of satisfaction is neither dramatic nor quick; but satisfaction does respond to changes in the organization. Investigators are expecting far too much if they are disappointed that changes in satisfaction scores are not big.

Certainly, there are many advantages to the creation and maintenance of a national database. The advantages will outweigh the disadvantages as long as users remember some of the important issues raised in this section. Of course, in addition to these conceptual and philosophical issues, there are also several crucial methodological and practical issues.

Methodological and Practical Issues

Three important methodological and practical issues will be discussed here. Two—ensuring the quality and equivalence of data, and whether to combine all the studies—pertain to constructing a database. The other pertains to the uses to be made of the information contained in such a database.

Constructing a Database

The first obvious problem in creating a database is to ensure quality and the equivalent nature of the information that goes into the database. As described earlier in this chapter, the survey of users of the IWS asked them to share their numerical data. The response to this request was very gratifying, with 50 people sharing data from 65 studies using the IWS in 88 separate administrations.

Respondents were asked to share the numerical scores they had calculated in the context of their own studies, not the actual raw data they used to calculate these responses. Each set of data was carefully scrutinized to make sure that the numerical scores fell into the established range of scores. A few of the data sets were eliminated because of such discrepancies. Respondents whose scores fell into the established ranges were assumed to have calculated the various numbers correctly. This assumption is necessary, but obviously may not be true. Since the differences in satisfaction levels may be small, variation in computation may mask changes in satisfaction levels.

The 65 studies represent a great many variations—size of hospital, size and type of nursing staff, and purpose of study, just to mention three. For example, the size of the hospital varied from less than 100 beds (in 12 percent of the studies) to more than 800 beds (in 13 percent). Because of the sampling criteria, no study was included if it had a sample of less than 50, but sample sizes range from less than 100 (45 percent) to more than 500 (8 percent). Some of the studies included only RNs, others also included LPNs; some included only full-time staff, others included all staff; and some studies included all the nursing staff, while others focused on one specialty within nursing. Some of the study sites had participative management models, especially shared governance, while others had the more traditional hierarchical type of management. Some investigators had as their major purpose the documentation and description of the level of satisfaction, while others were using the IWS to evaluate the change in satisfaction as a result of some type of job redesign. Some studies administered the IWS once; others administered it multiple times. Not all the studies calculated all possible numbers or analyzed the IWS in exactly similar ways. Not all studies were located in hospitals: a few were state, regional, or national surveys of nurses.

All of these variations present definitional problems for a database. Some are easier to resolve than others. For example, it is easy simply to use for each numerical score only those studies that calculated it specifically. For example, 26 different studies calculated mean scale scores for each component, while 43 studies shared their total scale scores. Thirty studies shared their IWS values. As a result, the number of studies used in each part of the database differs somewhat, as the figures and tables in this chapter demonstrate.

More problematic is the decision about whether to aggregate all the studies, regardless of sample, hospital size, setting, or purpose. Related to this is just how to present the results of the database. Should all studies be combined, or should only hospitals of a certain type (say, those with less than 200 beds and employing only RNs) be included?

The advantage of combining the studies is clear. The increase in numbers gives more confidence to the numerical values. Having numerical values available from other studies provides an important context for interpretating the values obtained in any particular study. As long as the computations are accurate, perhaps it can be assumed that the purpose, setting, and nature of the sample may not matter.

The disadvantage of such a large and all-inclusive database is that it violates some of the developing understanding of how to use level of satisfaction as a measure. Increasingly, it is obvious that level of satisfaction is sensitive to specific organizational changes; there is also some evidence that level of satisfaction is sensitive to type of nurse specialty. However, presenting and describing such specific information is not feasible in the format of this chapter. So, for the purposes of this chapter, the information has been presented as being one comprehensive database. It is probably this decision that contributes to the seeming lack of change in levels of satisfaction over time. In terms of actually using the database in practice-based research, it is obviously more meaningful to have comparisons that are more specific to one's own particular research setting. This is the suggested use of this database, which is described in Appendix D.

Using the Database

Obviously, the primary use of a database is in comparing the level of satisfaction of one group of nurses with that of another. This is undoubtedly the most common use that investigators have had in mind when they have requested such a database. Investigators want to know how their nurses compare to others. This desired comparison may be to nurses in similar hospitals, especially if the research interest is in analyzing the relationship of organizational structure to nurse satisfaction. An alternative focus for this comparative interest is more managerial. The comparison may involve following basically the same group of nurses over time to assess the effect of a management intervention, or the interest may be in evaluating the effect of some change in patient care delivery systems that has been instituted in only one part of a hospital. Several selections in Chapter 5 and Appendixes E and F use the IWS in this way. The ability to refer to level of satisfaction in other, similar organizational settings would increase investigators' understanding of their results.

Of course, these comparisons are best accomplished with a more specific version of the database than can be presented here. For example, if the hospital in which the original study is conducted is a 200-bed hospital, the investigator may find it most helpful to use comparative information only from hospitals of a similar size. It may be that the relevant variable is type of management, leading to comparisons with results only from these hospitals with shared governance. The interest of the study might focus on level of satisfaction of nurses working in specific settings, such as the operating room or the intensive care unit. Comparing these two groups with medical-surgical nurses might not be appropriate. This example highlights the fact that we do not know enough about what is satisfying to particular groups of nurses working in specific settings. The use of a comparative database will significantly increase investigators' ability to identify these satisfiers as well as to delineate organizational variables that affect level of satisfaction.

There are many other research uses of a comparative database. One example arises from examining the figures and tables appearing earlier in this chapter. In Figure 4.3, for example, there are several instances of studies that can be considered to be outliers, in the sense of having very different scores from the average. These outliers are in both directions. One study had a total score of 35 for task requirements; the average of all the studies for this component was 21.7. Something produced very high levels of satisfaction with this particular aspect of the job for the nurses in this study. The frequency distribution of scores for the organizational policies component shows outliers in both directions. The average of all the studies for this particular component was 23.8; two studies had scores that were 35 and above, while four studies had scores of 18 and below. It is important to study organizations that have either very low or unusually high levels of satisfaction, as this may lead to a much better understanding of the relationship between organizational structure and level of satisfaction.

No doubt other uses of this comparative database will be less research-oriented and more clearly managerial. As is obvious throughout this book, there is a significant overlap between research and management in the nursing field, which strengthens both practice and research. Perhaps the primary example of a use that would be clearly managerial is the need to document levels of satisfaction of the nursing staff in response to recent accreditation standards (JCAHO 1993). It is this use that will be most likely to cause a transition from doing comparative research to setting national standards for levels of satisfaction. Setting standards is not necessarily bad. In fact, as noted above, organizations may want to identify an acceptable level of satisfaction by using the quartiles suggested to aid in interpretation of the numerical scores.

What should be avoided is overreliance on the use of the numerical scores as absolute numbers capturing level of satisfaction. As experience with the IWS and use of a comparative database increase, it will be tempting to accept a given number—an IWS value of 13.0 for example—as being equivalent to the overall level of satisfaction of the nursing staff. This illustrates the tendency to reification, which was discussed at the beginning of this section. Even if standards are developed as part of an accreditation process, it is important to remember that the variable being captured by the standard is based on the perceptions of individuals and is hard to measure accurately. Use of the quartile method of interpretation suggested in the previous section will help prevent overreliance on the numerical scores.

Regardless of whether the interest in the comparative database is mostly research, mostly managerial, or a mixture of both, the use of the database will be enhanced by comparisons between specific groups of nurses. This chapter, of course, cannot present all the possible permutations required. Appendix D includes a description of the technical services available to support the database.

Conclusion

This section will offer a few concluding thoughts. It begins with technical issues related to scoring procedures and the structure of the IWS, then moves to the use of the IWS in the field and the place of the IWS in the general area of investigations about level of professional satisfaction of nurses.

Scoring the IWS

The single most frequent negative comment about the IWS concerns the scoring process. The weighting of the components by ranking of importance makes the scoring tedious. Calculating the Component Weighting Coefficient has always been viewed as tedious, if not complicated. However, it is the Component Weighting Coefficient (from Part A) that makes the IWS unique: no other scale that measures level of satisfaction also measures how important a particular component is. The theoretical literature strongly supports the importance of this analysis.

One of the objectives of the 1994–95 survey was to evaluate again whether it is necessary to use the Component Weighting Coefficients. (See Appendix B for a further discussion of this issue.) As illustrated in Figure 4.1 and Table 4.3, it can be tempting to view the values relating to expectations as constants. In fact, one would expect these values to be more stable over time than current level of satisfaction. However, Figure 4.1 also shows that there is some variability in the values calculated for the Component Weighting Coefficient, although the rankings of the components are quite stable. The range of values is small, only 1.0 for the largest, but this variation is large enough to matter in the computation of the overall Index.

There is a trade-off between the objectives of research and those of practice. It is clearly easier to use the second part of the IWS, creating only a measure of current level of satisfaction. The charts showing the separate scale scores for each of the components show that there is variation among these components, and they do seem to vary independently. However, the value of knowing the level of importance of a particular component remains. Once a baseline for level of importance is established for a particular institution, it would be appropriate to use just the second part in a monitoring design.

To Index or Not

The original conceptualization of the IWS was based on two important assumptions. The first is that a scale that measures level of satisfaction should be interpreted (or weighted) by information on what nurses value most (level of importance). The second assumption is that the best representation of level of satisfaction is one summary number that is weighted, that is, that considers both level of satisfaction and ranking of importance. Based on the 1994–95 survey, the first assumption remains valid: the level of information provided by the Component Weighting Coefficient is important in interpreting the meaning of the numerical scores that represent level of satisfaction.

The second assumption, however, is one that should perhaps be revisited, as suggested both by this research and recent research on physician satisfaction (Stamps and Cruz 1994). These results seem to indicate that the adjusted scores on each component and the Index itself are less sensitive to changes in level of satisfaction than are either the scale scores or the mean scores for each individual component. This makes sense from a mathematical perspective. If one component changes for the better while another changes in a negative way, these two changes are likely to balance out when represented in a total, weighted score. When one looks at the Index of Work Satisfaction, it seems that little or no change in satisfaction has occurred over time. However, when one looks at the level of satisfaction as represented by the mean scores for each component, some individual components have changed quite a bit. Research on physician satisfaction seems to indicate very different patterns of satisfaction on components based on specialty and practice patterns (Stamps and Cruz 1994).

Satisfaction is a multifaceted phenomenon. Hence, measurements divide satisfaction into different components. The IWS uses six components. Other scales have various numbers of factors, but all recognize the importance of separating satisfaction into its component parts. However, when the scores on the separate components are added together to create one summary number, this may obscure the importance of keeping the components different. In fact, it seems that these components vary independently; they are likely influenced by very different variables. Adding them together in one Index does not seem to add much, and it may obscure some information. As has been noted on other occasions in this book, there may be slightly different uses of the IWS for research than for practice, especially with efforts using the IWS to test the effectiveness of a particular management intervention or a job redesign effort or for those involved with developing standards or goals for level of nurse satisfaction. An important research area is to investigate the relationship between the weighted and unweighted scoring procedures, and to examine the pattern of variation among the components themselves.

In the meantime, the most useful numerical value arising from the IWS is probably the mean score of each component, including breaking down the interaction component into its two distinct subscales. These mean score values are particularly useful in a monitoring system used in an organization to account for the process of organizational change. Two of the components—organizational policies and pay—have been shown to be very sensitive to changes in organizational structure.

If a weighted number is appropriate, the most useful one is the Index, not the adjusted scores. These, of course, measure the same thing, but more investigators use the Index, and is easier to use as a summary number. Of course, the Index is not as sensitive to change as are the mean scores, since it is a weighted summary number. However, as with most summary numbers, it is especially useful for comparisons.

Using the IWS: Where to Go From Here?

One obvious conclusion arising from this research is that people are using the IWS. They are eager to have comparative data available in order to understand better the meaning of numbers. The responses to this second survey of people using the IWS provide interesting insights into the nursing profession, suggestions for using the IWS, and direction for future research. Reflection on this process of surveying users of the IWS provides one last observation, which takes the form of a suggestion. The IWS is the most researched and most frequently used measure of job satisfaction in the nursing field. Its grounding in solid and careful practice-based research makes it particularly valuable. Based on experience with measuring level of satisfaction, it may now be helpful to separate research uses from practice uses a bit. In uses that are primarily management-oriented, it seems very appropriate to use the IWS—either the Index itself or mean scores for each of the components—because of the instrument's standardization and wide use, leading to comparative possibilities as well as to beginning a process of developing standards or goals for acceptable levels of nurse satisfaction. In research use, however, it may be appropriate to modify the IWS, to use additional scales, or to develop new measures based on the experience gained in analyzing levels of nurse satisfaction.

Increasingly, uses of the IWS involve evaluation of a particular management innovation in a hospital or other organizational setting. Many uses involve incorporating a measure of job satisfaction into an organizational monitoring system, with frequent data collection. In these application-oriented cases, it is only necessary to do one baseline analysis of level of importance; and then for subsequent measures to use individual mean scores for each component and to keep these separate, which makes for much easier scoring. (As noted before, each component is undoubtedly affected by different variables, and this is an important research area.) It may be more appropriate to develop what might be termed "satisfaction profiles" for nurses. In this way, changes in each component over time can be monitored. Using satisfaction scores in a monitoring system clearly demonstrates the level of importance of nurse satisfaction to an organization. Use of Part B of the IWS as the satisfaction measure is appropriate in this situation because of the ease and standardization of use and the instrument's general familiarity in the field. The database will also be helpful in this effort, permitting comparisons to other organizations.

There are many important issues raised here related to the need for continued research, which may or may not involve the IWS. One is to develop a better understanding of the process by which nurses identify areas of importance, involving both qualitative and quantitative studies. For example, researchers need to clarify what nurse respondents mean when they rank autonomy as being most important to their professional satisfaction. Does this mean nurses have high expectations for this or that they value its existence? Although autonomy is very important to nurses, it seems only moderately satisfying. More information is needed to identify exactly what nurses mean by "professional autonomy," and then to identify ways in which their jobs might provide higher levels of it.

Research is also needed on what it means to rank one component higher than another. The paired-comparison technique is very quantitative, but the understanding of the phenomenon behind the choice needs to be clearer. Also, we need to test periodically whether these rankings of importance continue to remain stable, especially as the healthcare environment changes. Understanding the expectations of nurses is an important piece of being able to design jobs that provide high levels of satisfaction. The ability to evaluate the effectiveness of innovations is critical. Practice-based evaluations will be served well by using the IWS;

however, further research needs to examine the relationship between the individual job and the organization itself. New measures may be needed.

Use of the comparative database described in this chapter and in Appendix D implies general acceptance of the IWS as the measure of work satisfaction of nurses. Although the IWS is used with increasing frequency, this should not slow the development of other measures of work satisfaction. Statistical validation of the IWS took ten years, and the instrument has now been in use for ten years. While it has remained a sensitive measure over time, questions remain about what it measures. More research to refine it or create other measures is necessary to expanding the understanding of nurse satisfaction and the ability to measure this extremely important variable. Just one example is to test the results of several measurements of satisfaction against each other. As shown in Chapter 3, several measures exist, ranging from other scales to global measures using only one item. At the moment, it is not known whether or not these are all measuring the same construct.

There are also a great many unanswered questions about variables that affect nurses' level of satisfaction. For example, organizational policies are not ranked as being very important, but they also do not provide much satisfaction. There are several examples in Chapter 5 and Appendixes E and F in which administrative changes have positively and significantly affected level of satisfaction with organizational policies. How the job is designed clearly affects job satisfaction. More research is needed to identify the relationship between organizational policies and level of satisfaction.

Finally, it is important to increase the dissemination of information about nurse satisfaction, especially with respect to investigating the effect of organizational variables on perception of satisfaction. As shown in Chapter 3, this is an obvious area of interest in the published literature. However, as this second survey has demonstrated, there is a significant amount of research being done that is not represented in the literature. In some cases this is because of methodological problems, with small sample sizes and poor response rates being the primary examples. However, in other cases it is because the focus of research-oriented journals is often on development of new measures rather than uses of existing ones. As a result, many examples of using the IWS to measure level of satisfaction are not shared with other investigators. In many cases, the level of satisfaction is being measured to assess an innovation in patient care services, a change in nursing practice, or even a redesign of the management climate of an entire organization. So what is lost are not just uses of the IWS, but also some fascinating organizational innovations. An important part of the decision to conduct a second survey of those using the IWS was the desire to provide a mechanism for sharing the results of these practice-based research studies with investigators interested in similar questions. The next chapter presents a few examples of research studies that have a specific organizational focus. Appendixes E and F contain many other examples of studies using the IWS to investigate level of nurse satisfaction.

References

Blegen, M. A. 1993. "Nurses' Job Satisfaction: A Meta-Analysis of Related Variables." *Nursing Research* 42: 36–41.

Chappell, N. C., and M. Novak. 1992. "The Role of Support in Alleviating Stress among Nursing Assistants." *The Gerontologist* 32: 351–59.

Joint Commission on Accreditation of Health Care Organizations. 1993. *1994 Accreditation Manual for Hospitals. Volume 1, Standards*. Oakbrook Terrace, IL: The Commission.

Schaefer, J. A., and R. A. Moos. 1996. "Effects of Work Stressors and Work Climate on Long-Term Care Staff's Job Morale and Functioning." *Research in Nursing and Health* 19: 63–73.

Stamps, P. L., and N. T. B. Cruz. 1994. *Issues in Physician Satisfaction: New Perspectives*. Chicago: Health Administration Press.

5

PRACTICE-BASED RESEARCH: USING THE IWS TO INVESTIGATE THE RELATIONSHIP OF SATISFACTION AND ORGANIZATIONAL VARIABLES

hree places in this book offer examples of practice-based research projects using the IWS as a measure of satisfaction. This chapter contains five examples, each of which uses the IWS in a specific organizational setting to implement either a management intervention or an ongoing monitoring system to track changes in nurse satisfaction over time. Appendix E presents another 15 contributions. Some of these share the organizational emphasis of the studies in this chapter, but have fewer data collection points or smaller samples. Others in Appendix E investigate specific specialties or particular settings in which nurses work. The selections in Appendix E are research briefs. Their authors submitted full-length contributions, but space constraints restricted what could be included in this volume. Appendix F contains the third group of examples—20 contributions, all included as abstracts. The authors of all of the 40 selections, having provided their addresses and, in many cases, telephone numbers, are available to provide more information about their studies.

Even though these examples are termed practice-based research, the term does not mean that they are necessarily weak in research methodology. It merely denotes that each research project occured in a healthcare organization in which the patient care objectives were ongoing simultaneously with the research project. As a result, none of these organizations remained unchanging throughout the study period. These contributions also represent a mix of academic and professional interests, as is frequently the case among investigators using the IWS. An example of this close integration of research and practice is the research team involving Pat Martin and her coinvestigators (Appendix E, Selection 2) who had financial support both from the hospital in which they did their work and from an academic institution. Their work resulted in three separate master's theses, two of which are included as selections in this book—Gustin et al. (Selection 2 in this chapter) and Schmidt and Martin (Appendix E, Selection 1).

The central theme of the five selections in this chapter is that job satisfaction is an important variable affected by organizational setting or management. Some of these studies focus on specific types of interventions that change the nurses' roles, while others have a more general concern, with an emphasis on the effect of participative management (especially a shared-governance model) on the level of nurse satisfaction. The studies take place in a variety of hospitals—large and small, urban and rural. Three of the selections feature multiple data collection efforts over time and emphasize use of the information in a monitoring system.

Selection 1 by Ingersoll et al. involves an elaborate sampling plan to determine the effect of an enhanced professional practice model over time. Data were collected in three different hospitals. Five experimental units and five matched comparison units were studied at baseline and yearly for three years after the implementation of the model. Unit-based incentives encouraged high response rates. In addition to job satisfaction (measured by the IWS and the Price-Mueller Job Satisfaction Survey) and demographic and organizational data, the study measured the extent of model implementation. As might be expected from an attempt to measure complex organizational variables over time, the findings are mixed, with an excellent discussion of the problems of showing change in a complex organizational structure. Four specific examples of changes are included here, along with comments on the nature of the effort to evaluate these changes. Two insights stand out from this contribution. The first is that it is important to try to assess change over time. Ingersoll et al. notes, "Although satisfaction is considered to be a stable indicator of perception of work environment, no other studies have measured its stability for the length of time that was used in this study. This issue is an important one since short range studies are prone to misrepresentation of results when only pre-post measures are used. For example, had only one time point been used in this study, an erroneous effect would have been reported." The second insight concerns the discussion of the importance of fully implementing whatever model is being instituted. As the investigators note, in many evaluation studies, only part of the model is implemented, but rarely is that acknowledged. In this study, extent of implementation of the model was very important.

The selections by Gustin et al. (Selection 2 in this chapter), Martin et al. (Appendix E, Selection 2), and Schmidt and Martin (Appendix E, Selection 1) are from the same large research project. The purpose of that project was to provide a database over time to assist in policymaking and program decision making. Data were collected on job satisfaction, organizational climate, professional practice climate, communication, and demographic factors. Investigators administered the IWS eight times over three years, with data now being collected annually. There were several interesting ways of distributing the surveys, including with box lunches at meetings. These selections are based on the analysis of about 1,400 surveys at two hospitals, one with a shared-governance model and one with a more traditional organizational structure, which is the specific focus of the Gustin et al. selection. Overall work satisfaction scores increased between 1988 and 1992, and nurses working at the hospital with a shared-governance model had higher levels of satisfaction of autonomy, pay, and organizational policies. The finding with respect to organizational policies is important, since this component is usually so dissatisfying. Drawing on the large database, this research team also investigated the relationship of demographic variables to level of satisfaction and the relationship of satisfaction to organizational climate, with a discussion of these findings in the selections in Appendix E. Additionally, the investigators, particularly Martin et al. made suggestions for improvements in the IWS. Martin et al. examined the psychometric properties of the IWS and the relationship of the IWS to several other measures, including organizational climate, professional practice climate, the Schutzenhofer Nursing Activity Scale (a measure of autonomy), and a Satisfaction with Communication Scale. Appendix B, Section IV discusses some of the comments by Martin et al. about the structure of the IWS, as well as the comments of other investigators on the structure of the IWS.

Minnick, Pischke-Winn, and Thomas (Selection 3 of this chapter) describe another large-scale monitoring effort that used the IWS as part of quality-improvement activities. The setting for this investigation was Rush–Presbyterian–St. Luke's Medical Center in Chicago, which restructured patient care delivery. To evaluate the innovation, the investigators used the IWS and a Benefits and Schedule Scale they developed. The study used a pre- and postmeasure design, coupled with frequent data collection. One of the interesting aspects of the study is its discussion about keeping response rates up when doing frequent administrations. The importance of the work lies in its description of how to incorporate the IWS into an ongoing management system and in the way in which the organization effected change. Additionally, the investigators discuss insightfully the cost of incorporating the IWS into an ongoing management system.

Three other examples of hospitals using the IWS to evaluate a specific innovation can be found in Appendix E, Selections 11 (Ringer et al.), 12 (Pearson), and 13 (Joy and Malay). Ringer et al. evaluated the effect of a patient care redesign model involving Care Associates. Over a three-year period, there were large increases in satisfaction with autonomy and slight increases in satisfaction with professional status. Pearson investigated the effect of the use of a modification of the case management model in a rural hospital. Although there were no clear-cut answers on whether the case management model improved satisfaction, she noted that not enough time had passed for an appropriate evaluation. Joy and Malay describe a professional practice model developed and implemented at New England Baptist Hospital in Boston. Like Pearson, they felt that not enough time had elapsed to appreciate the effect of the model.

Mancini and McQuaide (Selections 4 and 5 in this chapter) focus on a slightly more general issue: participative management in the larger organization. Mancini studied a hospital that had a shared-governance model for seven years. As with the Gustin et al. study, where the shared-governance model had existed for ten years, Mancini found that the hospital with shared governance had higher levels of nurse satisfaction than the hospital without shared governance. The nurses were more satisfied especially with autonomy, organizational policies, and task requirements; which are the components of satisfaction Mancini felt should show the most change under this management model. Prock (Appendix E, Selection 14) studied two hospitals, one of which had shared governance. Her study could not determine any difference in satisfaction between the two hospitals, but she had problems with response rate and the shared-governance program had just started.

McQuaide enlarged the focus a bit more to include all types of "participative management." Her study involved medical-surgical units in five hospitals in southern New Jersey. For this research she developed a scale to measure level of satisfaction with decision making, the Nurse Participation in Decision Making Scale. In her analysis, she divided respondents into "high" and "low" satisfaction groups, based on their scores on the IWS. One of her major themes is the retention of nurses, a theme shared by many of the selections in Appendix E.

There are no earth-shattering findings presented here. There is, however, a clear dedication to the notion that job satisfaction is related to organizational structure and that job redesign can affect work environments for nurses, which in turn can provide more satisfying work experiences. The studies included in this chapter have made an effort to track such changes, albeit with mixed results. Methodological problems sometimes limit the nature of the conclusions that can be drawn. The researchers all note the limitation of the available time frame. The evidence is clear that participative management—such as shared-governance models—produces higher levels of satisfaction, as do several other types of innovation in the nature of the nursing practice model. However, it does take several years for the organizational culture to change so that this effect on satisfaction can be seen. Also, at the beginning of any particular innovation is a period of anxiety about change. This period may include expressed dissatisfaction. As Ringer and her associates from the Albany Medical Center note,

> As the project was implemented and revised over a three-year period, we often heard grumbling about the changes and the process of change itself. We administered the Index at yearly intervals to provide valid and reliable data about satisfaction. The yearly score along with ongoing unit-based focus groups helped us distinguish the grumbling that accompanies change from the thoughtful critique provided by the nursing staff in the analysis of the Index results. It helped keep us on track, and the Index scores presented in the form of bar graphs were immediately accessible to staff so they could see for themselves. (Appendix E, Selection 11)

Although the major theme of this chapter, as well as most of this book, is the importance of the organization in affecting job satisfaction, the last contribution in Appendix E (Koeckeritz) is a reminder that factors outside the organization affect job satisfaction also. She begins her selection with the thought that job satisfaction of nurses has declined over the past 20 years, while working conditions have improved. Her particular study is focused on issues related to the lives of women, especially what she calls the "second shift," the domestic responsibilities of women in their homes.

Although this enlarged focus presents a more complex model, Koeckeritz is not alone in this view. Several of the theorists discussed in Chapter 2 have also attempted to create more complex and realistic models. Newman (1989) and Grant (1986) both presented conceptual models of the relationship of satisfaction and motivation that included forces outside the control of the organization. Even Herzberg, Mausner, and Snyderman (1959) included what they termed "personal factors" in their model. Although it is important to retain this conceptual understanding,

the power of organizations to create working conditions that can positively affect satisfaction has been overlooked for too long. As noted in
both Chapters 2 and 3, the view of satisfaction has long been that it is
a characteristic of the nurse or perhaps of the individual job. The recent
trend to recognize the importance of involving the whole organization
is a recognition that work does not have to be dissatisfying. The five
selections that follow, as well as many others in Appendixes E and F, are
a clear testimony to the importance of trying to redesign organizations
to create more satisfying work environments.

1. A Longitudinal Study of the Effect of a Professional Practice Model on Staff Nurse Satisfaction

Gail L. Ingersoll, Alison W. Schultz,
Sheila A. Ryan, and Nancy Hoffart

Studies of staff nurse satisfaction have tended to use one-shot case studies or one-group pretest-posttest designs (Campbell and Stanley 1963) in which satisfaction is measured once and used to predict outcomes such as termination or absenteeism, or twice and used to measure short-term effects of an intervention. Although these studies have provided useful information about the role of employee satisfaction in work settings, little information is available about the long-term effect of organizational change on nurse satisfaction.

A recent study of the effect of a professional practice model on nurse and patient outcome measured satisfaction longitudinally over four years, using measurement instruments with established reliability and validity estimates. Data were collected from nurses exposed to the professional practice model and from nurses working in comparable patient care units who were not. The sample comprised nurses from four general medical-surgical units in an urban medical center, two general medical-surgical units in each of two community hospitals, and one general medical-surgical unit in each of two rural hospitals.

This selection describes the findings pertaining to nurse satisfaction. Reports of other outcomes may be found elsewhere (Ingersoll et al. 1996; Ingersoll 1996).

Description of Study

The effect of an enhanced professional practice model (EPPM) was measured over time in three hospitals, a 722-bed urban medical center, a 113-bed community hospital, and a 53-bed rural hospital. Five experimental

Gail L. Ingersoll, Ed.D., R.N., F.A.A.N., is Chenault Professor and Associate Dean for Research at Vanderbilt University School of Nursing, Nashville, Tennessee. Alison W. Schultz, Ed.D., R.N., is Associate Professor of Clinical Nursing at the University of Rochester School of Nursing, Rochester, New York. Sheila A. Ryan, Ph.D., R.N., F.A.A.N., is Dean and Professor at the University of Rochester School of Nursing, Rochester, New York. Nancy Hoffart, Ph.D., R.N., is Assistant Professor at the University of Kansas School of Nursing, Kansas City, Kansas.

This study was supported by Cooperative Agreement Award #U01 NR02156 from the National Institute of Nursing Research, National Institutes of Health, and the Division of Nursing, Health Resources and Services Administration. Funds also were provided by the Robert Wood Johnson Clinical Nurse Scholars Program.

For more information about this study, please contact Gail L. Ingersoll at Joint Center for Nursing Research, 327-A Goadchaux Hall, Nashville, TN 37201. Telephone (615) 343-4173; fax (615) 343-7711; E-mail: gail.ingersoll@mcmail.vanderbilt.edu units and five matched comparison units were studied at baseline (immediately prior to model implementation), and at one, two, and three years after model implementation. Two experimental units and two comparison units were selected from the medical center. Assignment to experimental or comparison status was determined by flip of coin. Because of the limited number of units available in the community and rural hospitals, two units in the community hospital and one in the rural hospital were used as experimental sites. These units were matched with comparable units in a 102-bed community hospital and a 49-bed rural hospital located in similar geographic areas and matched on multiple characteristics. A multivariate analysis of variance confirmed comparability of units prior to initiation of the study.

Experimental unit nurses were exposed to the EPPM, while comparison units continued according to existing practice patterns. No attempt was made to restrict organizational innovations in the comparison units, with the expectation that this approach would more accurately reflect the norm for regularly progressing care delivery environments. Participation in the study was voluntary, and nurses not wishing to remain on experimental units were given an opportunity to transfer to another unit in the hospital. None did so.

The design of the enhanced professional practice model introduced in this study drew from previous research concerning recruitment and retention of nurses. The model was composed of five interdependent conceptual elements (control over practice, compensation and rewards reflective of education and experience, continuity of care delivery, continuing education based on unit need, and collaborative practice among care providers). Introduction of the model was expected to result in early favorable changes in nurse perception of the work environment, which would ultimately result in improved retention of nurses, improved patient outcome, and reduced cost of care delivery (Ingersoll et al. 1996).

Nurse job satisfaction was measured with two scales, the attitude component (Part B) of the Stamps and Piedmonte (1986) Index of Work Satisfaction and the Price and Mueller (1981) Job Satisfaction Scale (JSS). A decision was made to use both tools since neither had been used previously in longitudinal studies, and both had some limitations in their appropriateness for measuring current work environments. The paired-comparisons (expectations) component of the IWS was not included because of the length of the overall questionnaire, which grew to 21 pages at several data collection points.

Data pertaining to characteristics of the nurse and the organizational environment also were collected. Each of the variables selected was reported as significant in previous studies of nurse satisfaction and retention.

Extent of model implementation was measured using an adaptation of a scale developed by Milton and colleagues (Milton et al. 1995). A score ranging from 0 (no evidence of model component implementation) to 8 (full implementation) was assigned to each component of the model. An overall model implementation score was then computed by summing the scores determined for each of the model components (Ingersoll et al. 1996). This approach to quantifying extent of intervention has been recommended by Basch et al. (1985) and Finnegan et al. (1989) to maximize the likelihood of assessing true cause-effect relationships between intervention and outcome.

Questionnaires with cover letters were distributed to all nursing personnel assigned to study units. Follow-up reminders were sent two weeks after the initial mailing, and repeat packets of questionnaire and cover letter were sent four weeks after the initial mailing to those who did not respond to first or second contact. In addition, an incentive offering was instituted to maximize return rates during the second, third, and fourth data collection periods. Units that met or exceeded their previous return rates were given $100 to use in any way they desired. The unit with the greatest return rate was given an additional $100; in several cases, more than one unit achieved 100 percent return rates, and all received the additional bonus.

Data were collected immediately prior to model implementation and at one, two, and three years after implementation. Complete psycho-metric testing procedures were performed for all instruments at each data collection point. Initial data analysis involved use of delta change scores to detect differences in pre- and postintervention outcomes. Type of unit (experimental or comparison) was compared for differences, as was type of hospital (medical center, community, and rural). Subsequent analyses included use of mean unit score. This approach was used because of increased appreciation for the group effect of the intervention and the recognition of the combined effects of the individuals involved.

Findings

Although data were collected from all staff in the study units, findings are presented for registered nurse staff only. This reporting practice was chosen to allow for comparison with other studies of nurse satisfaction reported in the literature.

No differences were seen for respondent characteristics between experimental or comparison unit nurses at any point in time. Consistent differences were seen according to hospital type, however, with nurses in the medical center being younger, less likely to be married, and more likely to be baccalaureate prepared. The majority of the sample was Caucasian and female (97.7 percent). The primary educational level for RNs was associate degree (49.5 percent), followed by baccalaureate (27.6 percent) and diploma (22.9 percent). Most were married (62.5 percent), with the next largest group those who never married (23.7 percent). Approximately two-thirds of those who were married had children, most of whom resided in the home (Ingersoll et al. 1996).

Instrument Testing Findings

The internal reliability coefficients (alpha) for the scales were .88 for the JSS and .73 for the IWS. Subscale reliabilities for the IWS ranged from .46 for professional status to .90 for promotional opportunity and are shown in Table B.3 (Appendix B).

Item to item, item to total, and scale to scale correlations were assessed for evidence of consistency or overlap within and across scales. The IWS and JSS were moderately and significantly correlated. All IWS subscales were moderately (organizational policies) to highly (interaction) correlated with the full work satisfaction scale. IWS autonomy and professional status subscales were highly and significantly correlated with the JSS. All other relationships between the two scales were weak to nonexistent.

Factor analysis of subscales for the IWS were consistent across data collection periods. As a result, one data point (Time 2) was selected to highlight findings pertaining to instrument validity estimates. The second data collection point was chosen because the questionnaire used to collect data at that time reflected modifications made to enhance clarity. Factor analysis findings partially supported previous reports of construct validity. Items were considered in the analysis if they loaded at greater than .30 on one or more factors (Nunnally 1994). The results of the factor analysis are described in Appendix B, Table B.5.

Nurse Satisfaction Findings

Some significant relationships were found between nurse characteristics and nurse satisfaction scores. Age was found to be significantly related to job satisfaction as measured by the IWS and the JSS, with older nurses being more satisfied than younger nurses. Income was significantly related to job satisfaction as measured by the IWS, but not by the JSS. Nurses with incomes at the extremes (highest and lowest) were more satisfied than nurses with midrange family incomes. Number of years worked in nursing was significantly related to IWS score, while educational level of the RN was significantly related to JSS score. Nurses who had worked in the hospital more than 15 years were most satisfied, followed by nurses who had worked less than one year. Diploma nurses were most satisfied, with associate degree and baccalaureate nurses showing comparable levels of satisfaction.

When delta change scores were used to assess differences between experimental and comparison units, no differences were seen for any of the subscale scores or for the overall job satisfaction score for the IWS. Some inconsistent differences were seen with the JSS, however, with individual scores for comparison unit nurses changing more favorably than experimental unit nurses between baseline and Times 2, 3, and 4. Because delta change scores are produced by substracting the second time period from the first, negative or minimal positive scores reflect improved outcome. (Details of this analysis are available from the author.)

When scores for nurses who remained in units throughout the study were compared for individual subscales, some differences between groups were seen at various data collection times. These changes were not consistent throughout the study, however. Moreover, there was no pattern of gradually improved or diminished response. For example, at Time 3, significant differences were seen for "organizational policies," with nurses in experimental units reporting more favorable responses. This finding is an isolated one, suggesting that factors other than the model contributed to this effect.

When unit means were used to detect change, some differences were seen. If the final data collection point is used (with the expectation of maximum effect at that point in time), experimental units show significantly greater levels of job satisfaction on both the IWS and the JSS. This finding may be a better indication of unit effect, since the number of individuals who were present on the units at the start of the study and remained throughout the duration was low (21.1 percent to 47.2 percent). Moreover, since the effort was directed at the group rather than the individual, the group's response may be more representative of true effect.

When only experimental units were included in the analysis, and extent of model implementation was used as a control variable, some differences were seen between units. All units implemented a portion of the model, but none of them implemented it fully. Of a maximum possible implementation score of 216, unit implementation scores ranged from 146 to 187. Mean total score for the units was 162.4 (plus or minus 15.08). Significant differences were seen for nurse satisfaction, using the IWS at Time 4, when extent of model was considered. Differences also were seen for the subscale organizational policies. Nurses from units that implemented greater amounts of the model were more satisfied.

Discussion

Although the level of job satisfaction of nurses in experimental units improved somewhat over the course of the study, it did not improve significantly more than that of nurses in comparison units. This negative finding may have been caused by several factors. First, professional practice models that focus on increased staff nurse control may not affect overall satisfaction with the work environment. Findings of previous studies are mixed, with some reporting positive effect and others reporting none. Second, job satisfaction is likely to be influenced by factors outside the unit. Consequently, the activities at the unit level may not be strong enough to overcome the negative influences of the external environment. This is particularly true if only a portion of the professional practice model is implemented, resulting in limited effect. Third, hospitals involved in the study (both experimental and comparison) introduced multiple retention strategies independent of the work underway in the experimental units. Because of the shortage of nurses during the period when the model was implemented, hospitals were introducing programs and practices that were consistent with the conceptual characteristics of the EPPM. As a result, favorable changes in perception of the work environment may have occurred in response to these more global improvements in work setting.

The absence of job satisfaction findings also may be a reflection of problems with the instruments used to detect change. The instruments used to measure job satisfaction, although widely used, were developed during the 1970s—a period in healthcare that differed considerably from the time in which this study was conducted. A review of the items used in the scales suggests that some of the constructs measured may be less relevant to current work environments than they were during the periods in which they were developed. The reliability and validity of both the IWS and the JSS were supported in this research, but there may be some indication for revision of individual items to reflect more accurately current workplace environments.

An additional factor contributing to the absence of more striking findings may be differences in time frame for longitudinal studies. Because previous studies have measured change over short periods, the absence of findings in this study may be an indication of the difficulties inherent in measuring a construct over time. Although satisfaction is considered to be a "stable" indicator of perception of work environment, no other studies have measured its stability for the length of time used in this study.

This issue is an important one since short-range studies are prone to misrepresentation of results when only pre- and postmeasures are used. For example, had only one time point been used in this study, an erroneous effect would have been reported. Longitudinal studies of nurse satisfaction and the effect of perception of work group on nurse satisfaction are needed.

The differences seen according to extent of model implemented highlight an important problem in evaluation studies. Frequently, interventions fail to produce a measurable effect on outcome. Rarely is any indication of the amount of intervention described. If only a portion of the intervention is introduced, the absence of findings may be an indication of insufficient amount rather than failure of the intervention to produce an intended effect. Without some indication of the extent of the intervention introduced, the potential for incorrect interpretation of findings is great.

Studies extending the method used in this study for quantifying extent of intervention are needed. The technique proposed here needs additional testing with different interventions and different populations.

2. A Descriptive Longitudinal Study of Work Satisfaction among Hospital Nurses

Tammy J. Gustin, Patricia A. Martin,
Phyllis B. Risner, and Therese C. Lupo

This study, which uses a longitudinal approach to data collection, is part of a larger research project entitled Organizational Dimensions in Hospital Nursing Practice, designed to build a database for secondary analysis and to assist in policymaking and program decision making based on monitoring perceptions of nurses over time. The study was collaborative and included four investigators from the hospital setting and two investigators from the university setting, a relationship facilitated by a long-term collaborative and contractual agreement between the two institutions. Funding for the project was obtained from the researchers' institutions and local grants. The Index of Work Satisfaction instrument by Stamps and Piedmonte (1986) was one of six instruments used to monitor nurses' perceptions over time. Other dimensions that were monitored included communication, organizational climate, professional practice climate, and professional nursing autonomy.

The IWS instrument was initially used in this institution in June of 1987, then again in 1988, and at seven more collection times from 1990 through 1995 in the same institution within the context of the larger study. Each administration involved the same population and the same statistical analysis. A total of 1,566 surveys were collected, with 1,403 surveys having complete data that could be statistically analyzed.

The purpose of the larger multiphase longitudinal research study was to increase the understanding of organizational factors that affect the provision of nursing care at Miami Valley Hospital. The longitudinal design was chosen to capture not only the employee's anticipation of

Tammy J. Gustin, R.N., M.S., is Administrative Officer at Miami Valley Hospital, Dayton, Ohio. This was part of her master's thesis. Patricia A. Martin, R.N., Ph.D., is Director of Nursing Research at Wright State University–Miami Valley College of Nursing and Health, Dayton, Ohio. Phyllis B. Risner, R.N., Ph.D., is Professor Emeritus at Wright State University–Miami Valley College of Nursing and Health, Dayton, Ohio. Therese C. Lupo, R.N., M.S., is Director, Nursing Administration at Miami Valley Hospital, Dayton, Ohio.

Acknowledgment is given to others on the research team: Gayle Jordan, R.N., M.S., Clinical Nurse; Linda Cox, R.N., M.S., Nurse Manager; Kimbra Kahle Paden, R.N., M.S., Clinical Nurse Specialist; Jean Corron, R.N., B.S.N., Infection Control Nurse; and Jayne Gmeiner, R.N., M.S., Project Manager, all at Miami Valley Hospital.

Funding for this research was provided by the Miami Valley Hospital Division of Nursing and a Faculty Collaboration Seed Grant from the Wright State University and Miami Valley Hospital Collaborative Agreement.

For more information about this study, contact Tammy J. Gustin at Miami Valley Hospital, One Wyoming Street, Dayton, OH 45409. Telephone (513) 208-8000.

change, but the employee's perception of the change once it occurs (Martin 1995).

Methodology

The population consisted of approximately 1,200 RNs in a 772-bed urban teaching tertiary and acute care hospital. The collection times were from March 1988 to January 1995 with a 10 percent to 20 percent response rate yielding a total of 1,566 surveys, with 1,403 being usable questionnaires.

In 1988, surveys were distributed to the nursing units in a large urban hospital with a traditionally based organizational structure and in a large religious-based hospital with a shared-governance model. The 1988 surveys were completed voluntarily and returned to the researcher within two weeks. The sample size for the 1988 study was 237 for the traditional hospital and 112 for the shared-governance hospital, with a response rate of approximately 20 percent.

The data collection, from 1990 through 1995, occurred in a single day at four one-hour sessions that included a box lunch for participants. All of the RN staff (approximately 1,200 nurses) received an invitation to attend. There were seven data collections conducted sequentially from December 1990 ($n=127$), May 1991 ($n=164$), November 1991 ($n=152$), September 1992 ($n=163$), June 1993 ($n=158$), January 1994 ($n=231$) and January 1995 ($n=222$).

Additional data acquired at the times of the data collection included information about concurrent organizational factors. Clinical nursing management completed a data sheet (Assessment of Organizational Factors) that included such items as unit census, staffing issues, new projects, major events, and any other key factors that might be relevant to the clinical nursing staff. Trending these factors at the time of the data collection gave the investigators the ability to interpret the job satisfaction data within the context of the organization. The IWS was one of six tools in a booklet that the participants were asked to complete.

Results

The results will be discussed as they relate to each of the major research questions. Only statistically significant findings will be reported here. The relationships with the demographics and correlation with the other instruments are discussed in the selection by Martin et al. (Appendix E, Selection 2).

Sample Characteristics and Demographics

The characteristics of the sample were identified by including demographic questions at the end of the survey booklet. Only the January 1995 data ($n=222$) are summarized here, as the demographic characteristics of the sample remained consistent over the eight collection times. Details of the demographic analysis are available from the author. The most important variables will be summarized here.

The majority of the respondents were between ages 30 and 39, with a close second in the 40-to-49 age group, for a total of 76 percent of participant total in these two groups. The year in which the respondent was licensed as an RN ranged from 1949 to 1994. The difference between the respondents' basic education and the highest degree earned is of interest. Respondents most frequently (40 percent) reported a diploma for the basic education but a B.S.N. degree (37 percent) for the highest degree earned, meaning that many of the associate degree and diploma graduates had returned to school. Fifty-seven percent of the respondents had worked in this institution for over ten years, and another 23 percent had worked in the institution for more than five years. Longevity is the norm, so retention and recruitment issues were not a primary concern; however, this is a good parameter to monitor as a means to evaluate changes in retention. As anticipated, the respondents were overwhelmingly from the Primary Nurse I job status group, meaning the majority of the participants were direct patient caregivers. Also reflective of the entire population, approximately 69 percent of the respondents were full-time employees. The most common shift worked by the respondents had a starting time of 7:00 AM. The respondents worked in a variety of areas of clinical practice including medical-surgical, maternal-newborn, critical care, behavioral, surgical service, ambulatory, and other. All areas of practice were represented, with maternal-newborn having the most participants at 25.7 percent. About 40 percent of the respondents identified some type of professional affiliation.

Work Satisfaction Results

The overall job satisfaction scores had an upward trend over the eight-year period from 1988 through 1995. The peak was in 1992, with a gradual decrease since that time (see Table 5.1).

The study of Job Satisfaction Related to Organizational Structure (Gustin 1988) examined the concept of shared governance and the relationship to work satisfaction utilizing the IWS tool (Stamps and Piedmonte 1986). As shown in Table 5.2, nurses in the hospital where the shared-governance model had been in place for ten years had significantly higher overall job satisfaction scores than the nurses in the traditional, more bureaucratic organization. Three components of job satisfaction were also found to be statistically significant higher in the hospital with the shared-governance structure: pay, autonomy, and organizational policies.

Table 5.1 Overall Job Satisfaction Scores for the Eight Collection Times at Miami Valley Hospital

Date	Overall Score
March 1988*	189.32
December 1990	192.29
May 1991	198.40**
November 1991	194.70**
September 1992	200.07**
June 1993	196.65
January 1994	192.32
January 1995	194.06

*Source: Gustin 1988.
**The overall IWS scores from May 1991, September 1992, and June 1993 are significantly higher than those from 1988 ($p < .0001$).

Table 5.2 Comparison Scores of Hospital Nurses with Traditional Governance and without Shared Governance

	Traditional Governance ($n=236$)	Shared Governance ($n=110$)
Overall Score	186.32	195.65
Pay	2.82	3.26
Autonomy	4.84	5.07
Organizational Policies	3.48	4.01

Source: Gustin 1988.

Summary of Longitudinal Results

There were no statistically significant relationships found between the overall job satisfaction score and the demographics in the longitudinal study; however, components of the IWS did have some relationships to the demographic data. There was a positive relationship between job status and the autonomy component, meaning the RN with a high autonomy score also had a high job status score. RNs with a high professional status score were more likely to be working in critical care. A high score on the organizational policies component indicated the RN was more likely to be long-term employee, have a higher job status, or work in a behavioral area of practice (i.e., psychiatry and chemical dependency).

The statistical analysis of Part A of the IWS found additional information related to the components. Over time the components judged as being most important were autonomy and pay, each being most important at different points of time. The pay component moved into first position when the last raise was further away from the survey time, and shifted to second place when pay raises were recent. The component found to be least important was organizational policies. The satisfaction results were consistent over time. Respondents consistently reported the highest satisfaction with professional status and the lowest satisfaction with pay.

Problems and Limitations

This research had some limitations. Investigators attempted to replicate the study exactly each time data were collected; however, minor changes were made to improve the process. For example, in an attempt to improve analysis by matching specific participants' perceptions over time, the participants' social security numbers were requested beginning in 1993. Because approximately 50 percent of the participants provided their social security number during the 1993 survey, analyzing comparisons of individuals is possible in the future.

A second limitation of this study is the method of participant selection. This study invited all RNs in the institution to participate in the survey, but participation was voluntary. In reality the respondents were self-selected and may not have been representative of the entire nursing staff.

The data collection methods were somewhat different in Gustin's (1988) original study. That study distributed the surveys and requested them back in two weeks, whereas the longitudinal study invited the participants for lunch to complete the questionnaire in a group setting. Another possible limitation is that the nature of a longitudinal study allows the same participants to take the same survey multiple times.

Summary and Conclusion

This research project focused on evaluating the effect of several different types of organizational change over a period of time, beginning in 1988. By 1990, six different measurement instruments were being used, among them the IWS (Stamps and Piedmonte 1986), the Professional Practice Climate Instrument, the Schutzenhofer Professional Nursing Activity Scale (Schutzenhofer 1983), and the Organization Climate Questionnaire (Duxbury, Henley, and Armstrong 1982). In 1993 the Communication Satisfaction Survey by Downs and Hazen (1977) was added. Currently, data collection for all of these tools occurs annually.

The administrative objective was to monitor nurse job satisfaction and other dimensions over a number of years to assist in evaluating the changes occurring in the institution. Some of the major changes that have occurred since 1988 include implementing a shared-governance model, a new layer of management, a new patient care model and work redesign, benchmarking efforts, and a revised clinical advancement system. This longitudinal study became very complex. The original vision was to examine one variable (shared governance) in relationship to job satisfaction. The reality has been, however, that many factors may influence nurses' perceptions of job satisfaction, such as benefits, size of hospital, geographic location of hospital, and others.

This descriptive, longitudinal study captured approximately 1,400 responses of hospital nurses' perception of work satisfaction utilizing the IWS tool. The overall satisfaction scores have trended in a positive direction and were statistically significant from 1988 to 1991, peaking in 1992. The overall scores have decreased since 1992, but not significantly.

The organizational policies component has consistently had a significantly lower score than expected for a hospital with over ten years of experience with a shared-governance model. However, the level of satisfaction with organizational policies is statistically significantly higher in the hospital with shared-governance than in the more traditional hospital.

The data indicate a relationship between work satisfaction and the demographics of the participants. Overall IWS, pay, autonomy, and organizational policies were all positively related to job status (e.g., Primary Nurse I, Primary Nurse II, Nurse Manager). This indicates that the higher the job status, the more satisfied nurses tended to be with overall IWS, pay, autonomy, and organizational policies. Additionally, the nurses who had longevity, worked in a behavioral area of practice, or in a higher job status were more satisfied with organizational policies. The nurses in the critical care area of practice reported greater satisfaction with professional status.

The value in studying and learning about nurses' perception of work satisfaction is that the information can be used in monitoring major changes in the institution and to provide a scientific rationale for making administrative decisions. While ideally the goal is to continue an upward trend in all components of work satisfaction, realistically the goal of maintaining the current level of job satisfaction of the hospital nurses during the rapidly changing environment of healthcare may be more achievable. The desire for a satisfied work group is based on the assumption that the benefits of high satisfaction include high productivity, low absenteeism, and low turnover. In this competitive environment, developing a database to assist in the decision-making process and giving registered nurses a forum to be heard are valuable strategies.

3. The Use of Nurse Satisfaction Data to Evaluate and Motivate Quality Improvement Activities During a Patient Service Restructuring Program

Ann Minnick, Katherine Pischke-Winn, and Charlene Thomas

Although the use of nurse satisfaction information as it relates to turn-over rates, recruiting opportunities, and labor organization potential is well documented, the use of such data in evaluating and motivating efforts to achieve quality improvements for patients has not been extensively explored. This selection describes the use of the IWS during the evaluation of the effect of a patient service restructuring program and the subsequent use of these data to act as a spur for further quality improvement efforts at the unit level.

Methodology

The Project

In the early 1990s, a large (25,000 annual admissions) academic medical center embarked on a program to provide patient-focused care, that is, care that is designed and implemented from the patient's perspective rather than the organization's. The planning process indicated that a number of different initiatives would need to be completed to attain this goal. Among these initiatives were the introduction of new types of workers including a unit-based multitask environmental worker, as well as the adoption of a case responsibility nursing model, clinical pathways, a patient point-of-view pharmacy delivery system, and new technology (wireless communication, bedside computers).

Key Decisions

The institution is nationally known for the quality of its nursing care. Locally, the quality of the nursing care is used by the hospital as a point for marketing. The satisfaction of nurse employees is thus especially important because it can influence the recruitment and retention of excellent

Ann Minnick, Ph.D., R.N., F.A.A.N., is Professor at Rush University and Director of Nursing Services Research and Support at Rush–Presbyterian–St. Luke's Medical Center, Chicago, Illinois. Katherine Pischke-Winn, B.A., R.N., is Assistant to the Director of Nursing Services Research and Support at Rush–Presbyterian–St. Luke's Medical Center, Chicago, Illinois. Charlene Thomas, Ph.D., R.N., is Associate Director in OR/Surgical Nursing at Rush–Presbyterian–St. Luke's Medical Center; Chicago, Illinois.

For more information about this study, contact Ann Minnick at Rush–Presbyterian–St. Luke's Medical Center, 1743 W. Harrison, 810SSH, Chicago, IL 60612. Telephone (312) 942-6990; fax (312) 942-3038.

nurses, activities that are two of the cornerstones of maintaining the quality of care. The institutional mission statement requires this emphasis on employees through its support for employee growth. It was deemed vital to monitor the effect of changes on employees, and especially on nurse satisfaction, during the implementation of the patient-centered care approach.

Variables and Their Measurement

Projected Use of the IWS. A team including staff nurses, nurse managers, and key hospital executives identified elements of nurse satisfaction that might be influenced by the project. These elements included satisfaction with the type and pace of work as well as the status of the work activities. The task requirements and professional status scales of the IWS were thus deemed important components of the evaluation. Although the other IWS scales were also judged to measure aspects of satisfaction that might be altered by the program, the chief reason for their inclusion was efficient use of resources and the assessment of unpredicted outcomes. For example, the organization has a continuing need to evaluate nurses' satisfaction with pay. The team decided administration of the pay scale with the others would eliminate the need for a second round of questionnaires.

Benefits and Schedule Scales. The survey that was used included two scales developed by Ann Minnick and Marc J. Roberts in 1991 to measure satisfaction with benefits and schedule (see Table 5.3). The rationale for the use of the benefits scale was similar to that noted for use of the pay scale. The schedule scale was used because changes in nursing positions might result in changes in satisfaction with schedules. Earlier studies had

Table 5.3   Items in Benefit and Schedule Scales*

Benefit Scale Items

   From what I hear about nursing personnel at other hospitals, our benefits package is fair.

   My present benefit package is satisfactory.

   An upgrading of the benefits package for nursing personnel is needed at this hospital.

Schedule Scale Items

   My present shift rotation (work schedule) requirements are satisfactory.

   I am satisfied with my ability to modify my work schedule.

   My present weekend work schedule is satisfactory.

   Modification of scheduling policies for nursing personnel is needed at this hospital.

---

*Developed by Ann Minnick and Marc J. Roberts, 1991.

indicated schedule and benefits were important to nurses' employment choices. The items were based on the IWS approach of asking about perceptions of fairness, comparability with other institutions, ascribed satisfaction, and personal satisfaction. These scales, as well as the IWS scales, were tested with three groups of registered nurses at two community hospitals to ascertain content understanding and appropriate reading level. In preliminary tests and a subsequent study of 1,269 registered nurses at 17 hospitals, the internal consistency for these scales was high (alpha range, .70 to .82). The correlates with the IWS scale scores were low.

The tool also included some individual items developed to measure opinions about specific aspects and outcomes of the patient-centered care initiative. For example, items relating to overall noise and overhead paging were included because one of the goals was to reduce noise. Items regarding the quality of nursing care were also included. The instrument distributed during the project included 93 items (12 were demographic) and took approximately 25 minutes to complete.

The strategic decision that the satisfaction of staff other than nurses should be examined simultaneously was made, consistent with the organization's emphasis on teamwork and decentralized responsibility as well as the organization's commitment to seek the satisfaction of all employees. The original items were altered to omit the word "nurse," and an alternative form was produced for distribution to employees who were unit-based non-nurses (e.g., clerks and multitask environmental workers).

Timing and Administration

Surveys were administered annually on pilot units. Concurrent with the decision to implement one portion of the initiative (the introduction of the unit-based multitask environmental worker) throughout the institution, the administration schedule was altered to 90 days pre- and postimplementation on every unit. Subsequently, data were collected annually on all units.

The investigators applied various publicity and administrative strategies to attain adequate response rates. The staff were informed that they could return surveys to a sealed box placed on the unit or through the institution's mail system to a central office. Anonymity was assured, and those responsible for processing the information were not administratively linked to any clinical area.

To emphasize further the message that all the initiatives of the patient-focused care project would be evaluated across a variety of variables, surveys and interviews with other stakeholders (patients, families, and physicians) were conducted simultaneously. This approach also allowed for comparison of the opinions of the stakeholders.

Results

Response Rates

The mean response rate of all units prior to implementation of the initiative was 62 percent, but there was wide variation across units, indicating that there were probably equally wide variations in the belief of unit staff that someone would respond to the findings. The data also indicate that achievement of an adequate response rate at one point in the program did not predict an adequate response rate at another time. Too-frequent administration may erode response rates to the extent that results are useless. Upon return to an annual administration, higher response rates were attained.

On most units the response rates of unit-based, non-nursing staff were disappointing. This was very problematic because on many units there were a small number of support staff. Two aspects identified during debriefings are being addressed currently to improve response rates for these staff. The first is time to complete the survey. Units that allowed these employees defined time to complete the questionnaire had higher response rates than those that did not recognize this need. The second issue is the general reading ability of the group. The annual questionnaire for unit-based support staff that is now used on all units has been shortened and simplified. Data concerning the effect of this modification on the response rate of non-nurses will be available in the future.

Reliability

The reliability of the IWS scales and the additional benefits and schedule scales was generally high, although the professional status scale reliability was low. Efforts to identify one item as the source of the low alpha scores obtained were unsuccessful. This is discussed further in Appendix B (see Table B.3).

Comment Analysis

Each questionnaire had a comment section. After an initial review for themes, categories were established for reporting purposes. The comment category format was a convenient way to group similar comments; comments were detailed once followed by a numerical notation indicating the number of times that particular comment was made. The comment categories were: quality of nursing care, quantity of nursing care, physical surroundings, charting, noise, other procedures, unit culture, unit management, administration, patient-focused care model, support services, and other or miscellaneous.

The majority of nurses took the time to write comments. Based on our postimplementation experience with 31 units, the mean proportion of staff who wrote comments was 71 percent. The range was 35 percent to 96 percent. The preimplementation rate was similar.

Nurses' comments were more likely to be negative than were patients' or physicians' comments. The higher the percentage of written comments, the more negative the tone. The most frequent negative comment themes revolved around: quantity of staff, the quality of supplemental staff, administration, a general mourning for the "old days," benefits, lack of appreciation, and scheduling issues. The pay, benefit, and schedule comments tended to emphasize the respondent, not the respondent's team. Their tone, however, was consistent with the individual IWS and Minnick-Roberts scale scores of the individual respondents. The "lack of appreciation" comments seemed to reflect concerns about executives' and managers' views of the nursing work force rather than generally poor professional status. "Lack of appreciation" was often connected within the same or following sentence to perceived declines in benefits and pay. In many cases, these perceived declines in pay and benefits were given as examples of the "lack of appreciation" of nursing by managers and executives. No nurse wrote, for example, that patients or support staff did not value nursing.

Organizational Response

The aggregate results were shared at the executive and department level twice a year. The response at the department level varied by area. Some department heads initiated extensive discussions and departmental projects or encouraged unit-level responses. The executive level responded not only to the scales related specifically to the project but also to those such as pay. The project staff noted that there was a need to present the results in concise, easily understood forms to busy executives. Requests for current, comparable data from other, similar institutions were frequent. The development of a benchmarking system using the IWS would increase the use of the IWS and its value to executives.

Effecting Change

The wide variation in some scores during the pilot and pre- and postimplementation data gathering periods seemed to indicate the need for unit-level rather than overall project readjustments. In addition, the informal responses to the results led some managers and administrators to consider how the results might be a reflection of issues that were outside of the scope of the patient-focused care project but relevant to quality concerns. The vice president of the division of nursing directed that the data continue to be collected and reported as part of the quality program (e.g., during Nursing Administration Council and via regular reports to the senior vice president). In addition, a unit-by-unit approach to results sharing was adopted.

Results Sharing at the Unit Level

The project staff discussed the results at a meeting with the unit leadership, which is composed of the unit director, the clinical nurse coordinators (CNCs), and the unit service manager (USM). CNCs are senior professionals who have responsibility for the care of groups of patients within a unit. A CNC is typically responsible for 7 to 12 patients and is assisted by other RNs and ancillary personnel. A USM is a non-nurse who is responsible for environmental quality on the unit as well as supervision of unit-based environmental workers. The USM reports to the unit director, a master's-prepared worker with clinical and administrative qualifications.

Typically the response rates and the effects of low numbers of responses on interpretation were discussed first. Two points were reinforced throughout the actual results discussion: (1) the need for the leadership to provide interpretation and (2) the need to communicate to the staff that the leadership had reviewed the data and that there was a commitment to being responsive. The majority of the unit leaders asked a member of the project team to give a brief (less than 20-minute) presentation of survey results to staff, followed by the unit leadership brainstorming with staff to identify unit quality-improvement projects.

Project Examples

One unit, following its postsurvey sharing of results, changed its entire process of staff scheduling. The survey results indicated staff dissatisfaction with the perceived fairness of scheduling and the rotation patterns used in individual staff schedules. When the unit leadership group reviewed the survey results, they had already attended three leadership-development programs that focused on communication, negotiation, and team building. They were prepared to attend to the staff's concerns and to lead staff in confronting issues in a positive manner and working to create a healthy work environment.

The unit director and a human resources employee skilled in group processes helped conduct staff focus groups to discuss both positive and negative survey results. These groups garnered feedback on staff perceptions of what the survey results meant to them and ideas for improvement projects. Dissatisfaction with scheduling was identified as an important issue that was adding to apathetic peer and leadership relationships. The leadership group took this opportunity to lay the foundation whereby staff could begin to work on a concrete issue (change in the scheduling structure). However, the underlying staff-development goals were team building, professional accountability, the importance of relationships, and employee empowerment.

The first step after the focus groups was writing and agreeing on a unit mission statement. This mission statement contained a section articulating the importance of developing staff to be strategic, self-developed, empowered employees. Next, unit leadership and staff decided that the staff would do self- and team scheduling. The unit leadership started to work with experienced employees on all three shifts to develop scheduling guidelines and establish clear deadlines for employee requests and the completed schedule. A train-the-trainer model was used, in which staff that had completed one month's schedule would work with the next month's team scheduler. The goal was that all staff would eventually rotate and learn the art of scheduling as well as accountability, communication, and negotiation with their peers. Unit leadership would review completed schedules, but the model was rooted in peer decision making.

It was a challenging transition for both leadership and staff. Managers worked to accept the relinquishment of this responsibility to staff and invested many hours in teaching and developing staff. The managers then had to trust that staff would grow and be accountable for the peer conflict resolution that is inherent with the initiation of self- and team scheduling. Staff had to deal with their fear of change and the idea that management "just did not want to do schedules anymore, which is really your job anyway" and move toward improving their communication and negotiation skills with each other.

After the first few self-schedule cycles were completed, the leadership group held "town hall" meetings for staff feedback. One shift experienced an easier transition to self-scheduling, so employees from that shift worked with peers on the other shift who were having a more difficult adjustment period.

Assessment and evaluation of the new scheduling system continue. A member of the employee satisfaction survey project is working with the unit's leadership group to select the next appropriate dates to distribute satisfaction surveys now that the new scheduling system is in place. Staff members are attending development programs aimed at improving communication skills. The leadership group hopes that this is the start of many projects that will lead to staff growth in communication and a sense of empowerment—the skills needed for *all* aspects of the patient-focused care project.

Another specific example was related to task requirements. Although the baseline score for this scale was acceptable for all the units within the surgical department, it was evident that, with the introduction of the multitask environmental worker to the unit's team and the incorporation of more unlicensed nursing personnel, there was an opportunity for improvement as well as a potential for decline.

The department's response focused on delegation. Having evolved through an era of primary nursing, during which nurses were educated and psychologically geared to do "everything for patients and families themselves," the essential elements of the strategy were (1) to teach and reinforce appropriate delegation skills to the professional staff and (2) to support staff as they learned to trust coworkers. All unit directors attended a half-day of training on the theory and practical application of delegation. They then transferred and reinforced this information to the staff through one-to-one developmental sessions between directors and CNCs.

A third example was related to scores obtained on the professional status scale. Clinical nurse coordinators and staff nurses were fully integrated into the development, implementation, and evaluation of critical pathways. The implementation of this strategy has enhanced the perception of the role of registered nurses on the healthcare team and has been reflected positively in follow-up job satisfaction data.

A final example concerns the surgical areas' response to findings about satisfaction with pay. A financial incentive bonus program was provided to nursing personnel. The bonus was implemented as a means of rewarding nursing personnel who not only contributed to the areas' fiscal success, but also met standards related to three specific criteria: quality performance, teamwork, and attendance. The change in the average score on the pay scale of the IWS was astounding; an 80 percent improvement. The ability to track the staff's response with the IWS pay scale helped management reach decisions about the future of the bonus program.

Resource Requirements

Although institutions may be interested in this approach to improvement, the constrained resources of today's hospital make it likely that many readers may dismiss using it due to perceived costliness.

Technical

Hospitals that use the IWS instrument for evaluation and improvement purposes require that results be available almost immediately. Our institution supports a data entry area, but many hospitals may find it more economical to use forms compatible with electronic scanning devices. Many institutions already own such devices, and their use in coding IWS data may actually make them more cost-effective, especially if they are currently underutilized.

The construction of a computer program that provides information in a report format also allows for timely and inexpensive data processing. Users of the reports and project staff need to discuss the meaning and use of data to determine the key statistics to be reported before completing such programming. This study has found a trend-type format especially helpful. Making the process as routine as possible by using methods such as a standard reporting format for talks reduces costs. Adoption of these strategies has enabled the investigators to construct reports for each unit with no additional labor and to complete feedback sessions within 30 days of data collection.

Personnel

Two types of personnel time are required to use the tool for monitoring and effecting change: project and unit personnel. Project staff activities include the duplication, unit preparation, distribution, and collection of instruments. The time spent in unit preparation is a key to a good response rate. Busy unit directors and senior clinical leaders need to be reminded of "start and close dates" for data collection. The support of key personnel for completion of the tool is invaluable. The average amount of time spent per unit on these activities is one hour. After the data are reduced, project staff time is required for basic interpretation and integration with other data. This work, which includes construction of an integrated summary statement, averages three hours per unit.

Unit personnel time in preparing for administration is minimal. Administration itself varies with the respondent and with the additional items an institution may choose to include with the questionnaire. The meeting time of project and clinical leadership staff to review the entire report (which includes all key variables for the project) averaged one hour during the first administration; subsequent reviews have averaged 45 minutes.

These resource data indicate that the expenditure is relatively small given the efficient targeting of quality improvement efforts that result. Beyond the effective quality improvement initiatives that have been launched because of the project, it is possible that resources were saved because they were not misdirected to units that did not need them. These are two points that can be highlighted in seeking the resources needed to support the approach.

4. The Relationship Between a Shared-Governance Management Structure and Registered Nurse Job Satisfaction

Valerie Mancini

In the past decade there have been radical changes in the healthcare delivery system. Increased technology and its resulting demands have changed the work environment, forcing a redefinition of nursing practice. Although demands are placed on individual nurses to respond to the challenging healthcare environment, responsibility and accountability are still invested primarily in other individuals (e.g., managers, educators, clinicians) who have been designated by the organization. Consequently, the members of the nursing staff typically do not participate in management decisions that affect their practice. Decision-making activities relevant to nursing care have been removed from the practitioner's span of control. This lack of control over professional autonomy has impeded the development of professional nursing practice (Prescott and Dennis 1985).

Not only has the progress of professional practice been hindered, but studies have indicated that lack of respect, low salaries, insufficient autonomy, and loss of control over the work environment have contributed to job dissatisfaction among nurses (Roedel and Nystrom 1988).

Change in organizational structure has been advocated as nurses attempt to increase their level of accountability as professionals (Porter-O'Grady and Finnigan 1984). A form of participatory management known as shared governance advocates a management structure in which communication channels cross hierarchic boundaries. This structure encourages a work environment that gives responsibility and accountability for both process and outcome to the individual practitioner. Shared governance is founded on the belief that the positive outcomes of participatory decision making, as seen in other environments, can be experienced in nursing as well (Peterson and Allen 1986). Shared governance proposes a system for maintaining an operational framework for an organizational structure that provides for the full utilization of nursing resources. Autonomy and accountability for establishing policy and participation in planning are fundamental to the professional's role. Shared governance, therefore, is designed to reflect the professional

Valerie Mancini, Ed.D., R.N., is Vice President of Nursing at St. Vincent Hospital, Worcester, Massachusetts.

For more information about this study, contact Valerie Mancini at St. Vincent Hospital, 25 Winthrop Street, Worcester, MA 01604. Telephone (508) 798-6344; fax (508) 798-1240.

character of nursing organizations. This emphasis aids in the cultivation of positive behaviors and practices (Porter-O'Grady and Finnigan 1984).

When the historical roots of participatory management are traced from Frederick Taylor to Porter-O'Grady and Finnigan, a radical change can be seen in the assumptions as to what motivates people to work. Today's major thinkers in the field of organizational theory have been far more generous in their assumptions about human motivation. They have come to see pay as but one of the variables that motivate people, not necessarily even the most important one. They assume fewer inherent differences between subordinates and supervisors. They assume that most people, workers and supervisors alike, have inherent needs to use their full capabilities, to be creative, to be responsible, to be involved in the decision-making processes at their workplace, and to do good work. This line of research and evolving theory flies in the face of much that goes on in the work of nurses today.

Many innovative changes such as primary nursing, case management, care and service redesign, and shared governance have been implemented in an attempt to increase job satisfaction and to reduce turnover among nurses. However, few studies have been conducted to measure levels of job satisfaction in response to changes in management structure. The purpose of this study, therefore, is to determine if a shared-governance management structure significantly affects the level of job satisfaction of registered nurses who work in hospitals.

The Index of Work Satisfaction was used to measure job satisfaction among two groups of nurses, one working in a hospital with a shared-governance management structure and the other working in a hospital without a shared-governance management structure.

Methodology

All registered nurses working in the hospital with no shared-governance structure (Hospital A) were requested to participate in the study. Introductory letters accompanied the questionnaire. Participants were told that the investigator was interested in measuring job satisfaction among registered nurses and that participation was voluntary. The consent form included a brief explanation of the instrument, an outline of the potential risks and benefits of participation, and that it took approximately 20 minutes to complete. A total of 442 surveys were distributed with paychecks in the spring of 1989 at Hospital A. Demographic data were collected from the subjects relating to age, sex, years of experience in nursing, level of basic education, highest degree completed, unit specialty, full- or part-time status, and shift most frequently scheduled. Subjects were asked to return questionnaires by mail within two weeks in a stamped addressed envelope. A total of 148 surveys were returned for a response rate of 33 percent.

In the hospital with the shared-governance management structure (Hospital B), 99 registered nurses, out of a total of 255, were randomly selected and scheduled to attend a session in which they were given the opportunity to respond to the Index of Work Satisfaction questionnaire. This represented a response rate of 39 percent. Demographic data were collected by another researcher.

The Index of Work Satisfaction was used as the measure for job satisfaction of nurses. Both Part A (expectations derived from the paired comparisons) and Part B (current level of satisfaction as measured by a Likert attitude scale) were used. Analysis of the IWS followed the guidelines provided by Stamps and Piedmonte (1986).

Results

Demographic Description

In both hospitals the sex distribution of respondents was predominantly female, with five or fewer males in each group. At the hospital without shared governance, the age range of the respondents was from 20 to 69, with a mean age of 34.8. In the comparison hospital with shared governance, the age range was 20 to 59, with a mean of 36. The mean length of time in the current jobs was 12 years at both hospitals. The range of years worked at the current hospitals showed distributions for both hospitals to be skewed, with the largest percentage of nurses working at their respective hospitals five years or less. There were no significant differences between the two hospitals with respect to length of employment.

The Index of Work Satisfaction

Table 5.4 shows the numerical results from the analysis of the IWS. This table shows the mean component scores and the total IWS scores for both Hospitals A and B. Table 5.5 presents the means of the six weighted satisfaction values and the IWS value for Hospital A and Hospital B. The components in both tables have been ordered from greatest to least for Hospital A. As shown in Table 5.5, except for the interaction component, all other satisfaction means were higher at Hospital B than at Hospital A. Although the mean score for the interaction component was higher at Hospital A (mean = 14.80) than at Hospital B (mean = 14.50), the mean adjusted IWS was not significantly higher (Hospital A, 12.78; Hospital B, 13.37). The differences in mean satisfaction for each component as well as for the total scale were tested for significance. Significant differences were found for three of the six components, autonomy ($p<.05$), task requirements ($p<.001$), and organizational policies ($p<.01$).

Results and Discussion

Shared decision making is a feature of a shared-governance management structure that enables the nursing administrator to begin to transfer

Table 5.4 Comparison of Mean Component Scores and IWS Weighted Scores at Hospitals A and B

	Hospital A			Hospital B		
	Mean Component Scores		IWS Weighted Scores	Mean Component Scores		IWS Weighted Scores
IWS Component	N	Mean	Mean	N	Mean	Mean
Professional Status	148	5.45	17.95	97	5.42	18.25
Interaction	147	4.95	14.80	97	4.60	14.50
Autonomy	145	4.80	17.40	97	5.00	18.28
Task Requirements	143	3.28	8.67	96	3.70	9.70
Organizational Policies	146	3.02	7.81	98	3.71	8.68
Pay	148	2.91	10.04	97	3.08	10.69
Total Scale	141	4.19	12.78	92	4.33	13.37

Table 5.5 IWS Component and Total Scale Scores, Hospitals A and B

	Hospital A[a]		Hospital B[b]		
IWS Component	N	Mean	N	Mean	t
Professional Status	148	17.95	97	18.25	1.03
Autonomy	145	17.40	97	18.28	−2.37*
Interaction	147	14.80	97	14.50	1.12
Pay	148	10.04	97	10.69	−1.12
Task Requirements	143	8.67	96	9.70	−3.55**
Organizational Policies	146	7.81	98	8.68	−2.82***
Total IWS Scale	141	12.78	98	13.37	−2.59***

[a] Subscale calculations based on 7, 8, 10, 6, 6, and 7 items, respectively. Data missing for 0 to 7 subjects per scale.
[b] Subscale calculations based on 5, 7, 8, 5, 5, and 5 items, respectively. Data missing for 1 to 7 subjects per scale.
*$p < .05$ **$p < .001$ ***$p < .01$

accountability to groups and individual members of the nursing staff. Accountability is invested in the practitioners of the profession; shared-governance management structures are designed to support these practitioners. It may be inferred, therefore, that since Hospital B had a shared-governance management structure in place for seven years, the mechanisms for decision making, autonomy, and accountability were firmly in place. For this reason the nursing staff at Hospital B may have responded more favorably to questions on autonomy on the IWS questionnaire than nurses at Hospital A.

Historically, nursing administrators in traditional clinical settings hold the major responsibility for the nursing care that takes place in the institution. They have tended to be much more task-oriented. These administrators often make the majority of decisions concerning task requirements of the staff nurses' role. Perhaps in Hospital B, the shared-governance management structure facilitated greater input from the staff concerning task requirements of the role. Since the nursing administrator supported the shared-governance model, it can be assumed that staff involvement was not only allowed but encouraged. Additionally, the vice president for nursing at Hospital B provided guidance and behaved as a role model to the staff. She had little actual control over decisions dealing with practice issues. If nurses at Hospital B believed they had more control over their practice by defining necessary tasks, it would be expected that they would respond more favorably to questions on the IWS that addressed task requirements.

Usually, nursing divisions require policy and procedure committees to formulate rules and policies that define nursing practice. Such rules have been believed to "protect the patient." Yet, if nursing is to be viewed as a profession, it should not be necessary to prescribe practice parameters so strictly. Instead, shared-governance management structures encourage practice standards to be written. These are used to guide sound practice judgment by providing a minimum baseline that defines the limits of behavior. They differ from policy and procedures in that they define basic expectations for performance against which judgment, activities, and processes can unfold (Porter-O'Grady and Finnigan 1984).

The nurses at Hospital B responded more favorably than nurses at Hospital A in the organizational policies component. Through a committee framework, decisions relating to appropriate clinical practice were made by those committee members at Hospital B. Their decisions became mandates of the organization. Perhaps because nurses at Hospital B had participated in decisions concerning organizational policy, their scores in this component showed a higher level of satisfaction than scores from nurses at Hospital A. The research question in this study was derived from the central premise that a shared-governance management structure in a nursing organization affects the level of satisfaction of its nurses. Underlying this study was the belief that registered nurses would be more satisfied with their job and work environment if the organization in which they worked was designed to promote better use of professional skills.

The results of this study offer some evidence that a shared-governance management structure provides an environment for registered nurses that supports professional behaviors, thus promoting job satisfaction.

Conclusion

Herzberg, Mausner, and Snyderman (1959) suggest that achievement, recognition, interpersonal relations, job status, and pay will affect satisfaction more than company policy, working conditions, and supervision. Unfortunately, many of these components that positively affect satisfaction are also difficult for management to control or improve. It may be for this reason that management often focuses on factors that seem to be more easily changed, such as personnel policy or working conditions. In fact, Stamps and Piedmonte (1986) report that investigators using the IWS sometimes add an additional component concerning specific organizational structure and managerial policy. They further report that, because staff studies have tended to be descriptive, the information gathered is rarely processed and attention is therefore not transferred to the work environment. In management-dominated organizations, the bureaucratic model dictates policy downward. Because hospitals function in this hierarchical system, they limit the independent behavior of staff nurses. Nurses who are unable to participate in decision making frequently become isolated; they experience dissonance between their ideal for autonomous practice as professionals and their powerlessness to control the environment in which they practice (Shidler, Pencak, and McFolling 1989).

Research related to shared governance is in an infancy stage. It is difficult, therefore, to determine how much participation or which shared-governance model would produce expected outcomes. Additionally, the question always exists as to how other factors, such as acuity levels of patients or staffing patterns, affect job satisfaction or dissatisfaction.

Future research should therefore consider other factors that may influence satisfaction, and should examine before-and-after comparison of satisfaction scores, as well as longitudinal studies comparing different models of shared governance. The results of this study offer some evidence that a shared-governance management structure may provide an environment for registered nurses that supports professional behaviors and thus promotes job satisfaction. Shared-governance management structures may also offer nurses opportunities for professional unity.

5. Satisfaction with the Decision-Making Process: Effect on Work Satisfaction and Tenure of Hospital Nurses

Jennie L. McQuaide

Purpose

Hospitals that have low turnover rates value their nurses and view them as professionals who are encouraged to participate in decision making (DeCrosta 1989). With its focus on nurse involvement in decisions and staff nurse empowerment, increased participative management often makes the difference between high and low retention rates (DeCrosta 1989; Trofino 1989; Volk and Lucas 1991).

While some researchers have studied factors leading to turnover among hospital nurses, others have explored the opposite perspective—factors leading to retention. One of the most outstanding studies on retention, "Magnet Hospitals: Attraction and Retention of Professional Nurses," describes factors that contribute to the magnetism of hospitals: participative management, open communication throughout the various levels of administration, knowledgeable leadership at all levels, and a strong commitment to high quality patient care (McClure et al. 1983). Identified as places in which people like to work, magnet hospitals have been described as successful because of radical decentralization (Kramer and Schmalenberg 1988; McClure et al. 1983). In a comparative study of satisfaction factors for nurses at magnet and nonmagnet hospitals, Kramer and Schmalenberg (1988, 1991a, 1991b) found that satisfaction levels at the magnet hospitals were higher than at the nonmagnet hospitals. At magnet hospitals, nurses reported greater satisfaction with staffing levels, with the degree of autonomy they have over their work, and with the range of salaries.

Collaborative Governance

Shared governance, collaborative governance, or self-governance is a representative form of governance involving the entire nursing department or the entire hospital (Jacoby and Terpstra 1990; Johnson 1989). A shared-governance model has been correlated with a 3 percent to 5 percent turnover rate; an increase in positive attitudes, trust, and

Jennie L. McQuaide is a consultant and an instructor at Gloucester County College, Sewell, New Jersey. This is part of her doctoral dissertation.

For more information about this study, contact Jennie McQuaide at 103 N. Jackson Avenue, Wenonah, NJ 08090. Telephone (609) 468-3001.

respect; more open communication; and decreased complaining (Jacoby and Terpstra 1990). After five years of shared governance, one hospital reported that 50 percent of its nurses had been employed there for five or more years, that nurses' satisfaction with working conditions had increased, and that doctors' satisfaction with the quality of patient care had increased (Johnson 1989).

Participative Management

Participative management usually refers to management strategies that are less comprehensive than in the collaborative governance model. Participative management may be unit-based, in which case it involves input from all nurses regarding the operation of the unit. Alternatively, participative management may be used to focus on a specific issue such as quality patient care, case management, or computerization; it may involve several units or departments. Input is sought from all who are involved; the staff of the units or departments work together to resolve the specific problem.

Controversy exists about the effectiveness of participative management as a strategy for increasing nurse satisfaction and nurse retention. In general, the nursing literature voices strong support for participative management, while the hospital literature questions the effectiveness of participative management (Schwartz 1990). Results of studies on participative management have been inconsistent (Stamps and Piedmonte 1986). A possible cause of the inconsistency is that the term "participative management" refers to a variety of management practices, which may be too diverse to be compared effectively. There has been little standardization in the methodology used or the questions asked (Stamps and Piedmonte 1986). Studies that support participative management use broad definitions that focus on the entire hospital culture (McClure et al. 1983). Studies that find no correlation between participative management and satisfaction (Counte et al. 1987) and no correlation between participative management and turnover (Alexander 1988) seem to use only a few specific questions as a measure of participative management. A possible explanation for their failure to obtain the anticipated results is the way in which participative management is operationalized.

The general literature on employee turnover reflects a similar controversy (Locke and Schweiger 1979). Lack of involvement in the decision-making process is a source of frustration and dissatisfaction to employees. Employees who perceive that they have higher levels of control over their work have greater satisfaction, lower intent to leave, and lower turnover (Spector 1986). In a review of studies on participation in decision making, Locke and Schweiger (1979) found that, as participation increased, satisfaction increased in 60 percent of the studies, remained the same in 30 percent of the studies, and decreased in 9 percent of the studies.

While nurse executives and hospital administrators have been involved in a debate about nurse participation in the decision-making process, there has been little direct input from nurses about what level of participation they want. Having an assessment tool that asks nurses to indicate the level of importance of an issue, as well as the level of satisfaction with their involvement in the decision-making process on that issue, can help to identify areas in which nurse participation is particularly important. Assessing both importance and satisfaction uses research strategies employed by Kramer and Schmalenberg (1991a, 1991b), Munson and Heda (1974), and Stamps and Piedmonte (1986).

The study described here focuses on participation in the decision-making process and the effect on overall work satisfaction and tenure of hospital nurses. The Index of Work Satisfaction (Stamps and Piedmonte 1986) was used to assess overall work satisfaction. The Nurse Participation in Decision Making Scale was developed as a means of directly asking nurses two questions: (1) what kinds of participation are important to you? and (2) how satisfied are you with the level of participation you have in the decision-making process?

Methodology

Survey Instruments

This study used two survey instruments, the Nurse Participation in Decision Making Scale (NPDMS) and the Index of Work Satisfaction (Stamps and Piedmonte 1986).

The ten-item NPDMS was developed for this study as a result of numerous personal interviews with nurses and nursing administrators and an extensive search of the literature. Respondents were asked to report on the level of importance of each item and their level of satisfaction with their participation in the decision-making process, using a seven-point Likert-type scale. Responses ranged from 1 (low) to 7 (high).

Turnover was assessed by respondent self-report on length of tenure in the present hospital unit. This provides a measure of retention. It is one of several different methods used to measure turnover. It is useful in this study because the information is obtained directly from the subject without breaching confidentiality. A high number of nurses with short tenure indicates high turnover.

The Index of Work Satisfaction was used to assess overall work satisfaction levels. It assesses six components of work satisfaction: pay, autonomy, task requirements, organizational policies, professional status, and interaction.

Survey Participants

During late 1993 and early 1994, surveys were distributed to all full-time registered staff nurses who were employed in medical-surgical units in five southern New Jersey hospitals. All participating hospitals were assured of confidentiality; consequently, no identifying demographic data are supplied here. The combined total of surveys distributed was 302; 110 surveys were returned. Of that number, 8 could not be used because of missing data. The overall response rate was 36 percent; the overall response rate for usable returns was 34 percent. The population for this study was a convenience sample.

Results

Nurse Participation in Decision-Making Scale

The items in the NPDMS and a frequency distribution of responses are shown in Table 5.6. Means for each item of the NPDMS were calculated for both importance and satisfaction (Figure 5.1). Looking at this information gives a picture of the level of importance and the level of satisfaction for each item of the scale as reported by the survey respondents. It also provides an assessment of the level of dissonance between the two scores. Items that rank high in importance and high in satisfaction are likely to contribute to overall satisfaction. Items that rank high in importance and low in satisfaction are likely to contribute to overall dissatisfaction.

Information from the NPDMS indicates that the four issues of greatest importance for the total study population were patient care, salary, staffing levels, and schedule. Mean scores for importance on these items were above 6.0 on a seven-point Likert scale. Five issues were ranked as moderately important: inservice topics, educational opportunities, procedures, peer review, and promotions. Mean scores for importance on these items were between 5.0 and 6.0. Developing the budget for the unit ranked lowest in importance, with a mean score of 4.2. With the exception of the budget item, all of the items of the NPDMS were moderately to highly important to nurses in this study.

While nurses ranked four items as highly important, they reported that no items provided equally high levels of satisfaction. Two items produced moderate satisfaction—patient care and the work schedule— with mean scores between 5.0 and 6.0. Four items fell in the middle range of responses for satisfaction—procedures, in-service topics, educational

Table 5.6 Frequency Distribution of Responses to NPDMS, Total Population ($N = 102$)

	Lowest			Undecided			Highest
IMPORTANCE							
1. Determining the work schedule for your unit	1.0%	1.0%	2.0%	4.9%	11.8%	28.4%	51.0%
2. Input regarding salary/benefits for nurses throughout the hospital	0.0	1.0	5.9	1.0	10.8	18.6	62.7
3. Choosing educational opportunities for nurses in your unit	2.9	1.0	0.0	10.8	15.7	25.5	44.1
4. Deciding about promotions for nurses in your unit	2.9	5.9	6.9	11.8	15.7	26.5	30.4
5. Setting minimum staffing levels for your unit	2.9	1.0	2.9	1.0	7.8	25.5	58.8
6. Participating on a peer review committed for handling nurse performance problems	1.0	4.9	8.8	8.8	18.6	28.4	29.4
7. Selection of topics for in-service training	0.0	1.0	3.9	5.9	19.6	29.4	40.2
8. Establishment of procedures for your unit	0.0	0.0	3.9	10.8	18.6	31.4	35.3
9. Developing the budget for your unit	15.7	12.7	10.8	10.8	14.7	15.7	19.6
10. Input in decisions about patient care	0.0	0.0	0.0	4.9	1.0	24.5	69.6
SATISFACTION							
1. Determining the work schedule for your unit	2.0	5.9	8.8	10.8	20.6	29.4	22.5
2. Input regarding salary/benefits for nurses throughout the hospital	14.7	20.6	17.6	12.7	14.7	15.7	3.9
3. Choosing educational opportunities for nurses in your unit	8.8	10.8	13.7	13.7	16.7	25.5	10.8
4. Deciding about promotions for nurses in your unit	15.7	13.7	11.8	24.5	13.7	14.7	5.9
5. Setting minimum staffing levels for your unit	20.6	11.8	17.6	7.8	21.6	12.7	7.8
6. Participating on a peer review committed for handling nurse performance problems	12.7	14.7	9.8	25.5	13.7	14.7	8.8
7. Selection of topics for in-service training	10.8	8.8	10.8	13.7	12.7	31.4	11.8
8. Establishment of procedures for your unit	4.9	3.9	10.8	12.7	23.5	33.3	10.8
9. Developing the budget for your unit	10.8	6.9	9.8	29.4	16.7	14.7	11.8
10. Input in decisions about patient care	1.0	5.9	4.9	7.8	23.5	35.3	21.6

Figure 5.1 Means for NPDMS, Total Population (*N*=102)

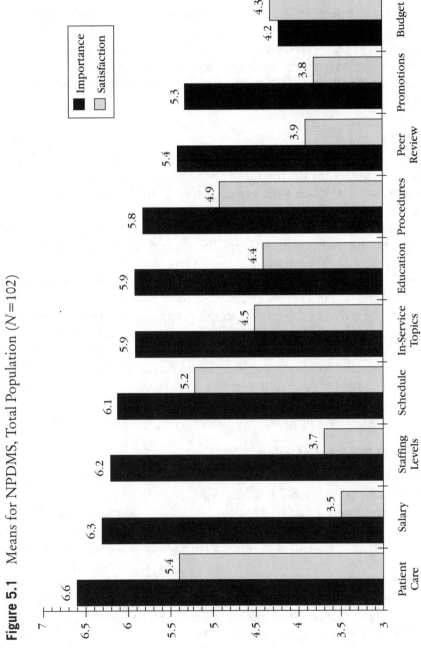

opportunities, and budget. The four items on which nurses expressed the lowest levels of satisfaction were peer review, promotions, staffing levels, and salary and benefits. Satisfaction scores on these four items were below 4.0.

It is interesting to note that of the four items ranked high in importance—patient care, salary and benefits, staffing levels, and work schedule—two were ranked first and second for satisfaction (patient care and work schedule, respectively) and two were ranked ninth and tenth for satisfaction (staffing levels and salary and benefits, respectively). The salary item reflected the greatest dissonance between importance and satisfaction.

Tenure

For the turnover measure, length of tenure was measured in months. The mean for tenure for the total study population was 52.9 months (4 years, 5 months); the range varied from 1 month to 310 months (25 years, 10 months).

In the current study, 29 percent of the 102 nurses were employed in the same unit for five or more years. By contrast, the New Jersey Hospital Association (1991) reported that in 1990, 38 percent of New Jersey hospital nurses had been employed for five or more years in the same setting, and that in 1991 this figure rose to 45 percent. Some discrepancy in these rates may be due to the specific question asked. The current study asked about length of employment in the same unit, while the New Jersey Hospital Association study asked about length of employment in the same hospital. In addition, some of this 16 percent difference may be due to the presence of some other unidentified factors. The 29 percent five-year tenure rate is considerably lower than the 50 percent five-year tenure rate for nurses at a hospital with shared governance (Johnson 1989).

Index of Work Satisfaction

The IWS was scored according to the instructions in the Stamps and Piedmonte (1986) book. For Part A of the IWS, component weighting coefficients were calculated for the total study population (Table 5.7). These coefficients provide information on the importance of the six components relative to each other. Part A also produces a rank ordering of the six components.

Part B focuses on level of satisfaction with various aspects of work. The frequency distribution of responses to the items is given in Table B.9, Appendix B. Component means were developed for the total study population, which are also shown in Table 5.7.

Table 5.7 IWS Satisfaction Component Scores, Total Population
(*N* = 102)

	Part A Component Weighting Coefficient	Part B Component Mean
Pay	3.6	3.3
Autonomy	3.6	5.0
Task Requirements	2.8	3.3
Organizational Policies	2.5	3.2
Professional Status	3.3	5.7
Interaction	3.0	5.0
Nurse-Nurse	5.7	
Nurse-Physician	4.3	

The six components of the IWS were rank-ordered by importance (as indicated by Part A) and by satisfaction (as indicated by Part B). For the total study population, the components of greatest importance were pay, autonomy, and professional status. The components of greatest satisfaction were professional status, interaction, and autonomy.

Both the NPDMS and the IWS scores supported the view that nurses valued autonomy and participation in the decision-making process; however, their level of satisfaction with autonomy and participation was lower than the level of importance they attached to these dimensions of their jobs. Both instruments also found that pay was highly important to nurses, but their level of satisfaction was lower than the level of importance they attached to pay and benefits. While nurses in this study viewed pay as important, it was not the issue of greatest importance.

Among the least important and least satisfactory aspects of their work were policies and procedures set by the hospital administration, and tasks respondents were required to do as part of their jobs. Nurses frequently reported dissatisfaction with the amount of paperwork involved in their jobs. They were also less satisfied when they were required to carry out many tasks that were not directly related to patient care. In addition, it is interesting to study the interaction component and the two interaction subscales. The score for interaction between nurses was higher than the score for interaction between nurses and physicians. In this study, communication and interaction between nurses were more satisfactory than between nurses and physicians.

While the importance findings of this study are consistent with those of Stamps and Piedmonte (1986), the satisfaction findings are slightly different. Stamps and Piedmonte found that organizational policies and pay usually produced the least satisfaction. Since nurse salaries have improved in recent years, the different findings may be due to the salary increases and the increase in the range of salaries currently available.

For Part B, total scale scores were developed. The range of scores was also calculated. The mean for total scale scores was 193; the range of scores varied from 101 to 279. The possible range for total scale scores varies from a low of 44 to a high of 308. A mean below 155 is considered a sign of major dissatisfaction. While the mean for the total study population was above 155, a few respondents had total scale scores below 155. For the total study population, 10 individuals, representing 10 percent of the study group, had total scale scores below 155. This indicates that a few respondents expressed low levels of satisfaction; however, the majority reported higher levels of satisfaction.

In order to obtain the final IWS score, the sum of the adjusted mean scores was calculated and then divided by six (the number of components). The mean for the IWS was 13.5; the scores varied from 7.1 to 19.7. Higher scores indicate higher levels of satisfaction.

Further Data Analysis

A review of the mean scores for importance for each item of the NPDMS indicates that nine items had mean scores equal to or above 5.0; they were retained as issues of moderate or high importance to the study nurses. Budget development was the only item whose mean was below 5.0. It was dropped, and all subsequent analyses were conducted using the revised nine-item NPDMS.

In order to investigate the two research questions, nurses who had a total scale mean for importance greater than 5.0 on the revised NPDMS were selected from the total population. This group consisted of 94 nurses (92 percent of the study population).

Next, the total scale means for satisfaction were assessed for this high importance group. Nurses from the high importance group whose total satisfaction means on the revised NPDMS were above 5.0 were placed in the high satisfaction group. This group consisted of 31 nurses (30 percent). These nurses perceived the items of the NPDMS as highly important, and they were satisfied with their level of participation in the decision-making process at their respective hospitals.

Nurses from the high importance group whose total satisfaction means were lower than 4.0 were placed in the low satisfaction group. This group also consisted of 31 nurses (30 percent). These nurses perceived the items of the NPDMS as highly important, and they were dissatisfied with their level of participation in the decision-making process at their respective hospitals.

A statistical test for correlation between satisfaction levels on the revised NPDMS and IWS scores was conducted. The results of the Mann-Whitney U test indicate that a significant positive correlation exists between satisfaction levels on the revised NPDMS and the IWS. Nurses in the high satisfaction group also had high overall work satisfaction as indicated by the IWS. Nurses in the low satisfaction group also had low overall work satisfaction as indicated by the IWS. Participation in the decision-making process was positively correlated with overall satisfaction, as anticipated.

A statistical test for correlation between satisfaction levels on the revised NPDMS and tenure was also conducted. The results of the Mann-Whitney U test indicate that no correlation exists between satisfaction levels on the NPDMS and tenure. It had been hypothesized that nurses in the high satisfaction group would have longer tenure than nurses in the low satisfaction group.

The results of this analysis support the results of the "magnet hospitals" study; participation in the decision-making process contributes to higher levels of satisfaction and greater acceptance of solutions to problems (McClure et al. 1983). Several other studies have found that autonomy, defined as participation in the decision-making process, is the best predictor of satisfaction (Curry et al. 1985; Hinshaw, Smeltzer, and Atwood 1987; Kramer and Schmalenberg 1991b; Stamps and Piedmonte 1986; Weisman et al. 1993).

The results of this study are also consistent with the existing research, which reports no relationship between participation in the decision-making process and tenure. Just as Alexander's (1988) study failed to support his prediction that increased centralization would result in increased turnover, the current study found no correlation between participation in the decision-making process and tenure. The absence of a relationship between satisfaction with participation in the decision-making process and tenure is contrary to what seems intuitive. Alexander speculated that increased participation in the decision-making process might be ineffective in reducing turnover if other structural changes were not also made in the organization. Perhaps additional variables need to be considered when examining the relationship between tenure and participative management. The magnet hospital of McClure et al. (1983) is a total hospital environment in which participative management is just one element. Perhaps the entire hospital environment or culture should be studied. The procedures used in this study may have been inadequate to identify any relationship between participation and tenure.

Another factor that must be considered as a possible explanation for the unexpected results regarding tenure concerns the type of unit studied.

Medical-surgical units are frequently the point of entry to the hospital system for beginning nurses. After spending some time in medical-surgical units, nurses often move on to specialty units within the same hospital or at another hospital. The decision to leave the unit may have little to do with overall work satisfaction or satisfaction with the decision-making process. Leaving may be the only way for a nurse to advance up the career ladder.

Limitations of this Study

This study should be viewed as exploratory in nature. A convenience sample was used; consequently, the findings cannot be generalized to other populations.

In three of the hospitals, response rates were low. There are several reasons why nurses may not have responded to the survey. The survey instrument was long, requiring approximately 30 minutes to complete. Some nurses may have declined to participate in the study because of the survey's length. In some cases, the method of distribution of surveys may have contributed to the low response rate. The researcher had no direct contact with staff nurses or nurse managers. Direct interaction between the researcher and staff nurses might have increased the response rate.

Implications

The findings of this study are important because they provide information directly from hospital nurses about the importance they attach to certain issues and their level of satisfaction with their participation in the decision-making process in relation to those issues. This information can be used in two specific ways: first, as a guide for making administrative decisions within the nursing department and within the hospital; and second, as a basis for future research.

Hospitals are highly complex organizations that deal with countless crises on a regular basis. To be effective and efficient, hospital administrators must be responsive to more or less constant turmoil. Management strategies that facilitate communication between hospital administrators and staff can be advantageous because information about current conditions is transmitted in timely fashion.

The NPDMS is a concise instrument that provides a systematic method of studying participative management in hospitals. It quickly produces information that can be used in the administration of the hospital. By rank ordering the items, a list of priorities can be developed based on the responses of all nurses or a random sample of nurses in a particular hospital. In addition, the responses to the NPDMS can be tabulated by unit or department, and priorities can be developed within the unit or department.

Research has shown that turnover is a process, not an isolated event. Some period of dissatisfaction occurs before a nurse makes the decision to leave the hospital. Nurses have indicated that intervention early in that process would prevent their departure (Landstrom, Biordi, and Gillies 1989). Although the current study finds no direct relationship between participation in the decision-making process and tenure, the relationship between participation in the decision-making process and overall satisfaction is strong. By using the NPDMS several times per year, hospitals could identify the concerns of nurses as early as possible and intervene in the process in a timely fashion.

This study raises a number of questions for future research on participation in the decision-making process. Replicating the study using a random sample of nurses throughout the hospital, rather than a convenience sample, might produce some different findings regarding tenure. Tenure patterns in medical-surgical units may be different from tenure patterns in other hospital units. Replication could also lead to generalizations regarding nurse participation in the decision-making process.

Additional research should be conducted that explores both the cost of increased nurse participation in decision-making and the effect of that participation on the quality of patient care. Comparisons should be made of units using increased nurse participation in decision-making and units using other management strategies.

Another much needed piece of research is a longitudinal study covering a five- or ten-year period during which increased nurse participation in decision making is in effect. Since it is known that implementation of participative management is a process that takes considerable time, a long-term study is vital to full understanding of the effect of such a management model on cost and quality of patient care.

Finally, a large-scale study that explores multiple factors is needed in order to examine interaction effects. The current research supports other research that found that participation in the decision-making process is highly correlated with overall work satisfaction. Since others have found that satisfaction is inversely correlated with intent to leave and intent to leave is correlated with turnover, it seems logical that participation in the decision-making process would also be related to tenure. Numerous researchers have considered the connection, and yet the scientific support for this apparently logical connection has not been found. That seems to imply that participative management alone is not sufficient to predict tenure. A large-scale study might identify the missing pieces of the puzzle. Such a study should examine the governance structure and the culture of the entire hospital. In addition, factors such as individual preferences for autonomy (Dwyer, Schwartz, and Fox 1992) should be considered.

References

Alexander, J. A. 1988. "The Effects of Patient Care Unit Organization on Nursing Turnover." *Health Care Management Review* 13 (2): 61–72.

Basch, C. E., E. M. Sliepcevich, R. S. Gold, D. F. Duncan, and L. J. Kolbe. 1985. "Avoiding Type II Errors in Health Education Program Evaluations: A Case Study." *Health Education Quarterly* 12: 315–31.

Campbell, D. T., and J. C. Stanley. 1963. *Experimental and Quasi-Experimental Designs for Research*. Chicago: Rand McNally College Publishing Company.

Counte, M. A., G. L. Glandon, D. M. Oleske, and J. P. Hill. 1992. "Total Quality Management in a Health Care Organization: How Are Employees Affected?" *Hospital & Health Services Administration* 37 (4): 503–18.

Curry, J. P., D. S. Wakefield, J. L. Price, C. W. Mueller, and J. C. McCloskey. 1985. "Determinants of Turnover among Nursing Department Employees." *Research in Nursing and Health* 8: 397–411.

DeCrosta, A. A. 1989. "Meeting the Nurse Retention Challenge: An Interview with Connie Curran." *Nursing* 19: 170–71.

Downs, C. W., and M. D. Hazen. 1977. "A Factor Analytic Study of Communication Satisfaction." *Journal of Business Communication* 14: 65–73.

Duxbury, M., G. M. Henley, and D. Armstrong. 1982. "Measurement of the Nurse Organizational Climate of Neonatal Intensive Care Units." *Nursing Research* 31: 83–88.

Dwyer, D. J., R. H. Schwartz, and M. L. Fox. 1992. "Decision-Making Autonomy in Nursing." *Journal of Nursing Administration* 22: 17–23.

Finnegan, J. R., D. M. Murray, C. Kurth, and P. McCarthy. 1989. "Measuring and Tracking Education Program Implementation: The Minnesota Heart Health Program Experience." *Health Education Quarterly* 16: 77–90.

Grant, P. 1986. *The Performance Management Process: An Integrative Approach to Human Resource Management*. Dubuque, IA: Kendall/Hunt.

Gustin, T. 1988. "Job Satisfaction of Nurses in Relationship to Organizational Structure." Master's thesis, Wright State University, Dayton, Ohio.

Herzberg, F., B. Mausner, and B. Snyderman. 1959. *The Motivation to Work*, 2nd ed. New York: John Wiley and Sons.

Hinshaw, A. S., C. H. Smeltzer, and J. R. Atwood. 1987. "Innovative Retention Strategies for Nursing Staff." *Journal of Nursing Administration* 17: 8–16.

Ingersoll, G. L. 1996. "Organizational Redesign: Effect on Institutional and Consumer Outcomes." In *Annual Review of Nursing Research*, edited by J. J. Fitzpatrick and J. Norbeck 14: 121–43.

Ingersoll, G. L., A. W. Schultz, N. Hoffart, and S. A. Ryan. 1996. "Effect of a Professional Practice Model on Staff Nurse Perception of Work Group and Nurse Leader." *Journal of Nursing Administration* 14: 121–43.

Jacoby, J., and M. Terpstra. 1990. "Collaborative Governance: Model for Professional Autonomy." *Nursing Management* 21: 42–44.

Johnson, S. H. 1989. "Building Respect: The Key to Retention." *Dimensions of Critical Care Nursing* 8: 3–4.

Kramer, M., and C. Schmalenberg. 1988. "Magnet Hospital: Institutions of Excellence, Part 2." *Journal of Nursing Administration* 18: 11–19.

————. 1991a. "Job Satisfaction and Retention: Insights for the '90s, Part 1." *Nursing 91* 21: 50–55.

————. 1991b. "Job Satisfaction and Retention: Insights for the '90s, Part 2." *Nursing 91* 21: 51–55.

Landstrom, G. L., D. C. Biordi, and D. A. Gillies. 1989. "The Emotional and Behavioral Process of Staff Nurse Turnover." *Journal of Nursing Administration* 19: 23–28.

Locke, E. A., and D. M. Schweiger. 1979. "Participation in Decision Making: One More Look." In *Research in Organizational Behavior*, edited by B. M. Staw, 1: 265–339. Greenwich, CT: JAI Press.

Martin, P. A. 1995. "Evaluation of Shared Governance." *Journal of Shared Governance* 1: 11–16.

McClure, M. L., M. A. Poulin, M. D. Sovie, and M. A. Wandelt. 1983. *Magnet Hospitals: Attraction and Retention of Professional Nurses*. Kansas City, MO: American Nurses Association.

Milton, D. A., J. A. Verran, R. M. Gerber, and J. Fleury. 1995. "Tools to Evaluate Reengineering Progress." In *Reengineering Nursing and Health Care*, edited by S. S. Blancett and D. L. Flarey, 195–202. Gaithersburg, MD: Aspen.

Munson, F. C., and S. S. Heda. 1974. "An Instrument for Measuring Satisfaction." *Nursing Research* 23: 159–66.

New Jersey Hospital Association. 1991. *1991 Hospital Nursing Services Survey*. Princeton, NJ: NJHA.

Newman, B. 1989. *The Newman Systems Model*, 2nd ed. Norwalk, CT: Appleton and Lange.

Nunnally, J., and I. Bernstein. 1994. *Psychometric Theory*, 3rd ed. New York: McGraw-Hill.

Peterson, M., and D. Allen. 1986. "Shared Governance: A Strategy for Transforming Organizations." *Journal of Nursing Administration* 16: 11–16.

Porter-O'Grady, T., and S. Finnigan. 1984. *Shared Governance for Nursing*. Rockville, MD: Aspen.

Prescott, P., and K. Dennis. 1985. "Power and Powerlessness in Hospital Nursing Departments." *Journal of Professional Nursing* 1: 348–55.

Price, J. L., and C. W. Mueller. 1981. *Professional Turnover: The Case of Nurses*. New York: SP Medical & Scientific Books.

Roedel, R., and R. Nystrom. 1988. "Nursing Jobs and Satisfaction." *Nursing Management* 19: 34–38.

Schutzenhofer, K. K. 1983. "The Development of Autonomy in Adult Women." *Journal of Psychosocial Nursing and Mental Health Services* 21: 25–30.

Schwartz, R. H. 1990. "Coping with Unbalanced Information about Decision-Making Influence for Nurses." *Hospital & Health Services Administration* 35: 547–59.

Shidler, H., M. Pencak, and S. D. McFolling. 1989. "Professional Nursing Staff: A Model for Self-Governance for Nursing." *Nursing Administration Quarterly* 13: 1–9.

Spector, P. E. 1986. "Perceived Control by Employees: A Meta-analysis of Studies Concerning Autonomy and Participation at Work." *Human Relations* 39: 1005–16.

Stamps, P. L., and E. B. Piedmonte. 1986. *Nurses and Work Satisfaction: An Index for Measurement*. Chicago: Health Administration Press.

Trofino, J. 1989. "Empowering Nurses." *Journal of Nursing Administration* 19: 13.

Volk, M. C., and M. D. Lucas. 1991. "Relationship of Management Style and Anticipated Turnover." *Dimensions of Critical Care Nursing* 10: 35–40.

Weisman, C. S., D. L. Gordon, S. D. Cassard, M. Bergner, and R. Wong. 1993. "The Effects of Unit Self-Management on Hospital Nurses' Work Process, Work Satisfaction, and Retention." *Medical Care* 31: 381–91.

Witzel, P. A., G. L. Ingersoll, A. W. Schultz, and S. A. Ryan. In press. A Cost Estimation Model for Measuring Professional Practice. *Nursing Economic$*.

6

A LAST WORD ABOUT MEASURING
NURSE SATISFACTION

S everal levels of research have contributed to this book. First are the many published studies that serve as the foundation for Chapters 2 and 3 as well as some of the selections in Chapter 5 and Appendixes E and F. These published works include theoretical as well as empirical studies; the research arises from a variety of academic and professional areas, including psychology, sociology, management, and nursing. Second are the 40 practice-based studies included in this book, most of them unpublished. Although not all of these studies meet the criteria designated for published research, each one makes a significant contribution not only to the use of the IWS as a measure of satisfaction, but also to a better understanding of the practice environments of nurses. Several also provide excellent reviews of the literature. These contributions provide a fascinating view of innovations in nursing practice that are currently being conducted in organizations, all of which are using level of satisfaction as an outcome variable. Space has limited detailed descriptions of these practice-based studies, but all of the authors are willing to discuss their specific findings as well as their interest in nurse satisfaction.

Taken all together, this represents a wealth of information about the nursing profession, nursing practice, and the type of research interests that are prevalent in the field today. This last chapter will present a summary of some of the most important insights that have been gained in the past ten years that the IWS has been extensively used. The focus of this chapter will be on both content and measurement. Although there is no intention to ignore research that uses other methods of measuring nurse satisfaction, this chapter will especially focus on the 40 contributions to this volume as well as the 18 published studies (see Table 3.1) that have used the IWS as a measure of satisfaction of nurses.

What Have We Learned about Research in Nurse Satisfaction?

The 58 different examples (published and unpublished) of research using the IWS as a measure of satisfaction are incredibly diverse. Although many of them use the IWS as a way to evaluate or monitor the effect of a particular organizational intervention, the type of intervention varies tremendously. Quite a few of the interventions involve some specific type of professional practice model, such as case management, primary nursing, clinical ladders, or patient-oriented nursing. Others address more general management concerns such as participative management or shared governance. Some of the studies have as a primary focus the better understanding of the needs of nurses. Some of these focus on particular types of nurses, such as nurse managers or those who work in operating rooms or critical care, medical-surgical, or neonatal intensive care units. Others study all nurses who practice in rural areas, for example, or use a random mailing list approach to query nurses about their perception of the profession independent of a particular job. Almost all of these studies (both published and unpublished) may be considered practice-based; that is, they occur in real-life organizations where nurses are working and patients are getting care at the same time as the research is going on. This of course means that not all important variables can be controlled, with a resultant diminution of methodological rigor. However, this also means that the research itself is an excellent reflection of practice concerns, probably a better reflection than some of the more "academic" research discussed in Chapters 2 and 3.

This said, it must immediately be noted that the contributions collected here do not lack a theoretical framework. In fact, the conceptual background of most of the examples is well developed. The space limitations of this volume prevent the sharing of this part of the research. Thus the phrase, "please contact the author," is all too common.

If anything, the unpublished studies contained in this volume demonstrate an interesting overlap between what might be characterized as management concerns on the one hand and academic or research concerns on the other. Among the contributions, at least half are a formal part of a graduate program—master's or doctoral. It is very common for researchers, while completing graduate work, to be employed at the hospital where the study is located. In some studies, the faculty of nursing schools are conducting research jointly with those working at the hospital. Several joint academic-hospital research groups are represented here. This overlap between management and practice enriches the field enormously, by ensuring that research is conducted on issues that are important to the nursing profession.

Use of Other Measurement Tools

Although this chapter focuses on studies using the IWS, satisfaction is not the only variable being measured. Many of the studies use other measurement tools: in fact, Gustin et al. (Chapter 5, Selection 2) and Martin et al. (Appendix E, Selection 2) use a total of six different measurement instruments. Examining the types of measurement tools used gives some insights into the types of variables that are viewed as being important. Table 6.1 shows a way to categorize the various measurement instruments represented in these two chapters. As can be seen from this table, there are two particularly large categories of these other measures. The first, organizational characteristics, includes measures of communication, collegiality, the climate of the organization, and esprit or morale. Although these measures are diverse (such as the effort by Ingersoll et al. to measure of extent of model implementation; Chapter 5, Selection 1), they have in common a concern for the effect of organizational characteristics on the level of satisfaction of the nursing staff. Even if the studies concern an innovation within a specific unit, the conceptual focus and measurement effort are concerned with the whole organization. A second large category of measures assesses the characteristics of the job itself, including tension and stress, professional activities, and autonomy. In this conceptual focus, it is the job or the unit that is the focus of measurement. (Chapter 3 discusses the distinction between an organizational focus and a job-specific level of analysis.)

Two other categories of measures that several investigators using the IWS have included are measures for personal characteristics (including personality) and social support systems. A few studies assess patient satisfaction, and some use multiple measures for satisfaction. These measures are representative of those used in other studies that are using measures of satisfaction other than the IWS (Stamps under review).

The types of measures used reflect what researchers think are important variables. A typical research process is to identify a variable of importance and then attempt to find a measure for it. Many of the

Table 6.1 Measurement Instruments Used in Conjunction with the IWS

Measurement Instrument	Author of Scale	Selection in Book/Article
Organizational Characteristics		
1. Organizational Climate Questionnaire	Duxbury 1982; modified by Martin 1995	Gustin et al. Chapter 5, #2
		Martin et al. Appendix E, #2
		Schmidt and Martin, Appendix E, #1
		Thompson et al. 1991
a. Esprit Sub-Scale	Duxbury 1982; modified by Martin 1995	
2. Nursing Organization Climate Questionnaire, Scale B	Duxbury et al. 1982	
3. Organizational Commitment	Porter and Smith 1970	Adams, Appendix E, #5
4. Extent of Model Implementation	Milton et al. 1985	Ingersoll et al. Chapter 5, #1
5. Communication Satisfaction Survey	Downs and Hazen 1977; Pincus 1986; Cox 1991	Martin et al. Appendix E, #2
		Gustin et al. Chapter 5, #2
6. Nurse Participation in Decision-Making	McQuaide 1996	McQuaide, Chapter 5, #5
7. NICU Nurse Collegiality Scale	Reeder and Stevens 1983; modified by Rush 1995	Rush, Appendix E, #9
8. Interdisciplinary Collaboration Questionnaire	Joy and Malay 1996	Joy and Malay, Appendix E, #13 (also Joy and Malay, 1992)
9. Collaborative Practice Scale	Weiss and Davis 1985	Baggs and Ryan 1990
10. Organizational Climate Description Questionnaire	Litwin and Stringer 1968	Gillies, Franklin, and Child 1990
11. Communication Scale (Feedback about Job)	Combination: Job Diagnostic Survey (Hackman and Oldham, 1975) and Downs-Hazen Measure of Communication (1975)	Tumulty 1992
Characteristics of Job		
1. Job-Related Tension Index	Kahn 1964	Burns Tuck, Appendix E, #6
2. Nursing Stress	Gray-Toft and Anderson 1981	Adams, Appendix E, #5

3. Professional Practice Climate	Miller 1989	Martin et al. Appendix E, #2 Gustin et al. Chapter 5, #2
4. Schutzenhofer Professional Nursing Activity Scale	Waltz and Strickland 1988	Gustin et al. Chapter 5, #2
5. Benefits and Schedule Scale	Minnick and Roberts 1996	Minnick, Peschke-Winn, and Thomas, Chapter 5, #3
6. Professionalism in Nursing Inventory	Adams 1996	Adams, Appendix E, #5
7. Control over Nursing Practice Scale	Gerber et al. 1990	Lancero and Gerber 1995
8. Nurse Case Manager Job Stress Index	Lancero and Gerber 1994	Lancero and Gerber 1995
9. Openness to Technology	Ball, Snelbecker, and Schechter 1955	Thompson, Ryan, and Baggs 1991
10. Professional Confidence Scale	Thompson et al. 1991	Thompson, Ryan, and Baggs 1991
11. Role Conflict/Ambiguity Scale	Rizzo 1970	Tumulty 1992
12. Nursing Role Conception Scale	Corwin 1960	Tumulty 1992
13. Job Stress Scale	Bailey and Claus 1977	Hinshaw, Smeltzer, and Atwood 1987
14. Control over Practice Scale	Harsley and Pelz 1976	Hinshaw, Smeltzer, and Atwood 1987

Personal Characteristics

1. Bem Sex-Role Inventory	Bem 1974	Adams, Appendix E, #5
2. Rosenburg Self-Esteem Scale	Rosenburg 1965	Adams, Appendix E, #5
3. Personality Hardiness Scale	Kobasa 1987	McCrea, Appendix E, #7
4. Crown-Marlow Social Desirability Scale	Crown and Marlow 1960	Rush, Appendix E, #9
5. Thomas-Kilman Conflict Mode Instrument	Thomas and Kilman 1974	Rush, Appendix E, #9
6. Reeder and Stevens Assertiveness Scale	Reeder and Stevens 1983; modified by Rush 1995	Rush, Appendix E, #9
7. Simplified Attitudes Toward Women Scale	Spence, Helmreich, and Stapp 1973; modified 1988	Koeckeritz, Appendix E, #15

Social Support

1. Norbeck Social Support Questionnaire	Norbeck 1981	Burns Tuck, Appendix E, #6
2. Caplan Social Support Questionnaire	Caplan 1980	Burns Tuck, Appendix E, #6

Continued

Table 6.1 Continued

Measurement Instrument	Author of Scale	Selection in Book/Article
3. Domestic Labor Responsibilities	Berk 1985	Koeckeritz, Appendix E, #15
4. Group Cohesion Scale	Good and Nelson 1973	Hinshaw, Smeltzer, and Atwood 1987
Other Nurse Satisfaction Measures		
1. Price-Mueller's Job Satisfaction Scale (JSS)	Price and Mueller 1986	Ingersoll et al. Chapter 5, #1
2. Nurse Job Satisfaction Scale	Brayfield and Rothe 1951, adapted	Hinshaw, Smeltzer, and Atwood 1987
3. Autonomy Subscale of Job Diagnostic Survey	Hackman and Oldham 1975	Tumulty 1992
Other		
1. Patient Satisfaction Instrument	Risser 1975	Joy and Malay, Appendix E, #13 (also Joy and Malay 1992)
2. Patient Satisfaction Survey	Hinshaw and Atwood 1983	Thompson, Ryan, and Baggs 1991
3. Turnover and Mobility	Hinshaw and Atwood 1980	Hinshaw, Ryan, and Baggs 1987

measures used are old, including several from the 1960s and 1970s. The investigators modified some of them; and, in at least three cases, the investigators developed new measures themselves (McQuaide, Chapter 5, Selection 5; Minnick, Pischke-Winn, and Thomas, Chapter 5, Selection 3; Adams, Appendix E, Selection 5; Joy and Malay 1992; Lancero and Gerber 1995 and Thompson, Ryan, and Baggs 1991). This shows a lot of activity in the field in terms of development of measurements, which is very appropriate. However, it should also be noted that the diversity of measures carries a significant problem in that it is not possible to compare results when such different measures are being used. Also, as can be seen in Table 6.1, several of these measures are old, some are significantly modified from their original use, and still others are combined into new measures. Of course, this raises validity issues.

The major conclusion that must be drawn is that the field is in need of reliable and valid measures for several variables that investigators view as being important. It seems obvious that variables related to the organization, to the nature of the job itself, and to the personal characteristics of the nurse are important: reliable and valid measurement instruments that will be generally accepted by researchers clearly need to be developed. This means that basic research is needed to develop such measures. This is obviously time-consuming, but is necessary. It is always easier to use measurement instruments developed by others, but if these are too dated—or too new—to have known reliability and validity, one can never be certain what is being measured. In many of these studies, the findings are mixed, or more ambiguous than the researchers expected. This may be due to the limitations of the measurement instruments themselves, rather than to the research setting.

One of the important roles of research is measurement development. This is an activity that is time- and resource-consuming, and difficult to do in combination with practice-based research efforts. Yet the effort should not be completely separated from the practice world, or the measurement instruments developed will be of limited use to the professionals in the field. One possible approach is to identify a couple of categories of variables that seem to be important and develop measures to be used by several researchers. If the measures are accurate, they will be applied, as is clearly shown by the wide utilization of the IWS. It is not necessary for every study to use the same measures, since that would cut down on the creativity of research efforts, but one of the roles of research is to identify measures that can be used with confidence in many different research settings. Only in this way will it be really possible to compare the results of different studies. This same need also exists with respect for measures of satisfaction, as will be discussed later in this chapter.

Rules of Research

Another of the contributions of the research model is the understanding of when findings can be generalized to other settings. In general, this is accomplished through a combination of large enough sample sizes and high enough response rates, together with using measures that have some known level of reliability and validity, as well as research designs that limit bias. Many of the studies included here have excellent discussions of the problems of trying to do research in real-life settings, when the respondent group may be affected by factors outside the experimental situation. Some multihospital studies, for example, used varying methods of data collection, sometimes to accommodate changing bureaucratic needs. In some cases, questionnaires were distributed at times of organizational tension, such as around times of layoffs or reorganizations, with a predictable effect on response rates.

As can be seen from Table 6.2, many of the studies have sample sizes and response rates that are too low. The investigators recognize these as problems, and most mention them as limitations, especially in terms of being able to generalize to other settings. Sample size and response rate are also problems for the published studies included on this table.

The studies administer questionnaires in many different—and creative—ways. Gustin et al. (Chapter 5, Selection 2) and Martin et al. (Appendix E, Selection 2) employed several methods of data collection, including providing a box lunch for those who responded. Some of the studies—Ingersoll et al. (Chapter 5, Selection 1) and Minnick, Peschke-Winn, and Thomas (Chapter 5, Selection 3) in particular—used a unit-based approach to increasing sample size and response rates. Ingersoll et al. for example, gave cash incentives to the units that had the highest participation rates. Some studies, such as Ringer et al. (Appendix E, Selection 11), obtained high response rates by focusing on small, specific units.

Part of the difficulty of generalizability is inherent in the approach taken by all these studies. Almost all of them are set in real-life situations that do not sit still just because somebody is studying them. Several of the studies, including Ingersoll et al. (Chapter 5, Selection 1), Minnick, Peschke-Winn, and Thomas (Chapter 5, Selection 3), Gustin et al. (Chapter 5, Selection 2), and Martin et al. (Appendix E, Selection 2), use the IWS in a monitoring sense. This means frequent data collection, with an increased chance that something might change within an organization. Of course, some of the studies are not able to demonstrate significant levels of change. It is hard to decide if this is because there actually is no change, or because the measurement tool may not be accurate, or because

Table 6.2 Sample Size and Response Rates for Published and Unpublished Studies

Published Studies Using the IWS as a Measure of Satisfaction	Sample Size	Response Rate
Hinshaw, Smeltzer, and Atwood 1987*		
• 7 urban and 8 rural hospitals	1597	82%
Blenkarn, D'Amico, and Virtue 1988		
• different units in psychiatric hospital	8; 9; 10	—
• pre/post implementation		
Baggs and Ryan 1990		
• ICU in a large hospital	68	100%
Gillies, Franklin, and Child 1990*		
• 4 units in 1 hospital	34	—
Houston 1990		
• ICU units in 7 hospitals using 12-hour staffing	—	—
Wells 1990*		
• nurse managers in 8 hospitals	95	69%
Williams 1990		
• medical-surgical unit compared to CCU	37	—
Bushy and Banik 1991		
• 8 rural hospitals	69	69%
Johnston 1991		
• 1 hospital	160	42%
Malik 1991		
• 2 hospitals, one with career ladder		
• ICU/CCU	17; 25	77%; 68%
Thompson, Ryan, and Baggs 1991		
• 4 units (2 experimental) in 1 hospital	58	—
Tumulty 1992		
• head nurses from 10 hospitals	110	78%
Kovner et al. 1994		
• 37 New Jersey hospitals		
• 86 pilot and 47 comparison units	858; 335	—
Lancero and Gerber 1995*		
• Nurse case managers, split between 2 models of case management	30	100%
Coward et al. 1995*		
• 26 rural and urban nursing homes in northern Florida	281	64%
Drews and Fisher 1996		
• children's hospital	45	29%
Studies Contained in this Book Using the IWS as a Measure**		
Ingersoll et al. Chapter 5, #1		
• 3 hospitals, 10 matched units		
• data colletion over time	255; 257; 235; 216	—

Continued

Table 6.2 Continued

Studies Contained in this Book Using the IWS as a Measure**	Sample Size	Response Rate
Gustin et al. Chapter 5, #2		
• rural hospital		
• monitoring with several measures over time	1403	10%–20%
Minnick, Pischke-Winn, and Thomas, Chapter 5, #3		
• 23 units over time	300–400	37% average
Mancini, Chapter 5, #4		
• 2 hospitals	99	39%
McQuaide, Chapter 5, #5		
• 5 hospitals	110	34%
Schmidt and Martin, Martin et al. Appendix E, #1, #2		
• rural hospital	61	86%
• 2 measurement points		
Klingshirn, Appendix E, #3		
• rural nurses in hospital setting	54	44%
Dunkin, Stratton, and Juhl, Appendix E, #4		
• multistate	3514	40%
• development of retention model		
Adams, Appendix E, #5		
• hospital-based	143; 583	25%
• development of statistical model		
Burns Tuck, Appendix E, #6		
• 14 hospitals	127	60%
• nurse managers and stress		
McCrea, Appendix E, #7		
• CCU nurses	90	59%
• 4 hospitals		
Hlavac, Appendix E, #8		
• CCU and medical-surgical unit in 1 hospital	87	75%
Rush, Appendix E, #9		
• neonatal ICU	100	75%
Cooley, Appendix E, #10		
• OR nurses	49	48%
Ringer et al. Appendix E, #11		
• 2 units	30	83%
• pre/post measures	18	45%
	12	71%
	14	61%
Pearson, Appendix E, #12		
• pre/post to test implementation of case management model	31	100%
	129	96%

Continued

Table 6.2 Continued

	Studies Contained in this Book Using the IWS as a Measure**	
	Sample Size	Response Rate
Joy and Malay, Apendix E, #13		
• pre/post measures on 2 units evaluating a professional practice model	—	—
Prock, Appendix E, #14		
• 2 hospitals, 1 with shared governance	60	40%
Koeckeritz, Appendix E, #15		
• 4 hospitals	315	43%

   * These studies used a modification of the IWS. (See Table 3.1)
   ** These studies are all contained in this book, either in Chapter 5 or in Appendix E. However, this does not mean they are all unpublished. Several of the studies have been published. See each selection for details.

the sample size is too small. It is obviously important to try to increase the sample size and the response rate as much as possible.

What Have We Learned about Satisfaction of Nurses?

The research into nurse satisfaction is seeking to understand what factors seem to be most related to nurses being satisfied with their jobs. In general, three large categories of factors thought to be related to satisfaction can be found in the published literature, as noted in Chapter 3. The first category of factors is related to the nurses themselves, including demographic and personality factors. The second category is related to the specific job a nurse has, and the third category of factors considers the organization itself—both its structure and its climate. These same factors are also found in the practice-based research studies, both published and unpublished, that constitute the focus of this chapter.

The Relationship Between Satisfaction and Demographic Characteristics

Demographic characteristics have always been included in studies of nurse satisfaction. In fact, it is this large group of factors that provides the main sense of continuity in research about nurses. As noted in Chapter 3, demographic factors were frequently the most important variables being studied in earlier research. In the current research environment, demographic variables often seem to be included primarily to increase the descriptive nature of the study or because "everybody else" includes these factors. When all of this research is evaluated, no clear picture emerges as to which of the demographic factors seem to be most related to satisfaction, and there has been little success using demographic factors to predict level of satisfaction. The more oriented a study is to management concerns, the less likely it is to consider seriously the role of demographic factors.

The studies contained in the latter part of this book reflect this trend: many included demographic factors, but in most cases, these were for descriptive purposes. And, typical of other studies, the results were mixed. For example, the sociological literature has long argued that older workers are more satisfied, although the reason for this seems arguable. Some propose that people reconcile their own personal career aspirations as they age, others observe a process of adapting to the organization's expectations, while still others note that with age comes greater life satisfaction also. Johnston (1991) and studies presented in this book (Ingersoll et al. Chapter 5, Selection 1; Martin et al. Appendix E, Selection 2; Ramsey and Henderson, Appendix F, Selection 6) found that older nurses were more satisfied, while Klingshirn (Appendix E, Selection 3) found no relationship between age and level of satisfaction. Bushy and Banik (1991) found that more experienced nurses were less satisfied, as did Walsh (Appendix F, Selection 4). Baggs and Ryan (1990) used demographic variables in their regression analysis to isolate better the effect of age and length of professional experience. They found that younger, more inexperienced nurses in the intensive care unit were more likely to be satisfied with the collaboration between physicians and nurses and also more likely to be satisfied than more experienced nurses.

Closely related to age is the length of professional experience, which is sometimes identified as total professional experience and sometimes identified as length of time at a particular institution. Several studies included this variable, which is probably more relevant than age anyway. As with age, however, the results were mixed. Both Ingersoll et al. (Chapter 5, Selection 1) and Dunkin, Stratton, and Juhl (Appendix E, Selection 4) found a relationship between longer professional experience and higher satisfaction. Dunkin, Stratton, and Juhl found a relationship between satisfaction and total years of nursing experience but no relationship between satisfaction and length of present employment; the relationship Ingersoll et al. found seemed to be present both for total years in nursing and for being at the hospital for more than 15 years. Schmidt and Martin, Martin et al., and Klingshirn (Appendix E, Selections 1, 2, 3) found no relationship between length of professional experience and level of satisfaction. Their studies focused on rural nurses, but so did Dunkin, Stratton, and Juhl (Appendix E, Selection 4). Several other studies examined this relationship in a more specific manner by focusing on one relevant component. Gustin et al. (Chapter 5, Selection 2), Martin et al. (Appendix E, Selection 2), and Burns Tuck (Appendix E, Selection 6) all found relationships between length of professional experience and level of satisfaction with organizational policies. Gustin et al. (Chapter 5, Selection 2) showed a positive relationship, while Martin et al. (Appendix E, Selection 2) found that long-term employees were less satisfied. Burns Tuck (Appendix E, Selection 6) found that, for nurse managers, more professional experience as a manager was positively related to higher satisfaction with both organizational policies and autonomy. For operating room nurses, Cooley (Appendix E, Selection 10) found that length of professional experience was only related to higher levels of satisfaction with interaction. Adams (Appendix E, Selection 5) found this relationship to be complicated. In her statistical model, length of time at the present job was not related to work satisfaction but was related to work commitment. As Adams notes, "Greater organizational commitment in the more tenured respondents may mean they have learned to operate within the agency to their advantage or may intend to stay in current positions because of economic factors."

The nursing literature has long investigated the notion that level of education is related to level of satisfaction. Perhaps because the types of educational paths available in nursing are diverse and the roles in practice may not be as directly related to level of education as one would hope, the relationship has never seemed especially strong. In this group of studies, Ingersoll et al. (Chapter 5, Selection 1) found that diploma nurses were more satisfied, Gustin et al. (Chapter 5, Selection 2) found that nurses with associate's degrees were more satisfied, and Klingshirn (Appendix E, Selection 3) found no relationship between education and satisfaction.

Ingersoll et al., Gustin et al., and Martin et al. (Appendix E, Selection 2) also explored other types of demographic factors that are at least partially related to the organizational structure. Ingersoll et al. found that nurses who had higher incomes were more satisfied, a relationship that seems obvious but does not hold for physicians (Stamps and Cruz 1994). Both the Gustin and Martin research teams found that nurses with a higher job status in the hospital seemed to have higher levels of satisfaction, especially in terms of being satisfied with organizational policies.

When reflecting on the mixed—and sometimes contradictory—findings of the relationship between level of satisfaction and demographic factors, one is not surprised that many studies include demographic variables only to help explain findings or to enable more precise comparisons. Analyzing demographic variables assumes that there is something about certain groups of nurses defined by specific characteristics (such as education or age) that helps to determine their level of satisfaction.

Increasingly, however, the paradigm is that, regardless of these factors, the organizational structure is more responsible for satisfaction than are demographic factors. Research reflects this trend in the field, and may have acted to lead the field to this conclusion.

The Relationship Between the Job, the Organization, and Level of Satisfaction

In some cases, there is overlap between a demographic analysis and a more organizational analysis. For example, several people studied whether different specialties of nurses have different levels of satisfaction. Hlavac (Appendix E, Selection 8) and Williams (1990) investigated whether there were differences in satisfaction between nurses working on medical-surgical units versus nurses working in critical care units; Burns Tuck (Appendix E, Selection 6) examined the level of satisfaction of nurse managers; Cooley (Appendix E, Selection 10) focused on operating room nurses; Rush (Appendix E, Selection 9) and Tranmer (Appendix F, Selection 15) examined nurses working in neonatal intensive care units, and McCauley (Appendix F, Selection 16) analyzed level of satisfaction of nurses in intensive care units, as did Baggs and Ryan (1990) and Houston (1990), who investigated the effect of 12-hour shifts. In all these examples, although the specific nurse specialties are examined because the investigators expect some variation as a result of belonging to one particular group (such as operating room nurse as opposed to intensive care unit nurse, for example), the specific focus of these studies is more organizational in that they examine the nature of the job of the nurse rather than the nurse's identity with the group. An especially good example of this is the study by Cooley (Appendix E, Selection 10) which found the level of satisfaction of nurses working in the operating room is at least partially dependent on the type of role they play: the greater the percentage of time spent in the role of circulating nurse, the lower the level of overall satisfaction. She also found that circulating nurses have lower satisfaction with pay, organizational policies, and autonomy.

This represents somewhat of a shift in conceptual thinking. More and more, the organization is viewed as being more important in affecting level of satisfaction of nurses. This can be seen both in a general way and in more specific ways that involve job redesign efforts. Several studies examined the effect of some general feature of the organization on level of satisfaction. McQuaid (Chapter 5, Selection 5) found higher levels of satisfaction among nurses who participated in the decision-making process at the hospital; Schmidt and Martin (Appendix E, Selection 1) found higher levels of satisfaction among nurses who thought there were higher levels of esprit in the hospital.

The basis for linking more specific job redesign efforts to level of satisfaction is that there is a general relationship between the organizational climate and how the nursing staff is treated. Many studies investigated the effect of a specific management intervention on the level of nurse satisfaction and used the IWS as the outcome measure. Three studies (Ringer et al. Appendix E, Selection 11; Pearson, Appendix E, Selection 12; Joos, Appendix F, Selection 9) investigated the institution of some type of case management; three studies (Minnick, Peschke-Winn, and Thomas, Chapter 5, Selection 3; Ingersoll et al. Chapter 5, Selection 1; Joy and Malay, Appendix E, Selection 13) described the institution of a professional practice model that involved something besides case management; and three studies (Mancini, Chapter 5, Selection 4; Prock, Appendix E, Selection 14; and the research team involving Martin, Appendix E, Selection 2, Gustin, et al. Chapter 5, Selection 2) investigated the effect of a shared-governance model on the level of satisfaction of nurses. Two studies specifically involved the Total Quality Management framework for the study, including Auerbach and Dornan (Appendix F, Selection 11) and Christy (Appendix F, Selection 13).

Naturally, one of the major interests is whether these studies were able to demonstrate that the specific intervention had an effect upon nurse satisfaction. Mancini (Chapter 5, Selection 4) discovered that all the satisfaction scores were higher in the hospital with shared governance than in the hospital without; and that the differences on the autonomy, task requirements, and organizational policies components were especially strong. The research team involving Martin, Gustin, et al. were also able to demonstrate that the nurses who worked in the hospital with a shared-governance model had significantly higher overall job satisfaction scores than nurses in the hospital without shared governance. In their study, the three components that showed the most change were autonomy, pay, and organizational policies. Not all studies investigating shared governance revealed positive findings. Prock (Appendix E, Selection 14), for example, did not find any difference in the level of satisfaction among nurses working in a hospital with shared governance as compared with nurses working in a hospital without shared governance. Even though all three of these studies compared the nursing staff of a hospital with shared governance to a hospital without shared governance, there were several important differences. Perhaps the most important difference is that in Prock's study, the shared-governance model had been in place for only a short time—18 months—while in the other two studies, the shared-governance model had been in place for much longer—7 and 10 years, respectively.

In most of the studies testing the implementation of a professional practice model, the results were mixed. In a small study utilizing only two units, Ringer et al. (Appendix E, Selection 11) showed an increase in level of satisfaction with autonomy, a nonsignificant increase in level of satisfaction with professional status, and a decrease in satisfaction with interaction in one unit and an increase in the other. Overall, the IWS itself showed a nonsignificant increase in one unit and a significant increase in the other unit. In the two larger studies, Ingersoll et al. (Chapter 5, Selection 1) showed a small (but not statistically significant) increase in satisfaction in their experimental group, and in Minnick, Peschke-Winn, and Thomas's study of 23 different nursing units (Chapter 5, Selection 3), some showed change and some did not.

Interest in whether alternative management strategies affect level of nurse satisfaction is very high, although the way in which the alternative management approach is described varies so much that comparisons are sometimes difficult. Sometimes studies will conceptualize an organization as having a more participative management style. Drews and Fisher (1996) found an increase in level of satisfaction with a more participative management style. Other studies conceptualize the management structure as either centralized or decentralized (Wells 1990). In a survey of 37 New Jersey hospitals, Kovner et al. (1994) found a variety of programs, and all innovations were related to an increase in some aspect of satisfaction.

The studies by Minnick, Peschke-Winn, and Thomas and Ingersoll et al. (Chapter 5, Selections 3, 1) provide several insights into the problem of demonstrating changes in the level of satisfaction of the nursing staff. Ingersoll et al. have an interesting and insightful discussion about how difficult it is to demonstrate that change in an organizational setting affects satisfaction levels. One of the most valuable lessons from their research is that it is important to implement fully whatever model is being tested. Far too often, either a management intervention or a professional practice model is only partly implemented. This decreases the likelihood of being able to demonstrate change. As Ingersoll et al. point out, there are organizational costs to change, and these are sometimes viewed as too high. Minnick, Peschke-Winn, and Thomas reinforce this idea of organizational costs. One of the costs is the time and personnel necessary both to analyze evaluative data and then to implement changes. This is especially true in programs that involve frequent data collection, which is inherent in monitoring programs. The institution in which Minnick and her team are collecting data view the organizational cost as worthwhile.

In their view, the IWS is useful in determining the effect of several efforts at work redesign, especially in terms of three of the components: task requirements, professional status, and autonomy. Schultz (1993) also explicitly addressed the organizational cost when evaluating the effect of a clinical advancement system. (This study is also referenced in Appendix F, Selection 12.)

Changing organizations is a very slow process. Sometimes, the nature of the work that a nurse does may change, but the way in which the nurse is treated does not change. In that situation, the IWS—like any measure—will reflect the mixed responses of the nursing staff. The importance of patience is strongly demonstrated in the shared-governance studies: in those hospitals where shared governance has been in place long enough to affect the organizational climate, there is a statistically significant effect on level of satisfaction. It is critical to recognize the conflict between how time is viewed in an academic and research orientation and in a complex, hierarchical practice setting. It may often be that change is not documented because the research timeline is not sufficiently long to capture it (Kovner et al. 1994). Or it may be that the nurses are not being treated any differently within the context of the larger organization. The body of literature addressing the relationship between organizational climate and satisfaction is beginning to come to consensus on a few conclusions, including the notion that organizations can change, although slowly. In addition to this, the importance of all levels of the organization being involved is increasingly recognized. In the 1995 study by Mularz et al., there were 21 task groups formed throughout the hospital to obtain "maximal vertical and horizontal participation throughout the organization," even though only one unit was actually being modified. McQuaide (Chapter 5, Selection 5) observes that increased participation in decision making is not sufficient to reduce turnover without other structural changes within the organization. This is not a new observation: the "magnet hospital" project described the importance of creating a new climate or culture within the hospital (McClure et al. 1983), as did Alexander (1988). However, in the recent climate, the concept of empowerment (see Chapters 2 and 3) reinforces the importance of involving all levels of the organization.

All of the studies that use the IWS demonstrate the importance of considering both the practice interests of the field and the rules of research. The failure of some studies to demonstrate change may be due to problems in sample size or response rates. One rule of research that may be followed too closely, however, is the notion of statistically significant levels of change. All of the studies contained here and in the published literature use the traditional 5 percent level to demonstrate statistical significance. This level is certainly appropriate for many situations, but in cases of trying to show changes in a variable such as satisfaction, especially change in response to complex organizational influences, this may well be asking too much. A level of 10 percent may be far more reasonable and better fit the reality of doing research in organizations.

One of the contributions of research is clearly the development of measurement instruments that are useful, generally accepted by the profession, and also reliable and valid. The ability to include level of satisfaction in a monitoring system, for example, requires a highly applicable measurement instrument. Many of the studies that use the IWS have made interesting observations about the measurement tool itself. These will be addressed in the next section.

What Have We Learned about the Index of Work Satisfaction?

One of the clearest messages that emerges from the various studies noted in this book is that the IWS is used in many different types of organizational settings and in many different types of research and demonstration projects. The measurement tool itself obviously fills a need to have a measure of nurse satisfaction. Its inclusion in ongoing quality assurance programs and as a variable to be tracked in a monitoring system speaks both to the general acceptance of the IWS as a measure of nurse satisfaction and the usefulness of the data in a monitoring situation. Over the decade in which researchers and managers have used the IWS, many lessons have emerged. This section will focus on some of the lessons that are specifically related to the measurement tool itself. Appendix B contains the technical data to which this section refers.

Integrity of the IWS

Several investigators have analyzed the statistical properties of the IWS. This process is very helpful in attempting to ascertain the parameters of the measurement tool and in identifying some of the limitations. Even with a well-established measurement tool, it is important to continue this validation process.

One of the less common statistical analyses done is a factor analysis to verify the validity of the scale. As may be seen in Appendix B, all of the factor analyses done by various investigators are supportive of the scale structure, which certainly increases the confidence in using the scale in a variety of settings.

The most common analysis is that of assessing the reliability of the six components that make up the IWS. As may be seen in Table B.3 in

Appendix B, four separate studies performed an analysis of the reliability of each of the components, and a fifth presented an overall reliability estimate. Two of the studies performed multiple analyses, and Ingersoll et al. (Chapter 5, Selection 1) present results of four different administrations. All these studies used Cronbach's alpha to analyze the reliability of the scale. In general, these statistical values are quite supportive of the scale. The estimate of overall reliability ranges from .79 to .89, which is considered to be a very strong value.

It is also very useful to examine the estimates of reliability of each of the components separately. Across all these administrations, pay is the strongest component, with alpha values of .83 to .89. It should not be surprising that this is such a strong component, since, of all the components, pay is conceptually the easiest to define. Autonomy, organizational policies, interaction, and task requirements all have alpha values in the .7 range, which is also acceptable. Both autonomy and interaction have a similar pattern: the range of alphas is quite small, from .70 to .79 for autonomy and from .72 to .84 for interaction. Organizational policies demonstrates a little more variation, with alpha values from .65 to .74, and task requirements has still more variation, with values ranging from .64 to .78. The professional status component shows the most variation by far, with values ranging from .29 to .63. Coward et al. (1995) created a shortened version of the IWS by using both factor analytic techniques and reliability estimates. The shortened professional status component had an alpha of .55. Gillies, Franklin, and Child (1990) used a shortened version of the IWS, which included only five components, one of which was professional status. The overall Cronbach alpha of this shortened scale was .91. However Baggs and Ryan (1990) did not include the professional status component because the alpha was too low. This component exhibits too much variation: some possible explanations are given in Appendix B, especially in Section IV.

In addition to the statistical analysis of validity and reliability, investigators used a variety of other ways to address whether the IWS is a "good measure" of level of satisfaction. One of the best examples of this is Dunkin, Stratton, and Juhl (Appendix E, Selection 4) who had 3,514 respondents in six different states. They asked the respondents to rate their overall satisfaction with their job on a five-point response scale. The correlation with that one global item and the IWS value itself was greater than .80. Another example of this type of analysis is found in Rush's study (Appendix E, Selection 9). In her analysis, Rush pulled out the interaction scale value and compared it to another scale that measured nurse collegiality. She felt these two scales were measuring similar constructs.

Developing and validating measurement instruments is one of the most important functions of research. As more measures are developed for variables such as organizational climate, social support networks, and empowerment, the need for research into new measures of satisfaction will increase. For some of these measures, there is a conceptual overlap with satisfaction. This confusion is evident in some of the published literature, as some researchers use satisfaction measures to assess organizational characteristics (Stamps under review). The prominent trend in nursing research is to incorporate into the research the organization in which nurses are working. Although this is clearly needed, it is important to delineate concepts carefully, so that different—and specific—measures will also be developed. Use of multiple measures in one study is one way to assess the specificity. For example, Ingersoll (Chapter 5, Selection 1) used two measures of job satisfaction in their research. They used both the IWS and the Price-Mueller Job Satisfaction Scale, and found them to be moderately and significantly correlated. More research of this nature needs to be done in order to develop the strongest possible measure of satisfaction.

It is also important to differentiate between satisfaction and other constructs. For example, Martin et al. (Appendix E, Selection 2) used the IWS to measure satisfaction, along with Duxbury's Organizational Climate Questionnaire and a Professional Practice Climate Scale (Table 6.1). Their results indicated that the IWS measures a different construct than the other two scales. This is important, since there is a small but noticeable trend in the published literature to use the IWS as a measure of "organizational satisfaction," which is not really what the scale is designed to assess.

Use of the IWS is clearly appropriate in studies of satisfaction that are practice-based, especially those that wish to evaluate an organizational innovation or compare their results to others' results. However, there is a clear need for research to continue in order to develop other measures of satisfaction. If there is one trend that is obvious in both the published and the unpublished literature, it is that nurse satisfaction is an important variable to be able to assess.

Although most people use the IWS exactly as it has been structured, some investigators have modified it slightly. The most frequent sort of modification is to change some of the wording of items. Another common way to alter the scale is to give only the second part, either using the component weighting coefficients that were suggested in 1986 (as Martin et al. did) or simply not calculating the IWS. The use of just the second part of the scale is fairly common. Some investigators have modified this second part by removing one component. Joy and Malay (Appendix E, Selection 13) deleted the component measuring pay, since they felt it was not relevant to their study, as did Coward et al. (1995). Dunkin, Stratton, and Juhl (Appendix E, Selection 4) modified the response mode of the second part. They asked each respondent to indicate the level of importance of each item, and used that rating to create a sort of expectation that is somewhat different from the paired comparisons.

These modifications raise an important issue, which is the relative value of having comparable studies at the expense of having studies that are specifically meaningful to a particular setting. This issue has always been important, and it becomes even more relevant with the increasing use of the IWS in quality assurance programs. Also, as the IWS is used more frequently, the desire for comparable results increases. With the establishment of a national comparative database, as described in Chapter 4, the need for comparability will become more problematic.

Component Scale Values Versus the IWS

Use of the IWS produces several possible numerical values, which are all described in Appendix B. The values fall into two general categories. One category is separate values, which measure the level of satisfaction with each individual component. The second category is numbers that are summed, allowing satisfaction to be represented by one number. There are two types of summed values. One is the IWS, which is a numerical value weighted by expectations. The second is the total scale score, which may be either a total score or a mean score of the current level of satisfaction. Which numerical score is used depends partly on the use being made of the information, as described in Appendix C. However, an assumption has always been made that it is desirable to have one summary number to represent satisfaction. The use of this one number has also been supported by the statistical analysis, since the overall reliability estimates of the total scale have been consistently high (see Table B.3).

The development of the IWS has followed the common custom of attitude scales. The first step is to identify separate components or subscales, each of which is unidimensional, which is the purpose of factor analytic techniques. The second step is to sum the values of these component parts into one score, which represents satisfaction. This same procedure was followed in attempting to develop a scale to measure the level of satisfaction of physicians (Stamps and Cruz 1994; Stamps 1995). In the analysis of the first version of this physician satisfaction scale, it was observed that each of the components did seem to measure different and distinct facets, but when these separate components were summed together into one numerical estimate used to represent satisfaction, the value did not perform as expected. Some of the studies in this volume reinforce this observation for nurse satisfaction. For example, in creating her statistical model, Adams (Appendix E, Selection 5) discovered correlations lower than expected for the total score from the IWS. Because of this, she used the scores from each of the subscales in her path analysis. She noted that this sacrificed a broader picture of work satisfaction, but she felt that using the subscales individually helped to determine which aspects of satisfaction were connected to other variables.

Some of the other investigators also found using the individual components provided more sensitive information. In Mancini's study (Chapter 5, Selection 4), which showed that nurses working in a hospital with shared governance had higher levels of satisfaction than nurses working in a hospital without shared governance, the investigator especially noted the effect of satisfaction with organizational policies. Level of satisfaction was higher with this component, a finding that is especially important because this is always a low satisfier. Mancini found that the three components showing the highest level of change were organizational policies, task requirements, and autonomy. She argued that these were exactly the components that were most desirable to change. Another example of the helpfulness of examining the components specifically is found in the work by Burns Tuck (Appendix E, Selection 6). She discovered a complicated relationship between stress and level of satisfaction for nurse managers. One of the strongest findings was the positive relationship between satisfaction with task requirements and satisfaction with an immediate supervisor. Several other researchers have noted that, while changes in overall satisfaction are not noticeable, changes in separate components are (Kovner et al. 1994; Ringer et al. Appendix E, Selection 11; Hodovanic, Appendix F, Selection 14; Napiello, Appendix F, Selection 2; Hinshaw, Smeltzer, and Atwood 1987).

Increasingly, one of the most common uses of the IWS is to evaluate how much change in satisfaction can be noted after a management intervention. It makes sense that the more sensitive the measure, the more likely that a change can be documented. It also makes sense that each of the facets measured by the subscales might be affected differently. When the data from the IWS are to be used to chart change in response to organizational interventions, it is probably more useful to analyze each component separately. Developing profiles of each component and tracking the changes over time may provide a more sensitive measure of change.

A Final Thought

The IWS is used in both academic and practice-based research, and this book has demonstrated the range and diversity of the type of studies being conducted. The most rapid rate of increase in studies lies in what might be termed the management area, but as has been repeatedly demonstrated, this does not mean that the studies are not research-oriented. There is a dynamic and beneficial overlap of management and research-oriented studies.

Although the IWS is not a perfect measure, it is well accepted in the field, as demonstrated by its use in monitoring systems as well as in statistical models. There is work that remains to be done on the scale itself: the professional status component should be revisited, and there should be more work done on the relative merits of using the IWS as a summed, weighted summary number and using the six separate component scores.

It is a mistake to want all the studies on nurse satisfaction to demonstrate the same thing. In fact, when all the studies in this volume are put together, a more comprehensive picture emerges. The first factor that must be considered when attempting to explain different levels of satisfaction is analogous to an "input" variable: this is the characteristics of nurses themselves. These characteristics may be demographic in nature, including age, race, or marital status. They may relate to professional preparation, including educational level, specialty, or role in the hospital, or to psychological factors, including perception of stress, or personality hardiness, as McCrea (Appendix E, Selection 7) terms it. The psychological factors may relate to self-esteem, gender roles, or to attitudes about feminism as Koeckeritz (Appendix E, Selection 15) shows. The importance of these factors is often overlooked. They may predict satisfaction or, more likely, some of these factors may help to explain the response of nurses to specific organizational situations.

The most prevalent factors being considered today fall into the category of "process variables." These include all those factors that the organization attempts to modify. In this volume, there are examples of specific management interventions, including case management, other types of change in the professional practice model, and more generic forms of participative management, including shared governance. Nurse satisfaction is increasingly being viewed as a dependent variable or an outcome variable.

Viewing level of satisfaction as something that is at least partly under the control of the organization provides a rationalization for the many innovative efforts at job redesign that are occurring in the nursing field right now. This is clearly an advance over previous models that viewed nurse satisfaction as something that could not be modified. This also accepts the level of nurse satisfaction as an important variable that needs to be accounted for carefully. Inclusion of nurse satisfaction in monitoring systems supports the centrality of satisfaction and its relevance as an outcome variable.

However, this is an oversimplification of the real world. Both Koeckeritz (Appendix E, Selection 15) and Dunkin, Stratton, and Juhl (Appendix E, Selection 4) provide important reminders that satisfaction levels are affected by factors that are outside the organization's control. Koeckeritz concentrated on those factors that are primarily related to the home environment and arise from the sociocultural environment. Her findings with respect to how domestic responsibilities are handled is a reminder of how complex level of satisfaction is. In Dunkin, Stratton, and Juhl's statistical model, one of the prominent explanatory variables was happiness in the community, another factor outside the responsibility of the organization.

These two studies in particular remind us that the world is a complicated place. Yet the fact that level of satisfaction is not totally determined within the organization is no reason for abandoning the effort to make the organizations in which nurses work more satisfying and responsive to their needs. The most powerful evidence on the effect of various organizational arrangements on level of satisfaction of nurses can be found in Chapter 5 and Appendixes E and F. When taken all together, it is clear that nurse satisfaction, which is remarkably low, can be improved by some relatively simple solutions within organizations. These solutions, however simple, must be carried out in their entirety and must affect not only the nature of the nurses' job requirements, but also the way in which organization treats the nursing staff. The IWS has obviously been a helpful tool in assessing these effects, as well as in designing new interventions. It is very important to continue the research in this area, both to improve on this measure and to create other measures for some of the other important variables. By using the IWS, an organization can deal concretely with nurse satisfaction so that both individuals and organizations can function more productively and in a manner that enhances personal development.

References

Alexander, J. A. 1988. "The Effects of Patient Care Unit Organization on Nursing Turnover." *Health Care Management Review* 13 (2): 61–72.

Baggs, J. G., and S. A. Ryan. 1990. "ICU Nurse-Physician Collaboration & Nursing Satisfaction." *Nursing Economics* 8: 386–92.

Blenkarn, H., M. D'Amico, and E. Virtue. 1988. "Primary Nursing and Job Satisfaction." *Nursing Management* 19 (April): 41–42.

Bushy, A., and D. Banik. 1991. "Nurse Satisfaction with Work in Rural Hospitals." *Journal of Nursing Administration* 21: 35–38.

Coward, R. T., T. L. Hogan, R. P. Duncan, C. H. Horne, M. A. Hilker, and L. M. Felsen. 1995. "Job Satisfaction of Nurses Employed in Rural and Urban Long-Term Care Facilities." *Research in Nursing and Health* 18: 271–84.

Drews, T. T., and M. C. Fisher. 1996. "Job Satisfaction and Intent to Stay: RNs' Perceptions." *Nursing Management* 27: 58.

Gillies, D. A., M. Franklin, and D. A. Child. 1990. "Relationship Between Organizational Climate and Job Satisfaction of Nursing Personnel." *Nursing Administration Quarterly* 14: 15–22.

Hinshaw, A. S., C. H. Smeltzer, and J. R. Atwood. 1987. "Innovative Retention Strategies for Nursing Staff." *Journal of Nursing Administration* 17: 8–16.

Houston, R. 1990. "Twelve-Hour Shifts: Answer to Job Satisfaction." *Nursing Management* 21: 88F–88H.

Johnston, C. 1991. "Sources of Work Satisfaction/Dissatisfaction for Hospital Registered Nurses." *Western Journal of Nursing Research* 13: 503–13.

Joy, L., and M. Malay. 1992. "Evaluation Instruments to Measure Professional Nursing Practice." *Nursing Management* 23: 73–77.

Kovner, C. T., G. Hendrickson, J. Knickman, and S. A. Finkler. 1994. "Nursing Care Delivery Models and Nurse Satisfaction." *Nursing Administration Quarterly* 19: 74–85.

Lancero, A. W., and R. M. Gerber. 1995. "Comparing Work Satisfaction in Two Case Management Models." *Nursing Management* 26: 45–48.

Malik, D. M. 1991. "Career Ladders: Position Enrichment vis-a-vis Tenure." *Nursing Management* 22: 120A–120F.

McClure, M. L., M. A. Poulin, M. D. Sovie, and M. A. Wandelt. 1983. *Magnet Hospitals: Attraction and Retention of Professional Nurses.* Kansas City, MO: American Nurses Association.

Mularz, L. A., M. Maher, A. P. Johnson, B. Rolston-Blenman, and M. A. Anderson. 1995. "Theory M: A Restructuring Process." *Nursing Management* 26: 49–51.

Schultz, A. W. 1993. "Evluation of a Clinical Advancement System." *Journal of Nursing Administration* 23: 13–19.

Stamps, P. L. 1995. "Physicians and Organizations: An Uneasy Alliance or a Welcome Relief?" *Journal of Family Practice* 41: 72–78.

———. Under review. "Meta-Analysis of Measures Used in Satisfaction Research."

Stamps, P. L., and N. T. B. Cruz. 1994. *Issues in Physician Satisfaction: New Perspectives.* Chicago: Health Administration Press.

Thompson, C., S. A. Ryan, and J. Baggs. 1991. "Testing of a Computer-Based Decisions Support System in an Acute Care Hospital." In *Nursing Informatics '91*, Proceedings of the Fourth International Conference on Nursing Use of Computers and Information Science, Melbourne, Australia, April 1991.

Tumulty, G. 1992. "Head Nurse Role Redesign: Improving Satisfaction and Performance." *Journal of Nursing Administration* 22: 41–48.

Wells, G. T. 1990. "Influence of Organizational Structure on Nurse Manager Job Satisfaction." *Nursing Administration Quarterly* 14: 1–8.

Williams, C. 1990. "Job Satisfaction: Comparing CC and Med/Surg. Nurses." *Nursing Management* 21: 104A–104H.

THE INDEX OF WORK SATISFACTION
QUESTIONNAIRE, 1997 REVISION

The Index of Work Satisfaction (1997 Revision)

Part A (Paired Comparisons)

Listed and briefly defined on this sheet of paper are six terms or factors that are involved in how people feel about their work situation. Each factor has something to do with "work satisfaction." We are interested in determining which of these is most important to you in relation to the others.

Please carefully read the definitions for each factor as given below:

1. Pay—dollar renumeration and fringe benefits received for work done.
2. Autonomy—amount of job-related independence, initiative, and freedom, either permitted or required in daily work activities.
3. Task Requirements—tasks or activities that must be done as a regular part of the job.
4. Organizational Policies—management policies and procedures put forward by the hospital and nursing administration of this hospital.
5. Interaction—opportunities presented for both formal and informal social and professional contact during working hours.
6. Professional Status—overall importance or significance felt about your job, both in your view and in the view of others.

Scoring. These factors are presented in pairs on this questionnaire. Only 15 pairs are presented: this is every set of combinations. No pair is repeated or reversed.

For each pair of terms, decide which one is *more important* for your job satisfaction or morale. Please indicate your choice by a check on the line in front of it. For example, if you feel that Pay (as defined above) is more important than Autonomy (as defined above), check the line before Pay.

_____ Pay or _____ Autonomy

We realize it will be difficult to make choices in some cases. However, please do try to select the factor that is more important to you. Please make an effort to answer every item; do not go back to change any of your answers.

1. _____ Professional Status   or   _____ Organizational Policies
2. _____ Pay   or   _____ Task Requirements
3. _____ Organizational Policies   or   _____ Interaction
4. _____ Task Requirements   or   _____ Organizational Policies
5. _____ Professional Status   or   _____ Task Requirements
6. _____ Pay   or   _____ Autonomy
7. _____ Professional Status   or   _____ Interaction
8. _____ Professional Status   or   _____ Autonomy
9. _____ Interaction   or   _____ Task Requirements
10. _____ Interaction   or   _____ Pay
11. _____ Autonomy   or   _____ Task Requirements
12. _____ Organizational Policies   or   _____ Autonomy
13. _____ Pay   or   _____ Professional Status
14. _____ Interaction   or   _____ Autonomy
15. _____ Organizational Policies   or   _____ Pay

Part B (Attitude Questionnaire)

The following items represent statements about how satisfied you are with your current nursing job. Please respond to each item. It may be difficult to fit your responses into the seven categories; in that case, select the category that *comes closest* to your response to the statement. It is very important that you give your *honest* opinion. Please do not go back and change any of your answers.

Instructions for Scoring. Please circle the number that most closely indicates how you feel about each statement. The *left* set of numbers indicates degrees of *agreement*. If you strongly agree with the first statement, circle 1; if you agree with it, circle 2; if you mildly or somewhat agree, circle 3. The *right* set of numbers indicates degrees of *disagreement*. If you strongly disagree with the first statement, circle 7; if you disagree, circle 6; if you mildly or somewhat disagree, circle 5. The *center* number (4) means "undecided." Please use it as little as possible.

Remember: The more strongly you feel about the statement, the further from the center you should circle, with agreement to the left and disagreement to the right.

	Agree				Disagree	
1. My present salary is satisfactory.	1 2 3 4 5 6 7
2. Nursing is not widely recognized as being an important profession.	1 2 3 4 5 6 7
3. The nursing personnel on my service pitch in and help one another out when things get in a rush.	1 2 3 4 5 6 7
4. There is too much clerical and "paperwork" required of nursing personnel in this hospital.	1 2 3 4 5 6 7
5. The nursing staff has sufficient control over scheduling their own shifts in my hospital.	1 2 3 4 5 6 7
6. Physicians in general cooperate with nursing staff on my unit.	1 2 3 4 5 6 7
7. I feel that I am supervised more closely than is necessary.	1 2 3 4 5 6 7
8. It is my impression that a lot of nursing personnel at this hospital are dissatisfied with their pay.	1 2 3 4 5 6 7
9. Most people appreciate the importance of nursing care to hospital patients.	1 2 3 4 5 6 7
10. It is hard for new nurses to feel "at home" in my unit.	1 2 3 4 5 6 7
11. There is no doubt whatever in my mind that what I do on my job is really important.	1 2 3 4 5 6 7
12. There is a great gap between the administration of this hospital and the daily problems of the nursing service.	1 2 3 4 5 6 7
13. I feel I have sufficient input into the program of care for each of my patients.	1 2 3 4 5 6 7
14. Considering what is expected of nursing service personnel at this hospital, the pay we get is reasonable.	1 2 3 4 5 6 7
15. I think I could do a better job if I did not have so much to do all the time.	1 2 3 4 5 6 7
16. There is a good deal of teamwork and cooperation between various levels of nursing personnel on my service.	1 2 3 4 5 6 7

Continued

	Agree						Disagree
17. I have too much responsibility and not enough authority.	1	2	3	4	5	6	7
18. There are not enough opportunities for advancement of nursing personnel at this hospital.	1	2	3	4	5	6	7
19. There is a lot of teamwork between nurses and doctors on my own unit.	1	2	3	4	5	6	7
20. On my service, my supervisors make all the decisions. I have little direct control over my own work.	1	2	3	4	5	6	7
21. The present rate of increase in pay for nursing service personnel at this hospital is not satisfactory.	1	2	3	4	5	6	7
22. I am satisfied with the types of activities that I do on my job.	1	2	3	4	5	6	7
23. The nursing personnel on my service are not as friendly and outgoing as I would like.	1	2	3	4	5	6	7
24. I have plenty of time and opportunity to discuss patient care problems with other nursing service personnel.	1	2	3	4	5	6	7
25. There is ample opportunity for nursing staff to participate in the administrative decision-making process.	1	2	3	4	5	6	7
26. A great deal of independence is permitted, if not required, of me.	1	2	3	4	5	6	7
27. What I do on my job does not add up to anything really significant.	1	2	3	4	5	6	7
28. There is a lot of "rank consciousness" on my unit: nurses seldom mingle with those with less experience or different types of educational preparation.	1	2	3	4	5	6	7
29. I have sufficient time for direct patient care.	1	2	3	4	5	6	7
30. I am sometimes frustrated because all of my activities seem programmed for me.	1	2	3	4	5	6	7
31. I am sometimes required to do things on my job that are against my better professional nursing judgment.	1	2	3	4	5	6	7
32. From what I hear about nursing service personnel at other hospitals, we at this hospital are being fairly paid.	1	2	3	4	5	6	7
33. Administrative decisions at this hospital interfere too much with patient care.	1	2	3	4	5	6	7

Continued

	Agree	Disagree
34. It makes me proud to talk to other people about what I do on my job.	1 2 3 4 5 6 7	
35. I wish the physicians here would show more respect for the skill and knowledge of the nursing staff.	1 2 3 4 5 6 7	
36. I could deliver much better care if I had more time with each patient.	1 2 3 4 5 6 7	
37. Physicians at this hospital generally understand and appreciate what the nursing staff does.	1 2 3 4 5 6 7	
38. If I had the decision to make all over again, I would still go into nursing.	1 2 3 4 5 6 7	
39. The physicians at this hospital look down too much on the nursing staff.	1 2 3 4 5 6 7	
40. I have all the voice in planning policies and procedures for this hospital and my unit that I want.	1 2 3 4 5 6 7	
41. My particular job really doesn't require much skill or "know-how."	1 2 3 4 5 6 7	
42. The nursing administrators generally consult with the staff on daily problems and procedures.	1 2 3 4 5 6 7	
43. I have the freedom in my work to make important decisions as I see fit, and can count on my supervisors to back me up.	1 2 3 4 5 6 7	
44. An upgrading of pay schedules for nursing personnel is needed at this hospital.	1 2 3 4 5 6 7	

DEVELOPMENT AND VALIDATION OF
THE INDEX OF WORK SATISFACTION

T his appendix is intended for those who may not be familiar with the development of the Index of Work Satisfaction and for readers who are interested in the more technical aspects of attitude scale construction. There are five sections in this Appendix:

I. History and Development of Validation Model

From the early development of the IWS in 1972 until the first publications in 1978 and 1979 (Stamps 1978; Stamps et al. 1978; Slavitt et al. 1978; Slavitt et al. 1979), serendipity dictated much of the work. Most of the scale's administrations were in hospitals that had requested assistance in dealing with what was usually termed a nursing "problem." No systematic revisions were made, but several times the items were altered to be more appropriate to the specific situation at hand.

During this early stage, all of the administrations of the measurement tool had dual purposes. The first was to collect data to measure work satisfaction in a specific setting, with the corollary managerial purpose of improving communication within the organization. The second was to revise and eventually to validate the scale using statistical analyses of the results. Most of the administrations were conducted by a University of Massachusetts (UMASS) research team which included, at that time, Professors Eugene B. Piedmonte and Ann Marie Haase, as well as many graduate students with training in nursing, public health, sociology, biostatistics, and epidemiology. The scale's initial 60 items were first increased to 72 and later reduced to 48. The 48-item scale is the one that was published in 1978 and is the version that was given to other investigators for use in their own settings.

Many positive responses and numerous inquiries followed the 1978 and 1979 publications, as well as increased requests for assistance in using the scale. It quickly became clear that both nurses and administrators were eager to have a practical tool that provided an accurate measure of occupational satisfaction of nurses. This positive feedback encouraged the continued research in the area.

From 1978 to 1986, the scale-development process involved other researchers. The UMASS team became the center of a network, receiving inquiries and specific technical questions as well as respondents' results. We also began receiving communications from other investigators who wanted comparative results, as well as expected norms. By this time, the potential for utilization in the field became obvious, as more and more researchers were willing to use what was actually a still-unvalidated research tool. We were reassured many times that, based on a review of the literature, ours was the "best available." Our research had indeed begun to direct the literature; there were many quotations not only of our technical work, but also of the conceptual thought underlying it.

Developing an attitude scale is both tedious and time-consuming. Besides that, it is not especially rewarded. This type of basic social sciences research was much more common in the 1920s, 1930s, and 1940s. The decision to attempt to validate this scale grew from the conviction that if the scale were to be used widely—as it seemed to be already— it would be important to have as valid a measurement instrument as possible. As with much social research, however, we were well into our investigation. It was neither possible nor practical to start anew, rejecting seven years of research and practical experience, both our own and others'.

So in 1978 we began a more deliberate process of validation, guided by the previous six years' experience. First, we reviewed the classical literature in attitude scale development, dating from 1929 to 1940. This search reassured us that the technical aspects of scale construction we had already completed were appropriate. We adopted a model of scale development that incorporated our previous research efforts and provided guidance for the next eight years of attempting to validate the IWS. This included five steps:

1. initial scale design, 1972
2. early revision process, 1972–80
3. statistical analysis, 1975–81
4. comparative analysis via a survey of users, 1983
5. a final validation study and revision of the IWS, 1985

II. Scale-Validation Process, 1972–86

This section describes the five stages of the Scale-Validation Process and gives the results for each stage. This will provide enough information for those interested in the technical aspects of scale design to replicate or process, if desired. As noted before, even though the initial design phase was formally begun after the publication of the 1978 and 1979 articles, it incorporated the earlier work.

Initial Scale Design, 1972

The first step in constructing an attitude scale is in many ways the most critical one. The classical literature reveals several possible ways of measuring attitudes, each of which relies on a particular theoretical framework. It is important to select one such framework for measuring attitudes and then to follow the specific design criteria for it. Otherwise it is not possible to proceed with statistical validation. Since a scale is quite different from a questionnaire, the issues of reliability and validity are important.

The design chosen in 1972 was the classic Likert scale. After an extensive review of the literature and many conversations with nurses, colleagues, and both nursing and hospital administrators, six important components of work were identified and defined: pay, autonomy, task requirements, organizational requirements, interaction, and job prestige. Attitude items relating to each component were designed and submitted to a panel of nursing judges who estimated whether the items were related in content to the particular component. The judges evaluated 250 such statements. This procedure resulted in the acceptance of 10 items per work component, and thus the original scale of 60 items.

Three important design decisions were made, all consistent with the Likert approach to attitude scales. The first was to arrange statements randomly by content area throughout the scale, so that respondents would not be aware of the component being tested. The second was to phrase half of the statements positively and half negatively, and to reverse the scores in such a way that a higher summed score represented a higher level of satisfaction. The responses of persons highly satisfied with their job situation should be evenly divided between "strongly agree" to positive statements and "strongly disagree" to negative statements. This accomplished the objective of being able to create one single summed score. The positively and negatively worded items were also distributed randomly throughout the questionnaire. The third design decision related to the response mode. We chose a seven-point response scale with a neutral midpoint, which allowed the respondent to make fine distinctions, but also enabled the investigator to collapse the data for presentation if appropriate.

At this point we made an important addition to the Likert method of attitude measurement. Many investigators had noted the importance of analyzing the effect of expectations on people's perceptions of their current level of satisfaction. Therefore, we created an additional aspect to the scale by measuring the relative importance of the six work components to the respondent. We did this by using the paired-comparisons technique developed by Edwards (1957), whereby respondents were asked to choose which of each of 15 pairs (e.g., autonomy or pay, task requirements or autonomy) seemed more important to their own level of work satisfaction.

From the beginning, then, the measurement instrument had two parts. Part A consists of the 15 sets of paired comparisons of the six work components; this measures the relative importance of each of the six components to the respondent, and describes the respondent's expectations. Part B is the Likert scale that measures the current level of satisfaction for each of the six components.

This two-part design allows flexibility in analysis and is one of the reasons that the scale is particularly useful. Since each of the six components is a conceptually separate dimension of satisfaction, each component yields a separate score. Thus, the rankings of level of current satisfaction (based on Part B, the Likert scale) may be compared with the rankings of relative importance (derived from Part A). This comparison helps in identifying the areas in greatest need of organizational or structural change.

One additional design step was then taken. A total weighted score—called the Index of Work Satisfaction—was calculated from Parts A and B. This score reflects both level of importance *and* actual current satisfaction. In order to do this, the average component score from Part B is multiplied by its appropriate weighting coefficient from Part A, thereby producing weighted component scores. These six weighted scores are then summed to produce one single number, the IWS, a total index that represents both the relative importance of the components and the current level of satisfaction. This creates a two-part measurement instrument that combines the strength of a classic way to measure attitudes (Likert) with a way to include expectations.

Early Revision Process, 1972–80

The original 60-item scale and the paired comparisons were first administered in 1972 to 246 nurses in a community hospital. Between 1972 and 1980, we also administered the scale in seven other settings, with each administration contributing to a revision of the original scale.

The revision process was really an effort to assess face validity and reliability. This involved repeated revisions, based on the results from each use and comments from respondents. These "eyeball tests" provide a good general estimate of the value of a scale, but they do not substitute for more deliberate statistical analysis, especially in terms of assessing validity.

The complete results of these seven administrations are available in detail elsewhere (Stamps 1978; Slavitt et al. 1979; Stamps and Shopnick 1981; Stamps 1981). In general, the rankings in Part A (the paired comparisons) remained similar for all seven studies. Autonomy and job status tended to be ranked as most important, while organizational requirements was almost always ranked as least important. As might be expected, there was much less consistency for the results in Part B (the Likert scale). This part of the scale is clearly more closely related to changes in the actual work situation. Among those hospital nurses included in these seven studies, the level of work satisfaction was higher for components central to their job (i.e., job prestige, autonomy, and task requirements) than for organizational or administrative aspects, including pay. The exception to this was a nursing staff in an ambulatory care setting: their extreme level of dissatisfaction with task requirements resulted in a rearrangement of their roles (Stamps et al. 1978).

Several revisions of Part B were made during these seven administrations. A few items were reworded or dropped, depending on the analysis of the frequency distribution of responses and the total number of items was increased to 72. The designation of two of the components changed somewhat: job prestige was renamed professional status, and interaction underwent several changes. The format for Part A remained unchanged.

It is common to make revisions of a scale based only on analysis of repeated administrations, and this is often the only step that investigators take. However, as we were making these revisions, other investigators also started using the IWS. Additionally, some of the organizational settings started to use the results to make policy and work-related changes. These applications seemed to us to exceed the power of informal revisions. Consequently we began to consider more rigorous quantitative methods of analysis.

Statistical Analysis, 1975–81

The most common statistical analyses that are performed in scale-development efforts pertain to reliability. These are clearly useful, but limited, especially if the scale in question shows some promise of applicability. In that case, it is also in everybody's best interest to analyze the validity, since this is a more stringent and necessary test of an attitude scale, especially for a scale that seems to have far-ranging applicability (Stamps and Finkelstein 1981). We used two analytic procedures to evaluate reliability and one to evaluate the validity of the scale.

Reliability

The first reliability measure is Cronbach's alpha coefficient, a very commonly used split-half reliability test that assesses internal reliability. This gives an estimate of the integrity of the six components themselves. A higher score indicates a closer association among those items that measure one component. Over seven administrations, Cronbach's alpha coefficient for each of the components ranged from .696 to .900, with an overall coefficient of 0.85. These values are all very acceptable and demonstrate a statistically strong scale.

The second measure of reliability is Kendall's tau. This was used to determine whether there were any significant differences between the use of the total weighted score (the IWS) and an unweighted score that used only the summed results of Part B. This issue came up primarily because of the two-part design of the scale, in which results from Part A are used to modify or weight the results from Part B. Such a two-part scale is conceptually sound, from both methodological and substantive perspectives. Its use is also supported both by Herzberg's and Maslow's theories, which suggest that different components of work satisfaction produce different amounts of satisfaction; they further suggest that linking incentives to more important and less satisfied needs leads to greater motivation and higher productivity. However, administration of both parts posed a practical problem because the scoring procedure is tedious. Kendall's tau was included as part of our analytic model to help assess the value of the weighted score approach. In the seven studies, this correlation was quite high—between 0.8 and 0.9—reinforcing the similarity of the two scoring approaches and also giving a strong indication that the items were accurately measuring the six components.

Validity

There are several methods for assessing the validity of the scale items, as well as their proper identification with one of the six components. We wanted to use the most understandable of the highly sophisticated statistical techniques, while also retaining a high degree of analytical power. We chose factor analytic methods, specifically using principal component analysis with a varimax rotation. This technique is widely available through packaged statistical analyses and is more easily understood than most of the other techniques.

The first factor analysis produced seven factors that accounted for 59 percent of the variance among the 72 items in this version of Part B. This factor analysis was then used to select the strongest 48 items, all of which were used in the subsequent analyses. The next analysis on a later study produced 13 factors that accounted for 70 percent of the variance. These two analyses were really quite similar, even though more factors were produced on the second. The extra factors were very similar subjectively to the original factor structure. Two more factor analyses were done, and these did show some differences, although not marked. One of these studies was on a non-nursing group, emergency medical technicians. This study produced 16 factors that accounted for 80 percent of the variance (Stamps and Shopnick 1981). Finally, our last study produced 15 factors that accounted for 82 percent of the variance. The results of these four factor analytic studies produced some items with lower factor loadings but also demonstrated a big group of items with higher factor loadings. Although the number of factors identified varied, careful analysis revealed many overlapping and similar factors.

An additional confirmation of the overall integrity of the scale was the Cronbach's alpha. The total alpha for the scale remained high, even after the reduction from 72 to 48 items. The total scale reliability declined very little, from .929 to .912. This is important, since it allows for the use of a shorter scale with no substantial loss of reliability.

At the conclusion of this third phase of the scale-development process, we had what we affectionately referred to as a "revised scale." It was this scale that we made widely available on request. In the context of many discussions with these "users" of the scale, it became obvious that they were still looking for more widespread application than we were comfortable with. In our minds, this was still a research tool, with some unacceptable factor loadings and some imbalances within the scale itself. It was this interaction with the users that led us to the decision to pursue the scale-development process yet another step, so that we could refine both the reliability and the validity estimates. This required a data collection effort solely for the purpose of evaluating the statistical integrity of the scale. Additionally, at the end of our previous administrations, we had no quantitative data for comparative purposes, since both the questionnaire and the scoring procedures had experienced several revisions. The rankings were comparable, but not the numbers. This was a serious drawback to developing any normative data. Therefore, we decided to make one last significant revision of the scale, based on information obtained from those who had used this revised scale.

Comparative Analysis: A Survey of Users, 1983

We had several objectives in mind for this phase of scale validation in addition to revising the scale, including comparing results with the hopes of developing some type of expected norms for level of satisfaction. We were also hoping to resolve the question of the necessity of giving the paired-comparisons part of the Index at every administration.

Surveys were sent out to 132 people who had requested information from us between 1978 (the year of the first publication of this scale) and 1983. The majority of requests (69) had come from graduate students, in either doctoral or master's programs, and 10 had come from people holding academic appointments in schools of nursing. The rest of the people who had written us were involved in nursing administration.

The survey questionnaire itself contained three categories of information. The first requested detailed information on the respondent's particular study or project, including setting, type of health professional studied, sample size, response rate, and methodology. Additionally, we asked exactly what parts of the IWS scale had been used. The second category requested comments on the scale itself, including the scoring procedure. The third category requested data from the respondent's study that might be compared with our results, as well as statistical analyses the respondent had performed. Finally, other open-ended comments were solicited. This section will summarize the findings from this first survey of users that were most relevant to the subsequent revision of the IWS scale.

Given the methodology of mailed surveys, coupled with a mobile target group of largely graduate students, we were satisfied with the 39 percent return rate. Of far greater concern was the extreme variability among the 51 studies that were returned to us. This variability affected completeness as well as accuracy. Most of the studies returned did not do any statistical analysis, tending to rely instead on our statistical evaluation of the scale.

An additional problem concerned the modification of the scale itself. A few respondents used only portions of the questionnaire, usually embedding one of our work components into a scale of their own design. Many studies used only an agree/disagree response mode, rather than the seven-point response mode we suggested. Ten of the 51 respondents sent us only rankings of the six components and rankings of current level of satisfaction rather than actual numerical calculations. Of those who did send the numerical calculations, many made scoring errors that we discovered when we recalculated their data. Very few respondents sent us frequency distributions of responses to the entire questionnaire, an aspect of the analysis on which we depended very heavily. Needless to say, this variability frustrated the objectives of comparing results and developing normative data. The situation underscored the need for more standardization to enhance the possibility of comparative research.

In order to make the best use of the 51 respondents' information, we set up criteria for including all or part of a particular study. Those studies most like our own in methodology became the "core studies." These 16 studies used all or most of the questionnaire, used the same seven-point response mode, and had primarily nurse respondents within the sample. Even using these minimal criteria, there was considerable variation. For example, only six of the core studies included the paired-comparisons section of the questionnaire; only four of these calculated the Index of Work Satisfaction. None compared the weighted versus unweighted scores. Only three studies calculated Cronbach's alpha, while four studies included a factor analysis. All others cited our statistical work within their study.

Added to these 16 studies were 5 studies conducted by the UMASS research team. These 21 studies were carefully analyzed, with the goal of determining what revisions needed to be made on the measurement tool. Only the results that most affected scale design will be summarized here. For ease of discussion, these results will be presented in several topics.

Part A (Paired Comparisons)

A total of 12 core studies, 5 of them done under our supervision, used the paired comparisons. The results of the ranking of level of importance were fairly consistent. The three components that were ranked as most important were autonomy, pay, and professional status. Interaction and task requirements were next, and organizational requirements was always ranked as least important.

Four studies involved other settings and other health professionals and had less consistent results, although autonomy was ranked no lower than third in importance and organizational requirements was consistently ranked sixth or fifth. Other than these two anchors, other rankings probably reflected conflicts specific to a given occupational group. For example, among emergency medical technicians, professional status and interaction, especially with physicians, were of primary importance.

Part B (Likert Scale)

All of the core studies used the Likert scale part of the questionnaire, but three modified this part of the analysis so much that their results were not comparable. Additionally, several of the studies computed scores for various subgroups, based on a variety of demographic factors. When these subgroups were analyzed, 35 different rankings were available for analyzing level of satisfaction. Taking all the studies together, nurses seemed most satisfied with autonomy, professional status, and task requirements. Interaction and organizational requirements were next, and pay was consistently noted as least satisfying.

In some cases, the variation in expressed level of work satisfaction could be explained by the setting. For example, in a teaching hospital, the highest level of satisfaction was found in interaction. However, in a more specialized setting (such as Shriner's hospitals), interaction did not seem as satisfying. It appeared from these data that the more technically trained nurses were least satisfied with interaction and most satisfied with autonomy and professional status. It was also interesting that the non-nurse professionals seemed to display a greater variation in their rankings of current level of satisfaction. This suggested some hesitation in generalizing use of this scale into other health professions before more standardized norms had been developed in nursing populations. Also, we were unable to suggest anything like expected norms, given the variability inherent in the studies producing these rankings.

Reliability Analysis

Very few studies completed any statistical analysis; most simply quoted ours. Also, none of the studies calculated Kendall's tau. This was expected, since few of the studies calculated the paired comparisons or the IWS. All the studies noted our previous high values (.86) as a justification for not using the paired comparisons part of the questionnaire. Three studies calculated Cronbach's alpha. One of those reported only the range of values (from .646 to .842), one reported an overall value of .91, and a third recombined items based on a factor analysis and thus produced alpha statistics on dissimilar subscales.

Validity Analysis

All of this reinforces the fact that the developers of any scale must take the time to conduct its statistical evaluation. What most people want is a scale that is ready to be applied in their setting. It is always very difficult to compare studies that use factor analytic techniques, since much of the final result is based on the investigator's interpretation of the appropriateness of any particular item on a component, and some variation occurs from the technique itself. A total of six data sets were analyzed, three of which were ours. The strongest and most consistent factor across all studies seemed to be pay, although the other components also demonstrated high levels of consistency. All of the factor loadings reported in the six studies were acceptable, and many were very high. The three strongest factors seemed to be pay, interaction, and task requirements. Two components that appeared to need revising included organizational requirements and autonomy.

Other Responses

Respondents to the survey made a wealth of comments on the questionnaire, both about uses of the scale and about possible revisions. Their general impression was quite favorable, although there were several negative comments about the scoring procedure and calculation of the IWS. Most found the scoring too difficult; many therefore elected to use only Part B, the Likert scale. Even so, our check of the data returned to us revealed that very few actually calculated Part B correctly. As might be expected, the most common modification suggested was to simplify the scoring procedures.

At this stage of the research, we were left with the feeling from our respondents that our scale was the "best available." However, it was not the best possible, as the factor analyses showed. Many respondents indicated the need for help in applying the scale, either in scoring it or in moving to the next stage of analysis and interpretation. Based on the results of this survey, we felt a minor revision of the scale was necessary, as was a final administration, one given in a community hospital setting, since the most consistent results had been obtained in community hospitals.

At this point, we realized that we could not meet the original objectives we had set for this phase of the scale development. Because of the diversity of responses to our survey, we could not make any comparisons, nor could we suggest any normative data. We also could not make any clear suggestions about the issue of using the paired comparisons, as so few people had actually used them. We decided to concentrate on a final validation of the scale, with an emphasis on presenting standardized scoring directions so that there would at least be comparability in scoring.

A Final Validation Study and Revision of the IWS, 1985

Based on these extensive analyses of both our own and other administrations, we revised the scale in preparation for the final validation administration. These revisions fell into two categories: (1) the mechanics of the scale, including scoring procedure, overall factor structure, and the issue of weighted versus unweighted score; and (2) changes in specific items on the scale. Because of their importance to the scale design, these will be described in some detail here.

Modifications in Scale Mechanics

Interaction Component   The interaction component has gone through several modifications. Its original designation was probably too broad, since it included both nurse-nurse and nurse-physician interaction. As a practical matter, however, we were reluctant to divide this into two separate components because that would lengthen the paired-comparisons part of the questionnaire. Of the 16 non-UMASS core studies used for data comparison, 11 used six components, in keeping with our original design. Six of the studies used six components for Part A and seven components for Part B, deriving the seventh component by scoring separately the three items that measured the specific interaction between physicians and nurses as suggested by our first factor analysis. Subdivision of interaction did provide a needed breakdown of this complicated and broad component. Factor analysis supported the subdivision, and most respondents noted the intuitive importance of these two separate areas of professional interaction. We decided to maintain six work components, but we created two subcomponents for interaction by increasing the number of items within this component. In this way six overall components are maintained, but nurse-nurse and nurse-physician interaction can be analyzed separately. When there is a big difference between the mean scores of the overall interaction component and the nurse-physician subcomponent, it suggests that substantial dissatisfaction with interaction is accounted for by the specific relationship between physicians and nurses.

Weighted Versus Unweighted Scoring Procedures   From the beginning of this research, an important distinguishing factor has been the ability of the IWS to weight current satisfaction with expectations or ideals. It is largely this feature that allows for differentiation between components of dissatisfaction for managerial use. Unfortunately, though, the scoring procedures for computing these weighted values are tedious. In addition, the comparison of weighted and unweighted scores consistently produced a Kendall's tau of .86 or .87, indicating no theoretical difference between weighted and unweighted scores.

For the validation study, the paired-comparison calculations were maintained.

Scoring Procedure Modifications The most important change in scoring procedure was the elimination of zero as a possible value for a component weighting coefficient (calculated from Part A). Originally, the lowest ranked component was assigned an automatic weight of zero. Although this clearly demarcated the lowest coefficient, it also complicated further scoring, since the computation of the IWS relies upon multiplication. Eliminating zero as a weight is accomplished by adding a constant.

Changes in Specific Items

As a result of the factor analysis and reinforcing comments from the survey, we made several changes in the wording of specific items on the attitude scale, reassigned some items to specific components, and reduced the overall number of items. This restructuring of the Likert scale part of the questionnaire used as a base the strongest parts of the previous questionnaire and was guided by the statistical analysis noted previously.

Final scale revision began by breaking the scale into its six work components and evaluating every item within each component. Four criteria were used. The first two relied on estimates of face validity and evaluation of the range of responses. We examined each item to see if it "seemed to fit" into the definition of the particular work component of which it was a part. Next we looked at the range of responses to each item. If the responses were all "agree" or all "disagree," the item was dropped, because it lacked the ability to differentiate adequately between positions. Then we reviewed the results of the factor analyses. Any item whose highest factor loading was .4 was dropped. We also examined the factor designation for each analytic technique. If the item identification switched from one work component to another, the item was dropped.

In constructing the revised scale, new items were created only when necessary. We tried to balance the number of items per component and also the positive and negative items per component. Various "ad hoc" revisions had created some imbalance in the scale on both of these criteria. Some new items were created in response to comments from our survey respondents. All these efforts tried to address apparent shortcomings in earlier versions of the scale. These changes are presented for each component.

Autonomy Although this component was usually rated as most important to the respondents, it has also had one of the weakest values of Kendall's tau (an average of .68, with a range of .54 to .80) and the weakest factor loadings on the individual items (with ranges around .3). Additionally, it had only five items. There also seemed to be some overlap with the organizational requirements component. To differentiate autonomy from organizational requirements, we dropped one item and added three new ones.

Organizational Requirements   This component formerly had ten items, most of which had relatively high factor loadings, an average Kendall's tau correlation of .78, and very little variation. We dropped the four weakest items, and added one new item to address an area not previously included: determination of work shifts. We changed the name of the component to organizational policies, and altered its description accordingly.

Pay   This has been a strong component in terms of both Kendall's tau (average of .80) and individual factor loadings. This may be because the concept of pay is relatively straightforward and easy to measure. We deleted one item.

Task Requirements   This component had moderately good Kendall's tau values (an average of .70) and moderately good factor loadings on the individual items. We dropped the lowest item, changed one from the professional status component to task requirements, and added one new item.

Job Status   This component had showed strong statistical analyses with high individual factor loadings and an average Kendall's tau of .77. We dropped two of the lowest items and switched one to task requirements. We also added two new items.

Interaction   Although this component had been the most troublesome conceptually, it had performed well statistically. As noted previously, we experimented with dividing this component into communication between nurses and between nurses and physicians. Although the nurse-physician subcomponent was well received and performed well statistically, we felt that increasing the number of components from six to seven would impede the practical use of the scale. Thus, this component was revised to include a total of ten items, half measuring nurse-nurse interaction and half measuring nurse-physician interaction. To do this, we dropped two items and added two new ones. Although interaction continues to be one single component, we suggested that the analysis separate the two subcomponents in addition to evaluating the total overall component.

These changes produced a 44-item scale, which was then administered for a final validation study in a 262-bed acute care community hospital. A total of 463 questionnaires were distributed with paychecks. Completed questionnaires were mailed back to us, and we used postcards to follow up nonrespondents. We received 246 completed questionnaires for a response rate of 53 percent (Kit 1985).

Results of 1985 Final Validation Study

Table B.1 shows the component weighting coefficients calculated from Part A. The rankings from this first part of the measurement instrument were very similar to those of earlier administrations. Component scores, mean scores, adjusted scores, and the IWS are also shown on this table, as are the ranges for each of these scores and the quartiles for each range. The total scale score for this sample was 173, the total scale mean was 3.93, and the IWS was 12.0. The overall satisfaction rate was only 56 percent of the total possible for this respondent group.

Table B.2 shows the frequency distribution analysis of the responses to the items on this 44-item scale.

In this final validation study, we performed the same statistical tests that we had throughout the scale-development process. Two of these statistics—Kendall's tau and Cronbach's alpha—are a measure of internal reliability, while the third—factor analysis—is a measure of validity.

Kendall's Tau

This statistic measures the strength of correlation between the weighted score (that is, the IWS) and the unweighted summed score of the attitude part of the questionnaire. This statistic had been consistently high in previous studies (.86 or .87). On this final study, it reached .92. This indicated that the correlation on the revised questionnaire was higher and the components even better defined than earlier versions.

Cronbach's Alpha

In previous studies, values for this split-half reliability technique ranged from acceptable to very high. In this latest version of the scale, the values were slightly lower on most of the components, but still well within the acceptable range (from .52 to .81), with the exception of the subcomponent of nurse-physician interaction. The total alpha was .82, which was slightly lower than the previous results but still very good.

Factor Analysis

A varimax rotation produced 12 factors that accounted for 62 percent of the variance. This factor analysis was supportive of the revisions made to the questionnaire. The lowest factor loading was on question 9 of the professional status component ("Nursing is a long way from being recognized as a profession"). All of the other loadings were above

Table B.1   Numerical Values for the Scale, Ranges, and Quartiles for Each Range

Component	Component Weighting Coefficient (Part A)	Component Scale Score (Part B), Range and Quartiles	Component Mean Score (Part B)	Adjusted Scores
Autonomy	3.61	35.2 Range: 8–56 20-32-44-56	4.4	15.8
Pay	3.5	16.2 Range: 6–42 15-24-33-42	2.7	9.4
Professional Status	3.3	37.8 Range: 7–49 17-28-38-49	5.4	17.8
Interaction	3.0	46.0 Range: 10–70 25-40-55-70	4.6	13.8
Nurse-Nurse	3.4	26.5 Range: 5–35 13-20-27-35	5.3	18.0
Nurse-Physician	2.8	19.8 Range: 5–35 13-20-27-35	3.9	10.9
Task Requirements	2.8	16.8 Range: 6–42 15-24-33-42	2.8	7.8
Organizational Policies	2.4	19.6 Range: 7–49 17-28-38-49	2.8	6.7
	IWS: 12			
Range: 0.9–5.3 Quartiles: 2.0-3.1-4.2-5.3	Range: 0.5–39.7 Quartiles: 10.3-20.0-29.7-39.7	Range: 1–7 Quartiles: 2.5-4.0-5.5-7.0	Range: 0.9–37.1 Quartiles: 9.9-19.0-28.1-37.1	

the .4 level with the exception of item 33 in the organizational policies component.

Based on these statistical analyses of the final administration, we made only a few revisions to the questionnaire. We changed the wording on the two items that had low factor loadings and we slightly changed the wording on a few other items to make them clearer. We also renamed some of the components and defined them more clearly. (For example, organizational requirements became organizational policies.)

This final validation phase produced the 44-item questionnaire that was included in *Nurses and Work Satisfaction: An Index for Measurement*

Table B.2 Frequency Distribution of Responses by Component, 1985 ($N = 315$)

	Strongly Disagree (%)	Disagree (%)	Moderately Disagree (%)	Undecided (%)	Moderately Agree (%)	Agree (%)	Strongly Agree (%)
Pay							
1.* My present salary is satisfactory.	28.7	22.5	9.0	1.2	10.7	25.4	2.5
8. Excluding myself, it is my impression that a lot of nursing service personnel at this hospital are dissatisfied with their pay.	2.1	7.0	5.0	4.5	12.8	27.7	40.9
14. Considering what is expected of nursing service personnel at this hospital, the pay we get is reasonable.	42.8	20.6	14.0	2.9	7.0	11.5	1.2
21. The present rate of increase in pay for nursing service personnel at this hospital is not satisfactory.	2.1	7.4	7.0	3.7	14.0	19.8	46.0
32. From what I hear from and about nursing service personnel at other hospitals, we at this hospital are being fairly paid.	12.4	16.2	13.7	9.5	23.7	19.5	5.0
44. An upgrading of pay schedules for nursing personnel is needed at this hospital.	0.8	2.9	2.4	4.5	14.7	24.9	49.8
Autonomy							
7. I feel that I am supervised more closely than I need to be, and more closely than I want to be.	35.7	23.8	14.3	7.0	7.0	6.6	5.6
13. I feel I have sufficient input into the program of care for each of my patients.	4.2	8.4	8.8	6.7	19.7	36.4	15.8
17. I have too much responsibility and not enough authority.	12.7	15.6	15.6	9.8	17.2	13.6	13.5
20. On my service, my supervisors make all the decisions. I have little direct control over my own work.	25.8	29.9	13.9	3.7	11.1	7.8	7.8
26. A great deal of independence is permitted if not required of me.	9.8	13.5	13.1	6.9	19.2	25.7	11.8
30. I am sometimes frustrated because of all my activities seem programmed for me.	8.2	19.6	10.6	9.4	20.3	18.4	13.5

Continued

Table B.2 Continued

	Strongly Disagree (%)	Disagree (%)	Moderately Disagree (%)	Undecided (%)	Moderately Agree (%)	Agree (%)	Strongly Agree (%)
31. I am sometimes required to do things on my job that are against my better professional nursing judgment.	19.6	15.8	12.5	5.0	23.3	13.7	10.1
43. I have the freedom in my work to make important decisions as I see fit, and can count on my supervisors to back me up.	21.9	21.5	11.6	6.2	17.4	14.8	6.6
Task Requirements							
4. There is too much clerical and "paperwork" required of nursing personnel in this hospital.	1.2	3.3	4.9	2.9	9.9	22.9	55.0
11. I feel I could do a better job if I didn't have so much to do all the time.	4.1	7.4	9.9	6.2	13.6	24.4	34.4
22. I am satisfied with the types of activities that I do on my job.	3.7	16.5	5.8	2.9	17.7	37.9	15.5
24. I have plenty of time and opportunity to discuss patient care problems with other nursing service personnel.	20.8	25.3	15.8	3.7	12.0	16.6	5.8
29. I would like to spend more time in direct patient care.	3.3	3.7	7.9	8.3	15.9	19.2	41.7
36. I could deliver much better care if I had more time with each patient.	2.1	2.1	1.7	5.0	12.9	26.6	49.6
Organizational Policies							
5. The nursing staff should be allowed to have more control over scheduling their own work shifts.	3.3	5.3	7.3	4.1	13.9	25.7	40.4
12. There is a great gap between the administration of this hospital and the daily problems of nursing service.	2.0	3.3	2.0	0.8	2.0	13.5	76.4
18. There are not enough opportunities for advancement of nursing personnel at this hospital.	2.5	7.8	7.0	7.4	15.2	22.4	37.7
25. There is ample opportunity for nursing staff to participate in the administrative decision making process.	62.9	15.9	7.3	3.3	5.7	3.7	1.2

33.	Administrative decisions at this hospital interfere too much with patient care.	5.4	7.4	12.4	7.9	12.4	22.3	32.2
40.	I have all the voice in planning policies and procedures for this hospital and my unit that I want.	30.8	17.9	17.1	4.2	12.9	10.8	6.3
42.	The nursing administrators generally consult with the staff on daily problems and procedures.	51.6	20.9	7.0	3.7	8.6	5.7	2.5
Professional Status								
2.	Nurses should be recognized as the most important component in providing care to the hospital patient.	3.7	2.9	2.9	1.6	7.3	25.7	55.9
9.	Nursing is a long way from being recognized as a profession.	8.6	15.6	9.9	2.5	11.9	23.0	28.5
15.	There is no doubt whatever in my mind that what I do on my job is really important.	0	2.5	4.3	1.6	8.0	18.4	65.2
27.	What I do on my job doesn't add up to anything really significant.	58.0	23.7	8.1	2.0	3.7	1.6	2.9
34.	It makes me proud to talk to other people about what I do on my job.	5.3	8.6	7.8	7.0	20.7	28.8	21.8
38.	If I had the decision to make all over again, I would still go into nursing.	18.8	9.2	2.1	10.8	10.8	20.4	27.9
41.	My particular job really doesn't require much skill or "know-how."	78.4	11.9	3.7	0.8	1.6	2.4	1.2
Interaction								
3.	The nursing personnel on my service don't hesitate to pitch in and help one another when things get in a rush.	1.2	3.3	6.5	.8	12.2	34.7	41.3
6.	Physicians in general don't cooperate with the nursing staff on my unit.	12.7	27.8	19.6	5.7	14.3	13.8	6.1
10.	New employees are not quickly made to "feel at home" on my unit.	30.6	16.5	7.9	2.5	14.9	12.4	15.2
16.	There is a good deal of teamwork and cooperation between various levels of nursing personnel on my service.	5.4	9.9	4.9	4.5	15.2	32.9	27.2
19.	There is a lot of teamwork between nurses and doctors on my own unit.	7.4	15.5	13.5	7.4	18.9	24.2	13.1

Continued

Table B.2 Continued

	Strongly Disagree (%)	Disagree (%)	Moderately Disagree (%)	Undecided (%)	Moderately Agree (%)	Agree (%)	Strongly Agree (%)
23. The nursing personnel on my service are not as friendly and outgoing as I would like.	33.6	28.7	11.5	2.5	9.4	9.0	5.3
28. There is a lot of "rank consciousness" on my unit: nursing personnel seldom mingle with others of lower ranks.	52.7	20.0	8.6	3.7	8.2	1.5	5.3
35. I wish the physicians here would show more respect for the skill and knowledge of the nursing staff.	1.5	6.1	9.6	5.7	15.5	19.2	42.4
37. Physicians at this hospital generally understand and appreciate what the nursing staff does.	9.8	16.4	11.9	4.5	26.2	25.5	5.7
39. The physicians at this hospital look down too much on the nursing staff.	6.1	13.9	18.4	8.6	22.1	18.2	12.7

*These numbers correspond to the item numbers on the validated questionnaire.

in 1986. This volume also included suggested scoring procedures and a strong message about using the scale as designed and following the scoring procedures.

Two issues remained unresolved. The first concerned whether the use of the paired comparisons was worthwhile, given the problems in scoring. The suggestion made in 1986 was to keep the paired comparisons if possible. A detailed scoring procedure was included to help with scoring problems. However, a caveat was included, indicating that if the respondents of a survey were hospital nurses, then numerical values for the component weighting coefficients from the final validation study (found in Table B.1) could be used to calculate the IWS. This retained the value of calculating an Index and alleviated the necessity of administering—and scoring— the paired comparisons every time. Related to this, it was suggested that interaction be maintained for computation as a single component, but that for internal analysis it be separated into its two subcomponents, nurse-nurse interaction and nurse-physician interaction. The interaction component was redesigned to have five items for each of these two subcomponents.

The second unresolved issue clearly involved the use of comparative values as well as developing norms or standards for nurse satisfaction. Because of the extreme diversity of responses to the survey of users, no comparisons could be made; neither could any norms be suggested. The publication of the 1986 book containing the scale and scoring procedures was recognized as the only way to begin this process. As a result, the book contained a strong caution about using the scale as it was presented and following the scoring procedures, even though this might result in a loss of flexibility for some investigators.

III. A Second Survey of Users, 1994–95

A second survey of people using the IWS was conducted in 1994–95, in preparation for this second edition. Chapter 4 described the survey process. As can be seen in that chapter, there was less variation in the way in which studies used the IWS. As a result, Chapter 4 presents the beginning of a general database that may be used to compare levels of nurse satisfaction in different settings and in different geographical regions.

Although the IWS is widely used, it is still not perfect. It is important that research into the statistical integrity of the IWS continue. Several of the investigators using the IWS have continued to analyze the structure of the scale, with particular attention to its reliability and validity. This section will present the results of these efforts, followed by a summary of respondent's comments.

As was the case in the first survey of users, most respondents to this second survey did not do any statistical analysis, since their main focus was the use of the IWS. This is certainly more appropriate now than previously, since the first edition of this book emphasized the fact that the scale was ready to use.

In any scale-development model, however, it is important to reflect on whether the scale is truly measuring what it seems to measure, especially with the passage of time. It is important, therefore, that a few people continue to address the issue of scale integrity, since this will help prevent the reification process discussed in Chapter 4.

Reliability Analysis

Only four investigators shared the results of their reliability analysis, and all of these used only Cronbach's alpha to help determine the internal reliability of each of the six components, as well as an overall estimate of reliability. Nobody assessed Kendall's tau to measure how close the weighted and unweighted scores are.

Table B.3 shows the results of these four studies in comparison to the last ones reported in 1986. Two of these studies—Minnick, Pischke-Winn, and Thomas (Chapter 5, Selection 3) and Ingersoll et al. (Chapter 5, Selection 1)—calculated reliability estimates in each of several administrations. This is especially helpful as it gives several reliability estimates over time.

As can be seen from this table, the overall reliability estimates are quite good and are similar to those from the first survey of users in 1985. The component with the highest reliability across all studies is that of pay, where the range is between .83 and .89. This is consistent with the earlier assessment and is not surprising, given that the concept of pay is perhaps the simplest of all to measure.

The autonomy and interaction components are also quite strong, with Cronbach's alphas in the .70 to .80 range and small variations in those ranges. The division of interaction into the two subcomponents seems supported, although fewer studies actually calculated this value.

Task requirements and organizational policies are also very acceptable components, although their ranges are a little more and both have a value of .65, which seems low in comparison to the others but which is actually very acceptable in terms of statistical criteria.

Most puzzling are the reliability estimates for the professional status component. Two studies produced very acceptable Cronbach's alpha values of .76 and .63, and the other three have values that are too low, between .29 and .49. This factor previously had been strong. In 1995,

Table B.3 Comparison of Reliability Analysis of the IWS, 1986 and 1995

Components	Stamps 1986	Koeckeritz[1]	Minnick, Pischke-Winn, and Thomas[2]	Ingersoll et al.[3]	Gustin et al.[4] Martin et al.[5]
Pay	.85	.86	.83; .87	.87; .89; .89; .86	.88
Autonomy	.69	.75	.75; .74	.70; .76; .74; .74	.76
Task Requirements	.69	.67	.73; .70	.69; .66; .64; .78	.70
Organizational Policies	.83	.73	.71; .70	.65; .67; .71; .72	.74
Professional Status	.76	.63	.29; .38	.47; .48; .49; .46	.45
Interaction	.82	.72		.77; .84; .81; .81	.79
• Nurse-Nurse		.71	.71; .71		
• Nurse-Physician		.84	.81; .83		
Overall	.91	.82			.89

[1] Appendix E, Selection 15.
[2] Chapter 5, Selection 3.
[3] Chapter 5, Selection 1.
[4] Chapter 5, Selection 2.
[5] Appendix E, Selection 2.

Coward et al. designed a shortened revision of the IWS to use with long-term care nurses. They kept three items from the professional status component (items 27, 34, and 41), which had a Cronbach's alpha of .55.

Validity Analysis

Two authors shared the results of their factor analyses. Table B.4 shows the results of Ingersoll et al. (Chapter 5, Selection 1). As can be seen from this table, all items identified in the pay subscale loaded heavily and consistently on the first factor. Four of the ten items identified for the interaction subscale loaded heavily on the second factor, while four interaction items loaded heavily and one loaded moderately on a fourth factor. The distinctions between these two factors appears to be the referent, which in factor 2 is nurse-physician interaction and in factor 4 is nurse-nurse interaction.

Four of the professional status items loaded heavily on the third factor, while one loaded moderately. An additional three items not associated with the scale loaded moderately on this factor, and two items associated with the scale failed to load. These two items loaded on factor 11, along with an additional item from the autonomy scale. Two of the three items in factor 11 appear to be related to recognition of the profession of nursing; the third is unrelated and appears to be problematic, since it loaded moderately in three other factors.

Table B.4 Sorted Factor Loadings for the IWS: Ingersoll et al. ($N = 257$)

	Factors*											
	1	2	3	4	5	6	7	8	9	10	11	12
Pay is reasonable.	.811											
Being fairly paid.	.780											
Upgrading of pay is needed.	.777											
Rate of pay increase is not satisfactory.	.775											
Present salary is satisfactory.	.769											
A lot are dissatisfied with pay.	.747											
Physicians cooperate with nursing staff.		.854										
Physicians understand and appreciate nursing.		.824										
Lot of teamwork between nurses and doctors.		.814										
Wish physicians would show more respect.		.507						.439				
What I do does not add up to anything significant.			−.716									
What I do is important.			.711									
Proud to talk about what I do on job.			.667									
I would go into nursing again.			.582							.301		
Good teamwork and cooperation among nurses.				.749								
Nursing personnel pitch in and help.				.735								
New employees not made to feel at home.				−.581								
Nursing personnel not friendly and outgoing.				−.536								
Required to do things against professional judgment.					.357							
Frustrated because activities are programmed.					.723							
Too much responsibility and little authority.					.638							
Freedom to make decisions and backup from supervisors.					.581	.652						
Great deal of independence permitted.						.630						
All the voice in planning I want.						.509				.307		
Could deliver better care if more time.							.731					

Item	Factor loadings
Have sufficient time for care.	.720
Have time to discuss patient care with nurses.	.572
What I do is important.	.538
Physicians look down on nursing staff.	.733
Administrative decisions interfere with care.	.681
Gap between administration and daily problems.	.763
Nursing has control over schedules.	.826
Nursing a long way from recognition as profession.	.335, .706
Too much clerical and paperwork.	.759
Most do not appreciate importance of nursing.	−.423, −.413
Lot of rank consciousness.	−.309
Not enough advancement opportunities.	.337
Little control over work.	−.335, −.320, .439, −.442
Satisfied with activities of job.	.481
Job doesn't require skill or "know-how."	−.486, .377
Ample opportunity to participate.	.366
Sufficient input into program of care.	.334, .360
Nursing administrators consult with staff.	−.358, .301
Am supervised more closely than necessary.	.389, .401

* Factor 1 = Pay; Factor 2 = Nurse-Physician Interaction; Factor 3 = Professional Status; Factor 4 = Nurse-Nurse Interaction; Factor 5 = Autonomy; Factor 6 = Independence; Factor 7 = Task Requirements; Factor 8 = Respectfulness; Factor 9 = Participation; Factor 10 = Mixed; Factor 11 = Professional Importance; Factor 12 = Mixed Negative.

Source: Ingersoll et al. Chapter 5, Selection 1 1996.

Factor 5 contains items associated with the autonomy subscale of the IWS. Only three items in the autonomy scale loaded heavily on this factor. Two additional items loaded moderately, while three items failed to load. Two of these items loaded heavily on factor 6, which in combination with several other items from the autonomy scale (which loaded moderately) and some from the organizational policies scale, appear to reflect independence of practice.

Four of the task requirements subscale items loaded heavily on factor 7. The other two items failed to load on this factor and were split between factors 3 and 12. Items loading on factor 8 appear to relate to respectfulness for the nurse, and items loading on factor 9 pertain to participation in decision making. Items in factors 10 and 12 are mixed and make little conceptual sense. Three items loaded on factor 11, which appears to pertain to professional importance.

As a further test of the construct validity of the IWS, subscales were compared to the overall scale by means of individual one-way ANOVAs. All subscales were significantly related to the overall scale at <.0001 level of significance.

Table B.5 shows the results of the factor analysis performed by Koeckeritz (Appendix E, Selection 15). This factor analysis produced 12 factors, explaining 52.4 percent of the variance. These results are very similar to those in the 1986 Stamps and Piedmonte study.

In 1995 Coward et al. modified the IWS to be more specific to the needs of nurses working in long-term care facilities. This shortened version was extensively reviewed by a panel of experts. Then the factor structure of the shortened version was verified by a factor analysis, which produced five factors that were "remarkably similar in structure and content to the original instrument" (Coward et al. 1995).

Item Analysis

A classic part of attitude scale development is the analysis of the pattern of responses to items, and this has always been an important part of the scale development process followed for the IWS. In terms of scale development, the frequency distribution of responses was part of the face validity procedure. Items that had all "agree" or all "disagree" responses were eliminated, as these items would not adequately discriminate between respondents.

In terms of analyzing results, the frequency distribution of responses to items can reveal much. In fact, we have never given mean values for each item, since we have always preferred to include the distribution in the analysis. Each aspect of the distribution is important and contributes its own piece to the interpretation, as discussed in Appendix C.

Table B.5 Factor Analysis of Job Satisfaction Measure:* Koeckeritz

Item	Factors							
	1	2	3	4	5	6	7	8
1 Pay	.79358	.03134	.17419	.09786	.11336	.06923	.10215	.02891
2 Status	.07209	.37707	.18261	.25283	.33744	-.16496	.03224	-.03530
3 N-N Interaction	.15601	-.01819	.18057	-.19996	.05836	.01563	.59590	.17955
4 Task	-.04511	.08593	-.14987	.43959	.02093	.15143	-.07713	-.00520
5 Policies	.22299	.20864	.11401	-.18297	.02439	.19090	.20467	.31122
6 N-P Interaction	.11906	.75595	.02886	-.06717	.00091	.20034	.07510	.06551
7 Autonomy	.14609	-.04791	.16319	.17912	.04131	.41823	.24370	-.30814
8 Pay	.61804	-.00269	-.01544	.23018	.26033	-.04931	.18734	-.05341
9 Status	.17557	.16470	.02384	.11135	.55074	-.05194	.07130	-.08360
10 N-N Interaction	-.08427	.03914	.13181	.17638	-.01384	-.02230	.65180	-.02392
11 Task	.11413	.00913	.13914	.69994	.02866	-.09077	.05974	.17941
12 Policies	.15624	.02188	.10233	.56409	.41750	.05290	.09492	-.03638
13 Autonomy	.03615	.26463	.15422	.13732	.04891	.56076	-.01002	.23407
14 Pay	.78064	.13208	.04049	.13260	.11605	.10421	.02355	.17715
15 Status	-.03028	.01679	.60103	-.23431	.04547	.30838	-.08906	.05874
16 N-N Interaction	.09604	.06734	.39216	-.07680	.11524	.26760	.46688	.20205
17 Autonomy	.20130	.12877	.15081	.37379	.18442	.33619	.07575	-.05355
18 Policies	.20922	.05084	.18224	.01573	.62730	.09288	-.05810	.00127
19 N-P Interaction	-.05382	.70737	.21951	.04282	.01670	.14337	.03054	.23315
20 Autonomy	.15574	.08125	.24007	.34606	.11144	.52503	.19683	-.05356
21 Pay	.67347	.06713	.05547	.13318	.31242	.03090	-.03085	.09279
22 Task	.05996	-.00510	.55237	.27847	.02930	.17151	.04705	.23671
23 N-N Interaction	.02648	.08261	.00806	.04901	.15722	-.00099	.78445	-.08287
24 Task	.08958	.13203	.03113	.26501	.16727	.06277	.04773	.64563
25 Policies	.01898	.05590	.07395	.11710	.55914	.20569	.00229	.49884

Continued

Table B.5 Continued

Item	*Factors 1	2	3	4	5	6	7	8
26 Autonomy	-.04804	.11053	.09425	-.03689	.07389	.70488	.06149	.13371
27 Status	.04286	.10905	.58777	-.05506	.13731	.15054	.19111	-.29118
28 N-N Interaction	-.01801	.07336	.02951	.02334	-.01132	.30588	-.66978	-.02472
29 Task	.18527	.14576	.00125	.51234	-.02681	.11722	-.01413	.51606
30 Autonomy	.16988	.09190	.30952	.26860	-.03066	.29939	.00274	-.00345
31 Autonomy	.12438	.26479	.18854	.31617	.13915	.33522	-.09726	-.17067
32 Pay	.74590	.17142	-.02017	-.00135	.02572	.10936	-.02998	.07379
33 Policies	.24809	.05676	.03052	.44846	.46473	.07858	.01902	-.04954
34 Status	.02170	.08635	.75609	.11334	.13695	.08398	.11048	.08483
35 N-P Interaction	.10539	.73229	-.08610	.16295	.15085	.01387	.05984	.06051
36 Task	.20529	.12401	-.08255	.64713	.05497	.07166	.04119	.21857
37 N-P Interaction	.09015	.75189	.12289	.03016	.07305	.12853	-.00043	.10204
38 Status	.04750	.08777	.57500	.09685	.20717	-.02767	.11965	.17401
39 N-P Interaction	.11063	.80053	.00686	.18221	.13913	.06496	.08056	-.14097
40 Policies	.10743	.05209	.10376	-.03233	.54138	.36262	.07207	.18998
41 Status	-.01386	.03976	.57858	-.12778	-.03083	.06592	.13827	-.25784
42 Policies	.18305	.09822	.06743	.05038	.54569	.16790	.20419	.23195
43 Autonomy	.10539	.13183	.12373	.03746	.36995	.54830	.24089	.04577
44 Pay	.78731	.02807	-.04176	.08479	.10934	-.01234	-.07010	-.06551
Eigenvalue	8.57781	3.45866	2.63944	2.11424	1.83196	1.63727	1.44989	1.36351
% of Explained Variance	19.5	7.9	6.0	4.8	4.2	3.7	3.3	3.1
Cumulative %	19.5	27.4	33.4	38.2	42.3	46.0	49.3	52.4

*Varimax rotation of factor matrix.
Source: Koeckeritz (Appendix E, Selection 15).

This Appendix (B) includes results from several frequency distributions. Table B.2 shows the results from the validation study reported in the 1986 book. Tables B.6 through B.9 show results from frequency distributions arising from some of the studies in Chapter 5 and Appendix E. Examination of these tables is supportive of the structure of the scale itself, which is the main concern of this appendix. The focus of Appendix C is interpretation of the various types of analysis that arise from using the IWS, including these frequency distributions.

Summary of Comments

The respondents to the 1995 survey made many comments pertaining to the overall usefulness of the IWS. These are contained in Chapter 4. Their comments about the structure of the scale follow here. In keeping with the intent of this appendix, all information pertaining to the more technical aspects of the scale is included here.

By far the most common comment of a technical nature concerned the professional status component. This is not surprising, due to the variable pattern of Cronbach's alpha, representing the internal reliability of this component. The three investigators whose results are shown in Table B.3 all made comments about the low reliability of this component.

The next most common technical comment concerned the scoring reversals that are an inherent part of constructing a Likert scale. A few investigators made specific comments about item 2 of the scale, which is part of the professional status component. It reads, "Nurses should be recognized as the most important component in providing care to the hospital patient." A few others questioned the direction of scoring on item 41, another item measuring professional satisfaction. ("My particular job really doesn't require much skill or 'know-how'.") It may be that the confusion regarding the direction of scoring for these two items contributed to lower than expected reliability values.

Another item that a few investigators have queried over the years is item 5, which reads, "The nursing staff should be allowed to have more control over scheduling their own work shifts." A few investigators questioned the direction of scoring for this item, while a few others changed the item to be more direct, as for example, "The nursing staff has sufficient input into their own schedule."

One investigator, Adams, (Appendix E, Selection 5), used separate values for the components in her statistical model rather than the overall reliability estimate because she felt that there were lower than acceptable relationships between the subscales.

Although these comments came from only a few of the many people who have used the IWS, it is important to acknowledge them because

Table B.6 Frequency Distribution of Responses by Component: McCrea (*N* = 249)

	Strongly Disagree (%)	Disagree (%)	Moderately Disagree (%)	Undecided (%)	Moderately Agree (%)	Agree (%)	Strongly Agree (%)
Pay							
1.* My present salary is satisfactory.	21.1	17.8	11.1	2.2	21.1	18.9	7.8
8. Excluding myself, it is my impression that a lot of nursing service personnel at this hospital are dissatisfied with their pay.	2.2	4.4	4.4	16.7	20.0	27.8	24.4
14. Considering what is expected of nursing service personnel at this hospital, the pay we get is reasonable.	18.0	27.0	21.3	3.4	10.1	18.0	2.2
21. The present rate of increase in pay for nursing service personnel at this hospital is not satisfactory.	1.1	6.7	6.7	11.1	16.7	25.6	32.2
32. From what I hear from and about nursing service personnel at other hospitals, we at this hospital are being fairly paid.	10.1	21.3	9.0	23.6	12.4	23.6	0
44. An upgrading of pay schedules for nursing personnel is needed at this hospital.	0	3.4	2.2	10.1	16.9	34.8	32.6
Autonomy							
7. I feel that I am supervised more closely than I need to be, and more closely than I want to be.	0	1.1	2.2	11.1	16.7	37.8	31.1
13. I feel I have sufficient input into the program of care for each of my patients.	2.2	2.2	5.6	6.7	25.8	39.3	18.0
17. I have too much responsibility and not enough authority.	11.2	21.3	25.8	11.2	23.6	4.5	2.2
20. On my service, my supervisors make all the decisions. I have little direct control over my own work.	23.6	38.2	15.7	7.9	3.4	9.0	2.2
26. A great deal of independence is permitted if not required of me.	0	0	5.6	9.0	25.8	37.1	22.5
30. I am sometimes frustrated because of all my activities seem programmed for me.	16.9	36.0	21.3	11.2	10.1	3.4	1.1

31.	I am sometimes required to do things on my job that are against my better professional nursing judgment.	21.6	37.5	9.1	9.1	18.2	0	4.5
43.	I have the freedom in my work to make important decisions as I see fit, and can count on my supervisors to back me up.	5.6	11.2	12.4	13.5	24.7	19.1	13.5
Task Requirements								
4.	There is too much clerical and "paperwork" required of nursing personnel in this hospital.	25.6	25.6	26.7	6.7	10.0	2.2	3.3
11.	I feel I could do a better job if I didn't have so much to do all the time.	5.6	17.8	25.6	11.1	20.0	14.4	5.6
22.	I am satisfied with the types of activities that I do on my job.	0	0	5.6	10.0	26.7	35.6	22.2
24.	I have plenty of time and opportunity to discuss patient care problems with other nursing service personnel.	8.9	11.1	22.2	4.4	21.1	26.7	5.6
29.	I would like to spend more time in direct patient care.	1.1	14.6	15.7	5.6	30.3	28.1	4.5
36.	I could deliver much better care if I had more time with each patient.	1.1	7.9	9.0	12.4	27.0	19.1	23.6
Organizational Policies								
5.	The nursing staff should be allowed to have more control over scheduling their own work shifts.	3.4	6.7	5.6	4.5	14.6	41.6	23.6
12.	There is a great gap between the administration of this hospital and the daily problems of nursing service.	0	4.4	4.4	7.8	26.7	27.8	28.9
18.	There are not enough opportunities for advancement of nursing personnel at this hospital.	4.5	13.5	12.4	20.2	18.0	14.6	16.9
25.	There is ample opportunity for nursing staff to participate in the administrative decision-making process.	23.3	27.8	15.6	16.7	13.3	1.1	2.2
33.	Administrative decisions at this hospital interfere too much with patient care.	4.5	12.4	22.5	14.6	24.7	16.9	4.5
40.	I have all the voice in planning policies and procedures for this hospital and my unit that I want.	10.1	20.2	20.2	11.2	13.5	12.4	12.4

Continued

Table B.6 Continued

	Strongly Disagree (%)	Disagree (%)	Moderately Disagree (%)	Undecided (%)	Moderately Agree (%)	Agree (%)	Strongly Agree (%)
42. The nursing administrators generally consult with the staff on daily problems and procedures.	32.6	30.3	9.0	9.0	9.0	7.9	2.2
Professional Status							
2. Nurses should be recognized as the most important component in providing care to the hospital patient.	0	3.3	10.0	5.6	15.6	30.0	35.6
9. Nursing is a long way from being recognized as a profession.	7.8	11.1	18.9	7.8	16.7	25.6	12.2
15. There is no doubt whatever in my mind that what I do on my job is really important.	0	0	2.3	1.1	6.8	25.0	64.8
27. What I do on my job doesn't add up to anything really significant.	68.9	23.3	6.7	1.1	0	0	0
34. It makes me proud to talk to other people about what I do on my job.	0	2.2	2.2	1.1	16.9	30.3	47.2
38. If I had the decision to make all over again, I would still go into nursing.	6.7	9.0	5.6	10.1	7.9	24.7	36.0
41. My particular job really doesn't require much skill or "know-how."	87.6	6.7	1.1	2.2	0	1.1	1.1
Interaction							
3. The nursing personnel on my service don't hesitate to pitch in and help one another when things get in a rush.	3.3	3.3	3.3	2.2	18.9	35.6	33.3
6. Physicians in general don't cooperate with the nursing staff on my unit.	0	2.3	2.3	5.6	36.4	40.9	12.5
10. New employees are not quickly made to "feel at home" on my unit.	16.7	22.2	13.3	7.8	21.1	13.3	5.6
16. There is a good deal of teamwork and cooperation between various levels of nursing personnel on my service.	1.1	4.5	8.0	5.7	28.4	27.3	25.0
19. There is a lot of teamwork between nurses and doctors on my own unit.	0	4.5	9.0	14.6	34.8	20.1	9.0

23.	The nursing personnel on my service are not as friendly and outgoing as I would like.	26.7	32.2	17.8	4.4	11.1	3.3	4.4
28.	There is a lot of "rank consciousness" on my unit: nursing personnel seldom mingle with others of lower ranks.	35.6	23.3	8.9	11.1	10.0	3.3	7.8
35.	I wish the physicians here would show more respect for the skill and knowledge of the nursing staff.	1.1	10.1	11.2	5.6	25.8	28.1	18.0
37.	Physicians at this hospital generally understand and appreciate what the nursing staff does.	2.2	10.1	12.4	14.6	29.2	27.0	4.5
39.	The physicians at this hospital look down too much on the nursing staff.	6.7	28.1	21.3	16.9	13.5	10.1	3.4

*These numbers correspond to the item numbers on the validated questionnaire.

Source: McCrea (Appendix E, Selection 7).

Table B.7 Frequency Distribution of Responses by Component: Hlavac ($N = 87$)

	Strongly Disagree (%)	Disagree (%)	Moderately Disagree (%)	Undecided (%)	Moderately Agree (%)	Agree (%)	Strongly Agree (%)
Pay							
1.* My present salary is satisfactory.	29.9	16.1	5.7	8.0	19.5	17.2	3.4
8. Excluding myself, it is my impression that a lot of nursing service personnel at this hospital are dissatisfied with their pay.	2.3	5.7	4.6	14.9	9.2	29.9	33.3
14. Considering what is expected of nursing service personnel at this hospital, the pay we get is reasonable.	40.2	12.6	12.6	8.0	14.9	10.3	1.1
21. The present rate of increase in pay for nursing service personnel at this hospital is not satisfactory.	0	1.1	5.7	8.0	4.6	23.0	57.5
32. From what I hear from and about nursing service personnel at other hospitals, we at this hospital are being fairly paid.	31.0	9.2	9.2	14.9	18.4	11.5	5.7
44. An upgrading of pay schedules for nursing personnel is needed at this hospital.	1.1	0	1.1	3.4	12.6	12.6	69.0
Autonomy							
7. I feel that I am supervised more closely than I need to be, and more closely than I want to be.	20.7	24.1	23.0	11.5	6.9	4.6	9.2
13. I feel I have sufficient input into the program of care for each of my patients.	5.8	3.5	8.1	8.1	19.8	29.1	25.6
17. I have too much responsibility and not enough authority.	4.6	6.9	18.4	10.3	12.6	21.8	25.3
20. On my service, my supervisors make all the decisions. I have little direct control over my own work.	12.6	23.0	19.5	11.5	11.5	6.9	14.9
26. A great deal of independence is permitted if not required of me.	5.7	11.5	9.2	17.2	24.1	26.4	5.7

30.	I am sometimes frustrated because of all my activities seem programmed for me.	5.7	19.5	21.8	16.1	6.9	12.6	17.2
31.	I am sometimes required to do things on my job that are against my better professional nursing judgment.	11.5	10.3	12.6	6.9	19.5	20.7	18.4
43.	I have the freedom in my work to make important decisions as I see fit, and can count on my supervisors to back me up.	24.1	11.9	16.1	9.2	18.4	16.1	4.2

Task Requirements

4.	There is too much clerical and "paperwork" required of nursing personnel in this hospital.	3.4	3.4	2.3	4.6	6.9	32.2	47.1
11.	I feel I could do a better job if I didn't have so much to do all the time.	3.4	10.3	5.7	8.0	17.2	18.4	36.8
22.	I am satisfied with the types of activities that I do on my job.	12.6	2.3	10.3	6.9	18.4	37.9	11.5
24.	I have plenty of time and opportunity to discuss patient care problems with other nursing service personnel.	32.2	17.2	18.4	8.0	12.6	10.3	1.1
29.	I would like to spend more time in direct patient care.	19.5	13.8	14.9	6.9	18.4	18.4	8.0
36.	I could deliver much better care if I had more time with each patient.	2.3	0	2.3	2.3	10.3	24.1	58.6

Organizational Policies

5.	The nursing staff should be allowed to have more control over scheduling their own work shifts.	29.9	8.0	6.9	3.4	21.8	23.0	6.9
12.	There is a great gap between the administration of this hospital and the daily problems of nursing service.	1.1	3.4	2.3	5.7	8.0	18.4	60.9
18.	There are not enough opportunities for advancement of nursing personnel at this hospital.	4.6	9.2	8.0	12.6	12.6	16.1	36.8
25.	There is ample opportunity for nursing staff to participate in the administrative decision-making process.	55.2	16.1	10.3	6.9	4.6	6.9	0
33.	Administrative decisions at this hospital interfere too much with patient care.	2.3	6.9	21.8	14.9	14.9	12.6	26.4
40.	I have all the voice in planning policies and procedures for this hospital and my unit that I want.	41.4	17.2	12.6	12.6	10.3	5.7	0

Continued

Table B.7 Continued

	Strongly Disagree (%)	Disagree (%)	Moderately Disagree (%)	Undecided (%)	Moderately Agree (%)	Agree (%)	Strongly Agree (%)
42. The nursing administrators generally consult with the staff on daily problems and procedures.	57.5	18.4	12.6	2.3	6.9	2.3	0
Professional Status							
2. Nurses should be recognized as the most important component in providing care to the hospital patient.	4.6	4.6	3.4	11.5	13.8	31.0	31.0
9. Nursing is a long way from being recognized as a profession.	16.1	9.2	17.2	5.7	19.5	16.1	16.1
15. There is no doubt whatever in my mind that what I do on my job is really important.	1.1	1.1	2.3	1.1	4.6	23.0	66.7
27. What I do on my job doesn't add up to anything really significant.	47.1	21.8	13.8	5.7	0	6.9	4.6
34. It makes me proud to talk to other people about what I do on my job.	8.0	3.4	5.7	10.3	21.8	27.6	23.0
38. If I had the decision to make all over again, I would still go into nursing.	11.5	5.7	3.4	6.9	8.0	23.0	41.4
41. My particular job really doesn't require much skill or "know-how."	73.6	9.2	9.2	2.3	3.4	1.1	1.1
Interaction							
3. The nursing personnel on my service don't hesitate to pitch in and help one another when things get in a rush.	5.7	6.9	4.6	6.9	18.4	35.6	21.8
6. Physicians in general don't cooperate with the nursing staff on my unit.	16.1	13.8	13.8	8.0	26.4	18.4	3.4
10. New employees are not quickly made to "feel at home" on my unit.	16.1	26.4	13.8	11.5	9.2	12.6	10.3
16. There is a good deal of teamwork and cooperation between various levels of nursing personnel on my service.	11.5	2.3	10.3	9.2	32.2	24.1	10.3

19. There is a lot of teamwork between nurses and doctors on my own unit.	27.6	14.9	11.5	8.0	23.0	13.8	1.1
23. The nursing personnel on my service are not as friendly and outgoing as I would like.	19.5	26.4	18.4	9.2	9.2	9.2	8.0
28. There is a lot of "rank consciousness" on my unit: nursing personnel seldom mingle with others of lower ranks.	31.0	20.7	11.5	9.2	9.2	11.5	6.9
35. I wish the physicians here would show more respect for the skill and knowledge of the nursing staff.	3.4	0	1.1	3.4	10.3	17.2	64.4
37. Physicians at this hospital generally understand and appreciate what the nursing staff does.	29.9	20.7	8.0	5.7	23.0	11.5	1.1
39. The physicians at this hospital look down too much on the nursing staff.	6.9	11.5	9.2	9.2	17.2	12.6	33.3

*These numbers correspond to the item numbers on the validated questionnaire.
Source: Hlavac (Appendix E, Selection 8).

Table B.8 Frequency Distribution of Responses by Component: Cooley (N = 50)

	Strongly Disagree (%)	Disagree (%)	Moderately Disagree (%)	Undecided (%)	Moderately Agree (%)	Agree (%)	Strongly Agree (%)
Pay							
1.* My present salary is satisfactory.	6.1	12.2	18.4	20.4	20.4	18.4	4.1
8. Excluding myself, it is my impression that a lot of nursing service personnel at this hospital are dissatisfied with their pay.	0	6.1	14.3	20.4	20.4	24.5	12.2
14. Considering what is expected of nursing service personnel at this hospital, the pay we get is reasonable.	10.2	12.2	34.7	24.5	8.2	10.2	0
21. The present rate of increase in pay for nursing service personnel at this hospital is not satisfactory.	2.0	8.2	16.3	10.2	20.4	16.3	24.5
32. From what I hear from and about nursing service personnel at other hospitals, we at this hospital are being fairly paid.	4.1	16.3	22.4	18.4	8.2	24.5	4.1
44. An upgrading of pay schedules for nursing personnel is needed at this hospital.	2.0	8.2	2.0	20.4	24.3	14.5	26.5
Autonomy							
7. I feel that I am supervised more closely than I need to be, and more closely than I want to be.	18.4	14.3	40.8	10.2	0	8.2	4.1
13. I feel I have sufficient input into the program of care for each of my patients.	2.0	2.0	10.2	24.5	34.7	26.5	0
17. I have too much responsibility and not enough authority.	6.1	16.3	24.5	28.6	14.3	4.1	4.1
20. On my service, my supervisors make all the decisions. I have little direct control over my own work.	6.1	8.2	42.9	20.4	12.2	4.1	6.1
26. A great deal of independence is permitted if not required of me.	6.1	2.0	4.1	18.4	24.5	34.7	10.2
30. I am sometimes frustrated because of all my activities seem programmed for me.	14.3	14.3	26.5	28.6	12.2	2.0	2.0

31.	I am sometimes required to do things on my job that are against my better professional nursing judgment.	28.6	21.4	26.5	14.3	4.1	4.1	2.0
43.	I have the freedom in my work to make important decisions as I see fit, and can count on my supervisors to back me up.	10.2	12.2	24.5	16.3	18.4	12.2	6.1

Task Requirements

4.	There is too much clerical and "paperwork" required of nursing personnel in this hospital.	0	2.0	4.1	20.4	34.7	28.6	10.2
11.	I feel I could do a better job if I didn't have so much to do all the time.	8.2	12.2	26.5	26.5	16.3	0	10.2
22.	I am satisfied with the types of activities that I do on my job.	2.0	0	6.1	14.3	28.6	38.8	10.2
24.	I have plenty of time and opportunity to discuss patient care problems with other nursing service personnel.	8.2	10.2	30.6	26.5	18.4	6.1	0
29.	I would like to spend more time in direct patient care.	4.1	2.0	24.5	34.7	16.3	14.3	4.1
36.	I could deliver much better care if I had more time with each patient.	6.1	14.3	6.1	36.7	20.4	10.2	4.1

Organizational Policies

5.	The nursing staff should be allowed to have more control over scheduling their own work shifts.	22.4	24.5	16.3	16.3	10.2	10.2	0
12.	There is a great gap between the administration of this hospital and the daily problems of nursing service.	18.4	18.4	36.7	12.2	2.0	10.2	0
18.	There are not enough opportunities for advancement of nursing personnel at this hospital.	4.1	10.2	16.3	22.4	24.5	12.2	10.2
25.	There is ample opportunity for nursing staff to participate in the administrative decision-making process.	6.1	14.3	34.7	16.3	24.5	4.1	0
33.	Administrative decisions at this hospital interfere too much with patient care.	6.1	14.3	16.3	32.7	22.4	6.1	2.0
40.	I have all the voice in planning policies and procedures for this hospital and my unit that I want.	12.2	10.2	28.6	28.6	10.2	6.1	4.1
42.	The nursing administrators generally consult with the staff on daily problems and procedures.	12.2	16.3	34.7	14.3	16.3	6.1	0

Continued

Table B.8 Continued

	Strongly Disagree (%)	Disagree (%)	Moderately Disagree (%)	Undecided (%)	Moderately Agree (%)	Agree (%)	Strongly Agree (%)
Professional Status							
2. Nurses should be recognized as the most important component in providing care to the hospital patient.	4.1	14.3	14.3	14.3	16.3	24.5	12.2
9. Nursing is a long way from being recognized as a profession.	2.0	18.4	22.4	20.4	14.3	16.3	6.1
15. There is no doubt whatever in my mind that what I do on my job is really important.	2.0	0	2.0	10.2	8.2	30.6	46.9
27. What I do on my job doesn't add up to anything really significant.	44.9	22.4	18.4	6.1	4.1	0	4.1
34. It makes me proud to talk to other people about what I do on my job.	2.0	2.0	0	10.2	20.4	38.8	24.5
38. If I had the decision to make all over again, I would still go into nursing.	12.2	4.1	14.3	8.2	14.3	22.4	24.5
41. My particular job really doesn't require much skill or "know-how."	6.1	0	0	6.1	4.1	18.4	63.3
Interaction							
3. The nursing personnel on my service don't hesitate to pitch in and help one another when things get in a rush.	32.0	2.0	4.1	12.2	24.5	34.7	20.4
6. Physicians in general don't cooperate with the nursing staff on my unit.	2.0	4.1	14.3	32.7	34.7	10.2	0
10. New employees are not quickly made to "feel at home" on my unit.	4.1	8.2	20.4	18.4	20.4	18.4	10.2
16. There is a good deal of teamwork and cooperation between various levels of nursing personnel on my service.	2.0	0	4.1	22.4	28.6	38.8	4.1
19. There is a lot of teamwork between nurses and doctors on my own unit.	2.0	0	16.3	40.8	16.3	0	2.0

23.	The nursing personnel on my service are not as friendly and outgoing as I would like.	14.3	18.4	24.5	20.4	16.3	4.1	2.0
28.	There is a lot of "rank consciousness" on my unit: nursing personnel seldom mingle with others of lower ranks.	4.1	6.1	18.4	12.2	20.4	18.4	18.4
35.	I wish the physicians here would show more respect for the skill and knowledge of the nursing staff.	2.0	2.0	4.1	16.3	34.7	18.4	22.4
37.	Physicians at this hospital generally understand and appreciate what the nursing staff does.	2.0	12.2	18.4	36.7	20.4	10.2	0
39.	The physicians at this hospital look down too much on the nursing staff.	2.0	14.3	34.7	12.2	28.6	2.0	6.1

*These numbers correspond to the item numbers on the validated questionnaire.

Source: Cooley (Appendix E, Selection 10).

Table B.9 Frequency Distribution of Responses by Component: McQuaid* (N = 102)

	Strongly Disagree (%)	Disagree (%)	Moderately Disagree (%)	Undecided (%)	Moderately Agree (%)	Agree (%)	Strongly Agree (%)
Pay							
1.** My present salary is satisfactory.	19	10	16	7	19	26	5
8. Excluding myself, it is my impression that a lot of nursing service personnel at this hospital are dissatisfied with their pay.	7	5	13	17	21	20	19
14. Considering what is expected of nursing service personnel at this hospital, the pay we get is reasonable.	19	9	21	10	20	19	4
21. The present rate of increase in pay for nursing service personnel at this hospital is not satisfactory.	1	5	18	7	21	16	33
32. From what I hear from and about nursing service personnel at other hospitals, we at this hospital are being fairly paid.	11	14	15	10	18	28	5
44. An upgrading of pay schedules for nursing personnel is needed at this hospital.	0	5	8	8	26	18	36
Autonomy							
7. I feel that I am supervised more closely than I need to be, and more closely than I want to be.	36	28	24	9	3	0	1
13. I feel I have sufficient input into the program of care for each of my patients.	0	2	7	7	29	40	15
17. I have too much responsibility and not enough authority.	9	18	30	16	13	11	4
20. On my service, my supervisors make all the decisions. I have little direct control over my own work.	26	28	28	5	7	4	3
26. A great deal of independence is permitted if not required of me.	1	2	14	8	28	37	11
30. I am sometimes frustrated because of all my activities seem programmed for me.	5	20	24	13	20	12	8

31.	I am sometimes required to do things on my job that are against my better professional nursing judgment.	28	27	13	8	16	3	6
43.	I have the freedom in my work to make important decisions as I see fit, and can count on my supervisors to back me up.	9	11	14	8	28	21	10

Task Requirements

4.	There is too much clerical and "paperwork" required of nursing personnel in this hospital.	0	3	11	5	16	32	33
11.	I feel I could do a better job if I didn't have so much to do all the time.	5	11	11	9	26	19	21
22.	I am satisfied with the types of activities that I do on my job.	2	4	8	3	40	27	17
24.	I have plenty of time and opportunity to discuss patient care problems with other nursing service personnel.	5	16	30	10	19	14	7
29.	I would like to spend more time in direct patient care.	1	11	24	6	26	18	16
36.	I could deliver much better care if I had more time with each patient.	1	1	4	6	21	23	45

Organizational Policies

5.	The nursing staff should be allowed to have more control over scheduling their own work shifts.	3	15	19	7	15	14	28
12.	There is a great gap between the administration of this hospital and the daily problems of nursing service.	0	6	10	9	25	19	32
18.	There are not enough opportunities for advancement of nursing personnel at this hospital.	4	9	15	8	22	24	20
25.	There is ample opportunity for nursing staff to participate in the administrative decision making process.	34	17	20	12	17	0	1
33.	Administrative decisions at this hospital interfere too much with patient care.	14	17	21	19	14	9	8
40.	I have all the voice in planning policies and procedures for this hospital and my unit that I want.	23	21	21	10	17	6	4

Continued

Table B.9 Continued

	Strongly Disagree (%)	Disagree (%)	Moderately Disagree (%)	Undecided (%)	Moderately Agree (%)	Agree (%)	Strongly Agree (%)
42. The nursing administrators generally consult with the staff on daily problems and procedures.	34	11	14	7	18	8	9
Professional Status							
2. Nurses should be recognized as the most important component in providing care to the hospital patient.	5	6	12	7	19	23	29
9. Nursing is a long way from being recognized as a profession.	11	20	25	4	15	13	14
15. There is no doubt whatever in my mind that what I do on my job is really important.	1	2	0	5	5	26	62
27. What I do on my job doesn't add up to anything really significant.	68	19	7	4	3	0	0
34. It makes me proud to talk to other people about what I do on my job.	2	2	6	1	25	28	37
38. If I had the decision to make all over again, I would still go into nursing.	6	0	5	9	8	19	54
41. My particular job really doesn't require much skill or "know-how."	79	14	4	1	1	0	1
Interaction							
3. The nursing personnel on my service don't hesitate to pitch in and help one another when things get in a rush.	3	4	5	3	21	34	30
6. Physicians in general don't cooperate with the nursing staff on my unit.	5	36	38	7	8	4	2
10. New employees are not quickly made to "feel at home" on my unit.	34	28	17	2	10	7	3
16. There is a good deal of teamwork and cooperation between various levels of nursing personnel on my service.	4	2	10	3	22	34	26

19.	There is a lot of teamwork between nurses and doctors on my own unit.	2	7	15	11	35	26	5
23.	The nursing personnel on my service are not as friendly and outgoing as I would like.	41	27	16	7	7	2	1
28.	There is a lot of "rank consciousness" on my unit: nursing personnel seldom mingle with others of lower ranks.	58	18	11	4	6	3	1
35.	I wish the physicians here would show more respect for the skill and knowledge of the nursing staff.	2	7	12	8	27	18	28
37.	Physicians at this hospital generally understand and appreciate what the nursing staff does.	8	5	19	9	36	19	5
39.	The physicians at this hospital look down too much on the nursing staff.	10	28	26	10	12	8	7

*Percentages are rounded to nearest whole number. Due to rounding, some totals do not equal 100%.

**These numbers correspond to the item numbers on the validated questionnaire.

Source: McQuaide (Chapter 5, Selection 5).

not many investigators are actually examining the structure of the IWS. As noted before, it is important to keep the research-and-development phase active, even with respect to a widely used scale.

These comments as well as those shared by other investigators give a sense of the strengths and limitations of the IWS. Sections IV and V of this appendix will address these strengths and limitations.

IV. Limitations, Problems, and Other Caveats

Developing a valid measurement instrument to assess attitudes is a lengthy process at best. One of the first problems confronted is theoretical. An attitude scale must be anchored in a theoretical framework. As shown in Chapter 2, there are several different theories of work satisfaction, some of which are mutually exclusive. Second, the relationship between theory and precise measurement is sometimes troublesome. For example, Maslow's hierarchy of needs suggests that self-actualization is the most important need for many people, yet in the work situation few jobs provide fulfillment for this need. Herzberg's Dual-Factor theory suggests that achievement, recognition, work itself, interpersonal relations, factors in personal life, job security, status, and pay will affect satisfaction more than organizational policy and administration, supervision, and working conditions. Koeckertiz (Appendix E, Selection 15) provides an excellent example of the importance of creating theoretical models that include social and cultural roles as well. However, many of these "satisfying" components are difficult for management to control or improve, since they lie outside the scope of the organization. Thus, while a questionnaire that measures these areas is theoretically important, it may have less practical value. This is why management's efforts to improve satisfaction often focus on factors that seem peripheral, such as personnel policy, working conditions, supervision, or organizational structure. The IWS is designed to measure those factors within the scope of the organization, and the components included are designed to measure a variety of factors that are central to the perception of satisfaction. It is important to be able to measure all aspects of satisfaction in such a way as to provide information that is of practical use to management.

The second general problem is more methodological. This scale has been developed over many years in multiple settings. Throughout the time of developing the scale, every study had dual objectives. At each site, the objective of research information paralleled the need for obtaining managerial information. The advantage of this is clear: this is a measurement instrument that has been developed in real-life situations, not in simulated or laboratory settings. In every setting in which the IWS has been administered, there has been very positive feedback regarding the usefulness of the information to management. The disadvantage is also clear, however. Little standardization has resulted. Often the need for managerial information overwhelmed the research objective related to improving the validity of the measurement. Lack of standardization created problems in comparing the results of our studies with those of others. Although many investigators have used this scale, the first survey discovered many variations in use, as well as inaccuracies and imprecision in scoring techniques. In the first edition of this book, this limited the possible comparisons to rankings, rather than any numerical comparisons. The second survey found much greater similarity of use and scoring, due in large measure to the easy availability of similar scoring techniques.

Another problem in both surveys was the difficulty of obtaining an adequate sample size and response rate. In 1983 and in 1994–95, response rates varied, at least partly dependent on the method used to distribute and collect the questionnaire. Mailed questionnaires had a range of responses from 15 percent to 89 percent. Studies that employed personal distribution of questionnaires had response rates ranging from 25 percent to 90 percent. Several studies that had especially low response rates mentioned that some organizational reason was responsible, including downsizing, union activity, or other administrative initiatives.

One of the major objectives of the first survey of users was to develop some sort of comparative ability. Because of the tremendous variation in the way the IWS was used and scored, it was not possible to develop that ability for the 1986 edition of this book. As a result of the second survey, reported in detail in Chapter 4, it is now possible to begin this comparative work. However, this does not mean that all the technical issues are resolved. In fact, there are three technical issues related to the design of the scale that need to be noted.

Professional Status Component

The professional status component is somewhat problematic. As may be seen in Table B.3, the Cronbach's alpha values are frequently too low. The item with the lowest factor loading on the entire scale is located in the professional status component: "Nursing is a long way from being recognized as a profession." Another of the items ("Nurses should be recognized as the most important component in providing care to the hospital patients") was mistakenly identified in 1986 as reading "Most people do not sufficiently appreciate the importance of nursing care to hospital patients." The first version is too extreme, and many people use the second version. The problem is that these two items are scored in different directions, which may partially account for some of the lower reliabilities obtained with this component.

Scoring Reversals

Some of the problems noted in the professional status component are related to the need to reverse the direction of scoring on half the items of a Likert scale. Inherent in the Likert design is the notion that it is desirable to be able simply to sum up the scores on a set of items so that a higher score represents a more positive attitude. This is only possible if the maximum for an individual item is always given to the most positive response possible to a particular statement. For example, a highly satisfied nurse would agree with the statement, "My present salary is satisfactory," and would disagree with the statement, "The present rate of increase in pay for nursing service personnel at this hospital is not satisfactory." Also inherent in the Likert design is the notion that half of the items in an attitude scale should be positive statements and half should be worded negatively.

This design gives the developer of a scale flexibility as to the direction of the scale. The IWS is oriented toward satisfaction, which is a positive direction: those items that are positively stated are given the highest value. This means that when a respondent agrees with the statement "My present salary is satisfactory," that response is given the maximum value, which is 7 on the 1-to-7 response mode used with the scale. Likewise, if a respondent disagrees with a negative statement, such as, "The present rate of increase in pay for nursing service personnel at this hospital is not satisfactory," that response is also given the maximum value of 7. The consequence of this arrangement is that, for positive statements, the Strongly Agree response is given a 7, and for negative statements, the Strongly Disagree statement is given a 7.

Table B.10 shows another way of looking at this. The first column shows all the positive statements that are included on the IWS. A respondent who is perfectly satisfied would respond to each of these with a Strongly Agree response, which would be given a maximum score of 7. The second column shows all the negative statements: a perfectly satisfied nurse would respond to each of these with a Strongly Disagree response; this response would be given a maximum score of 7.

Some of the investigators who responded to the second survey of users, conducted for the purposes of this volume, noted that they had changed the direction of scoring for a particular item, because it made more sense to them. This, of course, interferes with the comparability of

Table B.10 Scoring Reversals in the IWS

Positive Statements Strongly Agree=7; Strongly Disagree=1	Negative Statements Strongly Agree=1; Strongly Disagree=7
Pay	*Pay*
1. My present salary is satisfactory.	8.* It is my impression that a lot of nursing service personnel at this hospital are dissatisfied with their pay.
14. Considering what is expected of nursing service personnel at this hospital, the pay we get is reasonable.	21. The present rate of increase in pay for nursing personnel at this hospital is not satisfactory.
32.* From what I hear about nursing service personnel at other hospitals, we at this hospital are being fairly paid.	44. An upgrading of pay schedules for nursing personnel is needed at this hospital.
Autonomy	*Autonomy*
13. I feel I have sufficient input into the program of care for each of my patients.	7. I feel that I am supervised more closely than necessary.
26. A great deal of independence is permitted, if not required, of me on my job.	17. I have too much responsibility and not enough authority.
43. I have the freedom in my work to make important decisions as I see fit, and can count on my supervisors to back me up.	20. On my service, my supervisors make all the decisions. I have little direct control over my own work.
	30. I am sometimes frustrated because all of my activities seem programmed for me.
	31. I am sometimes required to do things on my job that are against my better professional nursing judgment.
Task Requirements	*Task Requirements*
22. I am satisfied with the types of activities that I do on my job.	4. There is too much clerical and "paperwork" required of nursing personnel in this hospital.
24. I have plenty of time and opportunity to discuss patient care problems with other nursing service personnel.	15. I think I could do a better job if I didn't have so much to do all the time.
29. I have sufficient time for direct patient care.	36. I could deliver much better care if I had more time with each patient.

Continued

Table B.10 Continued

Positive Statements Strongly Agree=7; Strongly Disagree=1	Negative Statements Strongly Agree=1; Strongly Disagree=7
Organizational Policies	Organizational Policies
5. The nursing staff has sufficient control over scheduling their own work shifts in my hospital.	12. There is a great gap between the administration of this hospital and the daily problems of the nursing service.
25. There is ample opportunity for nursing staff to participate in the administrative decision-making process.	18. There are not enough opportunities for advancement of nursing personnel at this hospital.
40. I have all the voice in planning policies and procedures for this hospital and my unit that I want.	33. Administrative decisions at this hospital interfere too much with patient care.
42. The nursing administrators generally consult with the staff on daily problems and procedures.	
Professional Status	Professional Status
9.* Most people appreciate the importance of nursing care to hospital patients.	2.* Nursing is not widely recognized as being an important profession.
11. There is no doubt whatever in my mind that what I do on my job is really important.	27. What I do on my job doesn't add up to anything really significant.
34. It makes me proud to talk to other people about what I do on my job.	41. My particular job really doesn't require much skill or "know-how."
38. If I had the decision to make all over again, I would still go into nursing.	

Interaction

Nurse-Nurse Interaction

3.* The nursing personnel on my service pitch in and help one another when things get in a rush.

16. There is a good deal of teamwork and cooperation between various levels of nursing personnel on my service.

Nurse-Physician Interaction

6. Physicians in general cooperate with the nursing staff on my unit.

19. There is a lot of teamwork between nurses and doctors on my unit.

37. Physicians at this hospital generally understand and appreciate what the nursing staff does.

Interaction

Nurse-Nurse Interaction

10.* It is hard for new nurses to feel "at home" on my unit.

23. The nursing personnel on my service are not as friendly and outgoing as I would like.

28.* There is a lot of "rank consciousness" on my unit: nurses seldom mingle with those with less experience or different types of educational preparation.

Nurse-Physician Interaction

35. I wish the physicians here would show more respect for the skill and knowledge of the nursing staff.

39. The physicians at this hospital look down too much on the nursing staff.

The numbers correspond to the item numbers on the IWS.
*These items have been reworded and/or renumbered in the revised questionnaire, as shown in Appendix A.

the scale since it changes the scoring. As may be seen in Table B.10, some of the items needed to be stated more clearly. Accordingly, we revised the wording of these items slightly, in the hope that these minor revisions will eliminate the confusion with scoring direction. The revised questionnaire appears in Appendix A.

Paired Comparisons

The original idea of using Edwards's (1957) technique of paired comparisons in conjunction with the Likert scale arose in response to the several theories indicating that people's satisfaction with their jobs is mediated by their expectations. This made the IWS a unique measurement instrument, but also increased the scoring requirements. Using the paired comparisons in the scoring procedure allowed the creation of an index, a summary number representing satisfaction that was weighted by expectations. Early on, we were concerned about the relationship between the weighted and unweighted scores. The computation of the Kendall's tau was an effort to decide if the weighted score and the unweighted score seemed to be measuring the same thing. That they were was a reassurance about the validity of the construction of the Index. However, if the weighted and unweighted scores are really measuring the same thing, then perhaps using the weighted score is not worth the extra work in the scoring. This became a balance between theoretical strength and easy applicability.

In the 1983 survey, it was discovered that very few studies calculated the value for the paired comparisons themselves. In fact, in the first edition of this book, we encouraged people to use the paired comparisons only in situations in which the expectations were unknown. The values for community hospital nurses were so similar in the various administrations that we wondered if there weren't some type of normative values.

In the 1994–95 survey, more investigators calculated the values for the paired comparisons, primarily because the first edition of the book contained directions for scoring. As shown in Chapter 4, there are now several studies to compare. There are obvious similarities in the component weighting coefficients, but the variance is enough that these should not be taken as normative values. As more experience is gained with the paired comparisons, more information is also being gathered about what is important to nurses. This is a very valuable piece of information, as demonstrated in the Appendix C discussion about analyzing the discrepancy between what is viewed as being important and what is viewed as being highly satisfying.

However, the price for this is still a more tedious scoring procedure as well as a longer questionnaire. Questions about the applicability of using this weighted measure are still arising. Experience with developing a physician satisfaction scale has prompted considerable reflection about the appropriateness of using one summary number to represent satisfaction as opposed to several individual component-specific numbers. (Stamps and Cruz 1994). As noted in Chapter 4, the whole idea of separating satisfaction into its component parts may not be compatible with putting these parts back together into one summary number. Adams (Appendix E, Selection 5) uses the separate component values in her statistical model of organizational commitment because these values seem more reliable than the overall summary number.

V. Recommendations

Several specific recommendations arose from consideration of these issues.

1. As a result of analyzing the frequency distributions of responses to the items as well as both the reliability and validity estimates, it seemed that some minor changes needed to be made on the scale. One of the outcomes of the survey process that led to the revision of this book was renewed confidence that the IWS is basically a useful and accurate measurement instrument. Given this reassurance, it was important not to make major changes since to do so would compromise comparability. However, the survey process highlighted some problems that could be easily remedied. Table B.10 identifies the items that have been reworded and/or renumbered. Most of the changes state the item more clearly to reduce confusion about the direction of scoring. Appendix A shows the Index of Work Satisfaction scale with these changes and with some additional modification of the format and instructions to help clarify the general purpose of the questionnaire. This is the version of the scale that should be used. Using this version of the scale should not jeopardize using the data reported in Chapter 4 for comparative purposes, but should result in higher reliability and validity estimates relating to the integrity of the scale itself.

2. In 1986, the interaction component was expanded and slightly redesigned to include two separate subscales, but only one scale was maintained for the paired comparisons. This suggestion is retained here. Dividing the interaction component is very helpful in terms of improved understanding of the responses of the nursing staff; adding this as another choice in the paired comparisons does not add enough information to be worth the trouble.

3. Although it may be tempting to do so, it is not appropriate to give up the paired comparisons part of this measure. Only by using the component weighting coefficients can the Index itself be

created. This is a unique aspect of the scale and should be retained. However, using the paired comparisons is not appropriate in every situation. In some settings, the IWS is being used to monitor nurse satisfaction. In such cases, it is appropriate to include the paired comparisons in the initial measure, but it is not necessary to do so with every administration, since expectations do not vary that much. In addition, the most valuable number to use in a study whose major purpose is managerial, especially when monitoring is involved, is the mean score for each individual component, rather than any one summary number. In this way, specific changes can be noted in response to organizational initiatives. For research purposes, the expectations of the nurses should still be measured, since this adds a rich dimension to the knowledge base of what provides satisfaction to nurses. Appendix C provides a discussion of some of the differences between a study whose major purpose is managerial and one whose major purpose is research.

4. As the usage of the IWS increases in the field, there will be even more pressure to find a way to compare scores across settings and to create some type of norms. This is appropriate, within the caveats presented in Chapter 4, but it is very important that the same scoring procedures are used and that exactly the same questionnaire is used, with minimal changes in wording. This clearly represents a loss of flexibility, but the trade-off is the ability to develop norms and conduct comparative analyses. More assistance is now available in scoring, as described in Appendix D, which should increase the comparability of studies using the IWS.

5. It is important to keep doing research on the IWS, even as it is being used in the field. Just because it is used widely does not mean that it should be accepted as it is. It is critical to continue research on the integrity and structure of the scale itself. More investigators need to do both validity and reliability analyses in order to continue to improve the scale and to ensure that its relevance is maintained. Also, many other content areas need to be investigated. It is clear, for example, that more work needs to be done on defining expectations. What does it mean for a nurse to say that autonomy is more important than task requirements? What is the relationship between these two and how can it be modified by the organization?

This appendix has described the scale-development process and some technical issues related to the structure of the scale. Appendix C gives some guidelines for using the IWS, including interpretation of the numerical findings.

References

Coward, R. T., T. L. Hogan, R. P. Duncan, C. H. Horne, M. A. Hilker, and L. M. Felsen. 1995. "Job Satisfaction of Nurses Employed in Rural and Urban Long-term Care Facilities." *Research in Nursing and Health* 18: 271–84.

Edwards, A. L. 1957. *Techniques of Attitude Scale Constitution*. New York: Appleton-Century Crofts.

Kit, M. E. 1985. "An Analysis of the Stamps-Piedmonte Index of Work Satisfaction as a Tool for Measuring Job Satisfaction of Nursing Personnel." Master's thesis, University of Massachusetts–Amherst.

Slavitt, D. B., P. L. Stamps, E. B. Piedmonte, and A. M. Haase. 1978. "Nurse's Satisfaction with Their Work Situation." *Nursing Research* 27 (March/April): 114–20.

———. 1979. "Measuring Nurses' Job Satisfaction." *Hospital & Health Services Administration* 24 (3): 232–42.

Stamps, P. L. 1978. "Satisfaction of Direct Care Provider." In *Ambulatory Care Systems*, Volume 3, *Evaluation of Outpatient Facilities*, 75–106. Lexington, MA: D. C. Heath.

———. 1981. "Job Evaluation Through Measures of Occupational Satisfaction." In *Handbook of Health Care Human Resources Management*, edited by N. Metzger, 133–56. Rockville, MD: Aspen.

Stamps, P. L., and N. T. B. Cruz. 1994. *Issues in Physician Satisfaction: New Perspectives*. Chicago: Health Administration Press.

Stamps, P. L., and J. Finkelstein. 1981. "Statistical Analysis of a Patient Satisfaction Scale." *Medical Care* 19 (November): 1108–35.

Stamps, P. L., E. B. Piedmonte, A. B. Haase, and D. B. Slavitt. 1978. "Measurement of Work Satisfaction among Health Professionals." *Medical Care* 16 (April): 337–52.

Stamps, P. L., and B. Shopnik. 1981. "Emergency Medical Technicians' Perception of Acceptance by Nurses and Physicians." *Journal of Ambulatory Care Management* 4 (November): 69–86.

USING THE INDEX OF WORK SATISFACTION
IN AN ORGANIZATIONAL SETTING

his appendix is divided into two sections. The first section discusses the process of preparing to conduct a study of nurse satisfaction. The second section discusses both data analysis and interpretation and offers some recommendations about interpretation.

Some of this appendix was previously included in Chapter 3 of the first edition. It has been modified to reflect the increased experience with the IWS in the decade since the publication of that edition.

Preparation for Use and Implementation

It is necessary to prepare adequately for the administration of the IWS. All levels of the organization should be involved in the preparatory steps. Lines of communication should be opened between the hospital administration, the nursing administration, and the nursing staff, especially with respect to any job redesign initiatives that might be implemented as a result of the study. An atmosphere of trust is important in the questionnaire's administration. A maximum response rate depends on the nurse respondents' belief that the administration really *wants* to make necessary changes to help them do their jobs better. Issues that need to be addressed in preparation for using the IWS include determining the motivation for assessing nurse satisfaction; instituting an appropriate planning phase that involves all levels of the organization; and implementing the findings of the satisfaction study.

Motivation

Paramount in this preparation process is the *honest* estimation of the motivation for assessing satisfaction, so that the potential for manipulation is minimized. Satisfaction with each component is compared with its importance (measured by the paired-comparison rank in Part A) to indicate which specific areas of the job need improvement. When a component receives high scores in both perceived importance and actual work satisfaction, it can be assumed that the respondents are satisfied with this component. (Professional status and autonomy often fit this category.) When a component receives high or moderately high importance by paired comparisons (Part A) but low satisfaction from Part B scores, it may be considered an area in need of improvement (often the pay component). When the component ranking is low, there are several interpretations depending on the actual work satisfaction score. If the factor has received high scores on current satisfaction, then it can be assumed that the respondents are satisfied with this area (as often is the case with interaction). When both importance and current work satisfaction scores are low, it may be that the factor is relatively unimportant and the respondents expect little satisfaction from it, or they may feel that satisfaction is unattainable in this area and have thus devalued it. The task requirements and organizational policies components may be interpreted in either of these ways.

Providing management with information about various areas of dissatisfaction may also enable management to manipulate the working environment in a manner that does not benefit the nursing staff. Discovering the relative importance and level of satisfaction of these work components, for instance, could lead to linking incentives to some of them while ignoring others. For example, if pay is a source of dissatisfaction but it is not valued highly, it may be easier to change scheduled work shifts than to deal with possible inequities in salary. This use is obviously to be avoided, as in the long run it does not contribute to anything but further alienation of nurses and all levels of administrators. When the scale is properly used, it can open channels of communication between various levels of health professionals and managers. It can also make possible specific changes in the organization by balancing administrative constraints with expectations and satisfactions of the clinical professionals.

As is true when using many management and evaluation tools, it is imperative to understand the motivation for wanting to use this scale. A measurement tool is only a technique. It cannot substitute for effective management. This technique does allow a sharing of perceptions from two important viewpoints: that of the nursing staff and that of the administrators. The IWS can be used to assist *both* groups in understanding their particular needs and constraints. The measurement tool will be most productive in those organizations that want to increase communication between nurses and administration but lack the technical ability to do so.

Planning

The successful administration of the IWS depends on an appropriate planning phase, the first part of which is clear delineation of motivation at all levels within the organization. To ensure maximum success, all levels of personnel within the administrative hierarchy should be involved. For example, if nurses in a hospital are to be surveyed, not only should hospital administrators be involved, but nurse administrators, staff nurses, and nurse leadership in the union (if any). Ideally, the use of this scale should arise from a concern to translate often ubiquitous staff dissatisfaction into discrete areas so that specific remedies may be identified. The more that all levels are involved in the planning phase, the more successful the venture will be. Additionally, other areas of concern specific to the organizational setting may be included. This whole measurement process is best viewed as a way of obtaining organized and systematic input from groups not usually heard from.

A specific part of the planning phase is an explicit discussion of the objectives for wanting to measure level of nurse satisfaction. These objectives should be written down, and discussed by all members of the nursing hierarchy. Additionally, each level should develop its own objectives and compare them. For example, nursing staff and nursing administrators may have somewhat different objectives. Communication can be improved only when these objectives are shared and the scope of responsibility is identified.

The process of sharing objectives usually results in the identification of the importance of knowing more about the nursing staff. This generally includes demographic variables as well as many other—always interesting—variables. Whether this information should be included depends on the objectives of the study. In an academic study, it may be desirable to include several demographic variables; in a study whose major objectives are managerial, inclusion of demographic variables may not be productive. In any case, parsimony is the rule: as more items are included, the data collection process becomes longer and more time-consuming for the respondent. When demographic variables are needed, only those that are of immediate relevance or for which there is a strong rationale should be included. Too many apparently unnecessary questions offend the respondent and will decrease the response rate. A good guideline is whether the organization is willing to implement different management strategies based on the results of these demographic items. In some cases (such as differentiating between RNs and LPNs, or differentiating between the various educational tracks in nursing), this may be appropriate; in most cases it is not.

It is usually in the interest of the organization to gather additional information on specific issues that may be important to the nurse respondents and to the organization. Although this questionnaire can be used in that way, caution should be exercised; only those issues important to the group that is being surveyed—and those that have administrative remedies—should be included. To raise other issues may alienate the respondents and may also raise false expectations. For example, to ask a question about nurses' views of control of work shifts without being prepared to decentralize that decision is a form of manipulation and raises expectations unfairly.

Implementation

It is difficult to separate implementation issues from planning issues. The most important single thought about implementation is this: *The IWS is designed to be translated into some type of organizational action based on the understanding gained from the questionnaire.*

This has been true from the earliest days of using the IWS. In one of the earliest research settings, where the IWS was modified for use in an ambulatory setting, the findings of the study resulted in a significant redesign of the task requirements of the ambulatory nurses (Stamps et al. 1978). Work satisfaction is a relative phenomenon and may be quite specific to a particular work environment. The main reason for implementing a satisfaction study should be to create change or to evaluate change within an organization. This scale is designed to help identify organizational dissonance, so that management can provide mechanisms to alleviate the dissonance. Management's ability to build direct strategies on this scale is partly related to three more technical issues: adequate response rate, grouped data, and interpretation of the data. (Interpretation is discussed in the second section of this appendix.)

Adequate Response Rate

It is absolutely imperative to try to maximize the response rate. This issue is raised in several places in the text of this book, especially in Chapters 4 and 6. A larger and more representative sample will obviously allow for more valid statistical analysis and therefore make it possible to interpret subtle differences more accurately. A more practical concern, however, is related to the issues discussed above. If the information is to be used to make decisions, it is imperative that everybody be represented.

The questionnaire can be effectively distributed with paychecks, to individuals or in groups, in person, or by mail to homes. Retrieving the completed questionnaires is more complex and is related to another issue: confidentiality. The use of this data collection instrument triggers an increase in information flow and communication throughout the organization. Respondents must be assured that their responses will remain absolutely confidential. If this assurance cannot be made credible, the respondents may either refuse to answer the questionnaire or give only those answers that they feel are acceptable. Both will bias the data.

The seriousness with which the respondents answer the questionnaire is influenced by their estimation of management's respect for their candid opinions. Therefore, no one who has direct supervisory or administrative authority over the group being surveyed should handle the questionnaires or be involved in the data analysis. Those surveyed can mail their questionnaires back in an envelope that is provided. An alternative strategy is a data collection box that is locked and placed in a nonthreatening location. The best strategy is to have the questionnaires picked up personally by someone outside the hospital administration.

Grouped Data

Grouping data is an additional method of assuring a high response rate by dealing sensitively with the issue of confidentiality. It should be emphasized that no respondent will be identifiable. Most managers will want the measure to include some demographic or organizational characteristics, such as units, floors, work assignments, or shift assignments. To the extent that individual nurses cannot be recognized, these may add important information. However, any necessary compromise must be in the direction of increasing confidentiality rather than increasing data. All possible cross-tabulations of research and demographic variables should be arrayed in "dummy tables" with no fewer than seven persons in the most narrowly defined category, for example, full-time medical-surgical RNs on the fifth floor. In addition, no person who has supervisory authority should handle the raw questionnaires. It is also neither wise nor necessary to have identifying personal characteristics on the questionnaire.

Use of the Standardized IWS

Although the IWS has been designed for managerial use within an organization, the desire to compare one set of results with others has been one of the constant themes of the ten years since the first edition came out, as discussed in Appendix B.

This second edition will inevitably facilitate the comparative use of values obtained from using the IWS. Such comparisons of results of studies are obviously very helpful. For example, the question of whether participatory management systems such as shared governance increase satisfaction can best be answered by comparing a hospital with shared governance to one without such a model. Several practice-based studies included in Chapter 5 and Appendixes E and F do just this.

The only way to do such comparisons, however, is to use the IWS as designed (the revised form appears in Appendix A) and to score it as suggested (as described in Appendix D). This means a loss of flexibility for some investigators, but the benefit is in the increased ability to compare results from one setting to another.

Guidelines for Analysis and Interpretation

This section provides guidelines for both analysis and interpretation of the data collected by the IWS. Although there is a natural overlap between these two topics, there are some important differences, so they will be dealt with separately.

Data Analysis

There are several categories of analysis possible, including qualitative and more subjective analyses as well as the quantitative summary figures that arise from the scoring of the IWS.

1. Weighted Values of Components

The component weighting coefficient is derived from Part A of the questionnaire. It is especially valuable for developing a better understanding of what factors are most important to nurses, and in comparing level of importance to nurses in various work settings.

2. Rankings of Paired Comparisons

By using the component weighting coefficient it is possible to rank-order the six components. This rank order tells what the respondents regard as most important, thus providing information about level of expectations.

3. Mean Component Score

Calculating the mean score for each of the six components from the Likert scale (Part B) provides useful information about each of the components that contributes to level of satisfaction.

4. Ranking of Current Level of Satisfaction

These mean scores are used to create rankings of current level of satisfaction for each of the components.

5. Total Scale Score and Mean Score

The range of the total scale scores from Part B is 44 to 308. This may be conveyed by using a total score or by using a mean score.

6. Adjusted Component Scores

A weighted score for each component can also be calculated. This allows for rankings of components based on both importance and current level of satisfaction.

7. Index of Work Satisfaction

The final summary number available is the IWS, derived from the combination of the component weighting coefficient (Part A) and the mean component score (Part B), and then scaled to represent one summary score.

Three additional analyses that are slightly more qualitative in nature may also be included.

8. Comparison of Dissonance Between Rankings of Paired Comparisons (Part A) and Rankings of Level of Satisfaction (Part B)

The comparison of these two sets of rankings provides important information to help managers plan directions for the types of organizational changes that might be designed. This allows for the setting of priority areas.

9. Frequency Distribution of Responses to Individual Items

This extremely important analysis is too often overlooked. Data should first be examined with all seven possible responses; then the categories can be collapsed into three for presentation purposes if desired. Examination of responses to individual items will provide a lot of guidance to appropriate interpretation of the quantitative figures. In many cases, response to a specific item will provide suggestions for change. This is a more qualitative and subjective assessment, but it is a definite help in the interpretation of the quantitative summary figures.

10. Analysis of Other Data Gathered

It is always tempting to include items that are either of general interest ("curiosity value") or of specific interest to the facility itself. These are often demographic or other descriptive items: education, marital status, full- or part-time status, specialty, length of time worked, administrative responsibilities. It is extremely important to select only those items that seem important in the particular setting. In fact, there is probably no strong rationale for including many of these variables in most studies. The problem here is to remember the focus of the study: what applications may be made of these demographic factors? It may be that the factors will be used to further specify results to target groups, but this specification to small groups may be counterproductive because it increases problems with confidentiality. Additionally, unless management strategies are going to be targeted to specific groups, it is not appropriate to include the level of detail.

Work should not cease on the issue of determining the relationship between level of work satisfaction and demographic factors within the field of nursing. If anything, the ambiguous demographic findings reported throughout this book underscore the need for such basic research. It is important, however, to separate the management objectives from research objectives in the application of this measurement tool.

Of more value are issues of particular interest to a specific organization, including work shifts, availability of continuing education, availability of adequate parking, efforts at unionization, management models, and thoughts on appropriate role definitions, among others. When considering which, if any, of these issues to include, investigators should use only those items that are timely and about which organizational remedies can realistically be designed. To do otherwise promises the respondents too much, raises expectations, and may also create false issues of dissatisfaction. Including too many items "just because they would be interesting to look at" undermines investigators' ability to maximize the response rate. Encouraging open-ended responses on the survey process and the organization in general is also useful. These responses should be given serious weight in the analysis. They often contain valuable insights into the nurses' perceptions.

Interpretation: General Guidelines

The analysis process produces a wealth of numerical information, which immediately raises the question of what conclusions to draw as a result of the data. Generating the numbers—despite a tedious scoring process for those using both parts of the scale—is actually easier than interpreting what the numbers mean.

Table B.1 (in Appendix B) shows the numbers, their ranges, and the quartiles for the range for the scores from the paired comparisons and the attitude scale part of the IWS. These are the scores that were determined during the 1985 validation study and reported in the 1986 book. Chapter 4 gives ranges from the 50 studies contributed to this second edition. These obviously help set the context for a particular research site. They also raise the issue of making comparisons. Once comparisons start, setting acceptable standards for satisfaction will not be far behind. This edition will probably accelerate this process, both with the publication of the data in Chapter 4 and the availability of a specific comparative database, as described in Appendix D. Given the increased experience with the IWS in the ten years since the publication of the first edition, the move to comparative studies and to setting standards is appropriate. However, there are two important general issues that need to be remembered in this process.

Numbers Versus Quartiles

There are two ways in which the numerical scores can be interpreted. The first is obviously as absolute numbers. For example, the score for the autonomy component is 35.2. This is easy to use for comparisons, but to do so misses an important point, which is the possible range of the score. For the autonomy component, for example, the range of scores is from 8 to 56. This means that a score of 35.2 is just slightly above the fiftieth percentile, or in the second quartile. Knowing this is obviously important to the accurate interpretation of the numerical score of 35.2.

The data in Chapter 4 are discussed in this way because it is more appropriate to describe conclusions based on an understanding of the range of scores for each component than simply in terms of the absolute score. First of all, this gives a more complete understanding of exactly what a 35.2 means, since any number is meaningless without knowing the range. Second, since the ranges of the various components are not the same, using quartiles—or percentiles—allows for easy comparisons across all the components.

It is also more appropriate to set standards for level of satisfaction using quartiles rather than absolute numbers. This allows for a range of scores to be viewed as acceptable. An organization might decide to set a uniform standard across the board and say that scores on each of the components should be above the fiftieth percentile, or in the third quartile. Another organization might select one or more components for particular attention and decide that the satisfaction scores on organizational policies and task requirements should be at the top of the third quartile, for example.

It is an ironic quirk of our highly technological society to have a sense of dissatisfaction with our limited ability to do more with these numbers. However, until the development of the IWS, not much could be said definitively about level of satisfaction of nurses. With this second edition, because of the increased use of the IWS, it is possible to meet the objective of having comparative data, an objective initially set in the first edition. Even with this wide application, it is important to remember the difficulty of the concept that is being measured. Using quartiles for interpreting the data will reinforce a certain caution in the types of conclusions that can be drawn.

Purpose of the Study

As is obvious from the many practice-based studies included in this volume, one of the most positive aspects of the research going on now in the nursing field is that there is a blurring of the lines between academic research and managerial use of the IWS. This contributes to reality-based research that is very useful to the field. However, it should be recognized that it is sometimes quite appropriate to acknowledge the differences between more academic research and more applied research. In terms of using the IWS to measure satisfaction, both the types of calculations done and the nature of the interpretation accomplished are related in large part to the purpose of the study.

In studies whose major purpose is applied research, that is, managerial or specific evaluative purposes, the major emphasis of the analysis should be the mean scores of each of the components (analysis category 3 above). In this way, the effect of a specific job redesign effort can be more specifically assessed. For example, in Mancini's study (Chapter 5, Selection 4), the score on the organizational policies component increased after a hospital's long-term experience with a shared-governance model. Although the numerical change was small, it was important because this component is so dissatisfying. One of the most appropriate ways of interpreting these data is to develop a graphic profile of the mean score of each component. In this way, changes in each component can be tracked over time and easily compared. This is especially appropriate when the IWS is being used in a monitoring system, as described in Chapter 5, Selections 1, 2, and 3.

Another analysis that should be at the center of an applied use of the IWS is the frequency distribution of responses to individual items on the attitude scale (category 9). Although it seems tedious to interpret these results, the responses to the items very often assist both in understanding the perceptions of the respondents about the current situation and in creating appropriate job redesign strategies. Interpretation of these items should include a traditional social psychological approach, which preserves as much information as possible. This approach retains all seven response modes, especially in the initial interpretation. This is important because an attitude is more adequately represented by a range than by a specific point. This range is referred to as a latitude; it may be either a latitude of acceptance or a latitude of rejection. Someone who responds Strongly Agree (or Strongly Disagree) to a statement generally has a more narrow latitude of acceptance, which indicates a more intense feeling. A person responding either Moderately Agree or Moderately Disagree usually has a wider latitude of acceptance, indicating feelings that are not as intense. If one particular item on the attitude scale generates a pattern of responses that involve mostly Strongly Agree (or Strongly Disagree), this indicates a perception that is strongly polarized. Knowing the pattern of responses is of value to organizations that want to be able to change situations so that feelings of satisfaction will also change.

Additionally, it is particularly helpful for an organization to identify one or two specific items within each component to use as "indicator items." The responses to indicator items can be monitored over time as part of the profile used to keep track of the mean scores for the components. These items will most likely be specific to different organizations, which may preclude comparisons between sites. However, it should be recognized that an inherent part of the use of the IWS for mostly managerial purposes is that the focus is internal rather than primarily comparative. Although some comparison with other organizations is obviously helpful, the most important comparisons are those made over time in the same organization, especially when evaluating specific managerial interventions. Again, several of the practice-based research selections included in this volume provide excellent examples of this.

Studies with a managerial focus should not ignore the paired-comparisons part of the questionnaire, but should use it in a manner slightly different from studies with a more academic focus. It is valuable for managerial studies to give the paired-comparisons part of the questionnaire, but probably only one time, and usually the first time in a study which involves multiple data collection points. The major reason for collecting data on paired comparisons is to identify those components in which there is the most dissonance between what is viewed as being of highest importance and what is viewed as being most satisfying (category 8). This process will help identify those specific areas of the organization that need the most attention or the most immediate remedies. This is consistent with the original purpose of the measurement tool, which is to divide the concept of satisfaction into separate component parts.

As discussed in Chapter 4, this is also related to a recent reconsideration of the value of one weighted summary number rather than the designation of the separate components. This does not mean that the weighted or adjusted numbers are not relevant, but they are certainly less relevant for studies with a primarily managerial focus.

Those studies with primarily an academic focus are characterized by a desire for comparative information, and they are frequently associated with a one-time data collection process. Because of this comparative focus, the weighted aspect of the scale is probably more useful to these research efforts. These studies will be more likely to calculate the component weighting coefficient values from the paired comparisons and to use these values (category 1) rather than the rankings (category 2). Such use of the measurement tool allows for the development of a greater knowledge base about what is of highest importance to nurses. It also allows for comparisons by site. At present, for example, there is not enough known about whether nurses who practice in hospitals value different components than those practicing in home care or ambulatory care settings.

Just because the study is more academic in its focus does not necessarily mean it has no interest in how specific job redesign initiatives affect satisfaction. A still unanswered question, for example, is what effect organizational change has on level of expectations. Although these expectations probably change less rapidly than satisfaction levels, there is no indication that they remain stable throughout a nurse's professional career.

Studies that are more academic in purpose may also be concerned with the current level of satisfaction, and as such may use the component mean scores also. However, it is more likely that the total scale score and total mean score (category 5) may be especially appropriate because of the ease in comparison. Likewise, the weighted score of the Index itself is especially appropriate for such comparisons.

Demographic data (category 10) are particularly suited to studies with an interest in comparative research, as such information may not be critically important for evaluation of one specific organization but is clearly important for the continuing work to develop a better understanding of factors outside the organization that may affect satisfaction levels.

Naturally, the two types of research are not totally distinct from each other. It is impossible to separate completely an organization's concerns from larger professional issues. The practice-based research examples included in this book demonstrate this clearly. Even though demographic factors are more appropriate for academic research, there may be clear reasons for including them in a management-oriented study. For example, an ongoing question is whether levels of satisfaction differ by type of educational preparation for nursing. A hospital might change its role definitions or staffing patterns after doing a satisfaction study that included the variable of educational preparation. Another example is the total scale score (category 5) which, as a summary figure, is especially appropriate for comparisons, but also acts as a general warning flag to organizations in terms of predicting overall level of satisfaction.

These two general applications—research oriented, which has primarily an external focus, and management-oriented, which has primarily an internal focus—should not be overdichotomized. However, it is important for investigators to understand the differing values of the data to the specific internal needs of a particular organization, or to the ability to compare types of hospitals, or to the contribution to basic research within the nursing profession. Without this reflection, studies generate too much data and investigators or managers feel overwhelmed. In those cases, the data are often simply set aside. The losses from this are twofold. One is a generalized, long-term loss of knowledge that might be useful in better understanding what provides satisfaction to nurses. The second loss is at first glance more specific and immediate: that is the inability to determine whether a particular managerial initiative had any effect on either the performance or the satisfaction of nurses. This situation is too often generalized, when in fact the problem is either not completely implementing the intervention (as Ingersoll notes in Chapter 5, Selection 1) or not completely analyzing and interpreting the data. Identifying specific sets of information and completely analyzing and interpreting the data will be much more helpful, in both the short run and the long run.

References

Stamps, P. L., E. B. Piedmonte, A. B. Haase, and D. B. Slavitt. 1978. "Measurement of Work Satisfaction among Health Professionals." *Medical Care* 16 (April): 337–52.

GAINING PERMISSION TO USE THE INDEX OF WORK SATISFACTION AND OBTAINING SCORING ASSISTANCE

The Index of Work Satisfaction is a copyrighted scale and may only be used by permission. In the first edition of this book, the copyright was held by Health Administration Press, which necessitated that investigators interested in using the scale write two letters: one to the author and one to Health Administration Press. With this second edition, the process has been streamlined. The copyright is now held solely by the author. Researchers who wish to use this instrument should write a letter requesting permission, and as part of this letter, briefly describe the proposed study. The primary reason for this is to keep the author apprised of the type of research using the IWS. Permission to use the IWS will be given quickly, although investigators must allow time for the mail process, as fax or e-mail communication will not be used for this. Such letters should be sent to:

Dr. Paula Stamps, Professor
Community Health Studies Department
School of Public Health and Health Sciences
Arnold House
University of Massachusetts
Amherst, MA 01003

Please contact the author by telephone (413/545-6880) or fax (413/545-6536) with any additional questions or comments.

Because of the many questions about the scoring process, as well as some complaints, more technical assistance is now available to support this part of the process of using the IWS. Three objectives provided guidance in arranging for such technical assistance. The first related to necessity: as the IWS evolves into the next stage of wider applicability, one of the major issues will be the comparability of results. Using the questionnaire exactly as it is designed and using the same scoring procedure is critical for the comparisons to be meaningful. If norms or standards for satisfaction arise from this process—as is likely—their validity will depend on the data from which they arise. If there are many variations in the research process, these standards will not be well accepted in the field. The first survey of users (conducted in 1983 prior to the first edition of this book) discovered substantial variation both in using the questionnaire and in the scoring procedures. The second survey of users (conducted just prior to this second edition) revealed much less variation, in both the use of the questionnaire and the scoring procedures. However, there is still too much variation for the development of standards. The availabilty of technical assistance will provide enough standardization at least in the scoring procedures for more credible comparisons and the development of standards.

The second objective, however, was to recognize that not everybody either wants or needs such comparisons, nor is everybody interested in the development of standards for nurse satisfaction. A substantial number of users are primarily interested in their own results, which are usually specific to a particular organization. To force a standardized use on them would be inappropriate. Also, this would curb the revisions and changes in the IWS that are necessary for further refinement and development of the measurement instrument. This means that the technical assistance that is available must be flexible and provide support to a wide variety of studies using the IWS.

The third objective was to make sure the technical assistance was not so expensive that it curtailed the use of the IWS in the field. This would obviously be counterproductive to the increased application of this measurement tool. A substantial proportion of current users are graduate students, and their experience is valuable, as they are frequently working in areas that include both an academic and a more applied emphasis.

To meet all three of these objectives, a menu approach to technical assistance was developed. The following services are available, and investigators are urged to select only those that are applicable to their particular research. Services are available individually or in combination with one another.

1. **Questionnaires.** The copyrighted version of the IWS questionnaire is available on disk (as well as paper), formatted for the data collection process. Customized questionnaires may also be designed, either with additional items or with minor changes in wording.

2. **Scoring instructions.** A packet that gives the step-by-step instructions for scoring the IWS is available for a modest price. This is a simplified version that is easy to follow. The packet describes the method for scoring both parts of the questionnaire, but the instructions for each part are given separately for those who are using only one part of the scale. These instructions may be used to create computerized scoring programs. Although the scoring procedures are not difficult, they are tedious, so using a computer is obviously helpful.

3. **Scoring service.** For those who do not wish to score their own questionnaires, investigators can mail in their completed questionnaires, which will be scored for them. Prices for this will vary depending on the number and type of analyses desired.

4. **Data analysis and interpretation.** Two levels of analytic reports are available. The first is a brief technical report summarizing the results and presenting a brief comparison to general national data, similar to that presented in Chapter 4. The second is a more detailed analysis of the findings, including comparison of the results to a database that is specifically relevant to the particular setting of the study. For example, if the research involves respondents who are working in a 200-bed hospital with shared governance, the comparison will involve a hospital of similar size with a participative management model. The report will also include recommendations based on the analysis of the data from the satisfaction survey. Prices will vary depending on the extent and specificity of the report.

5. **Technical assistance in design.** Although many studies using the IWS are straightforward, some involve more complicated designs. Some studies using the IWS involve management or job redesign initiatives and are primarily concerned with evaluation. Assistance is available in designing these studies and interpreting the results. Management consulting, the creation of alternative managerial systems, and evaluation design are also available. Prices for this are determined based on individual requirements.

These services are being provided primarily for those who would like to use the IWS in an organization in an ongoing monitoring system or as a formal part of the accreditation process or in a large-scale evaluation. The services are available from Market Street Research, a full-service independent marketing research firm. Market Street Research has 20 years of experience in providing custom-designed research and evaluation services to clients in a wide range of health and human services organizations, including hospitals, HMOs, mental health providers, outpatient clinics, and a wide variety of nonprofit organizations, both large and small.

Market Street Research specializes in state-of-the-art research design with an emphasis on providing design assistance that is uniquely suited to a particular organization. Market Street Research has particular expertise in strategic planning, community image studies, member and patient satisfaction research, employee satisfaction research, and evaluation research. The costly, time-consuming, and routine aspects of market research have been computerized to reduce costs and to allow the staff more time to analyze and interpret findings.

The initial database described in Chapter 4 is now available at Market Street Research. As noted in Chapter 4, this involves comparing mean scores from studies. It is hoped that the database will evolve into one that can present comparisons on groups of respondents rather than groups of studies. This will occur as investigators send their questionnaires in for scoring. It will also be possible for those people who wish to score their own questionnaires to have access to the database; they will be able to receive comparisons based on groups of studies, similar to those presented in Chapter 4.

Regardless of whether the data are shared after the investigator calculates the scores or Market Street Research scores the raw questionnaires, it is important that all data be entered into the database so it will be current. Any time an investigator uses any of the technical services, their data will be entered into the database. No data set will ever be available individually to anyone but the investigator, and once entered into the database, individual data sets will not be identifiable.

The exact nature of the database and the range of technical services available will vary and no doubt change over time, as will the prices for each of the possible technical services.

When contacting Market Street Research for a description of all support services available, as well as prices, simply indicate your interest in obtaining information about the IWS and you will be referred to the appropriate person. Market Street Research can be contacted at:

Market Street Research
26 Market Street
Northampton, MA 01060
Phone (413) 584–0465
Fax (413) 582–1206
E-mail: MarketSt@crocker.com

APPENDIX

USING THE IWS IN PRACTICE-BASED RESEARCH

As noted in Chapter 5, this book contains 40 different examples of practice-based research using the IWS as a measure of satisfaction. The five selections in Chapter 5 have a particular emphasis on using the IWS to evaluate changes in level of satisfaction as a result of some organizational innovation.

Some of the 15 contributions included in this appendix and the 20 included in Appendix F share this interest but with fewer data collection points or smaller samples. The format of these 15 contributions is that of a research brief: the investigators submitted full-length contributions, but space constraints restricted what could be included here. In many cases what was left out was data, but in other cases it was an analytic literature review. The investigators' addresses, and often telephone numbers, are included here (as well as in Appendix F) to facilitate the reader's ability to contact them for more information.

The process of selecting the contributions to be included in this book, including the most appropriate format for each one, has clearly been the most difficult part of preparing this second edition. The range of these studies is impressive, as are the variety of ways in which they include satisfaction as a variable. Although many of these studies— but not all, by any means—are unpublished, the main reason for this does not necessarily lie in their methodology, as the sample sizes and response rates of published studies using the IWS are not substantially different (see Table 6.2). It is important to increase the dissemination of knowledge about measuring satisfaction, both the process of the research as well as the results. The 15 studies contained here and the 20 studies in Appendix F substantially improve the knowledge base about how to change organizations to improve nurse satisfaction as well as how to understand the complexities of conceptualizing satisfaction and the role of organizations in its determination.

If one theme can be identified for the studies in this appendix, it is a concern for ways to increase the ability of healthcare organizations, especially hospitals, to retain nurses. This theme is represented over many different settings and several specific types of nurses.

The first two contributions are part of the large research project that is a joint effort between Miami Valley Hospital and Wright State University. (See also Gustin et al. Chapter 5, Selection 2.) Schmidt and Martin (Selection 1) and Martin et al. (Selection 2) investigated the relationship between work satisfaction and esprit, which is a way to measure morale and is viewed as a component of organizational climate. Their design involved measures over two points in time in a hospital located in an Ohio town of 8,000 people. They were able to show a moderate relationship between esprit and work satisfaction.

More important, perhaps, is their finding of relatively high levels of work satisfaction, which Schmidt attributes to the small size of the hospital. As Schmidt points out, there are few levels of administration in this small hospital. She also discusses the close relationship between the nurses and the community: "Interaction of nurses not only occurs in the facility, but also among their children and spouses in school, area industry, church, and other community activities. Many of the persons growing up in this community return to this area after time, thus facilitating extended family relationships."

In Selection 3, Klingshirn reinforces some of these themes, since her research also focused on rural settings. "Within a small rural hospital where employee numbers are low, RNs are viewed as leaders and this gives them a sense of self-esteem." Her study, which also showed high levels of work satisfaction, especially with organizational policies, a relatively dissatisfying component, took place in three separate hospitals in northern lower Michigan.

All three of these selections are concerned with special problems that exist in rural areas that influence the ability of healthcare organizations to maintain nurses in their facilities. Dunkin, Stratton, and Juhl (Selection 4) also focused on this problem. With funding from the Office of Rural Health Policy located in the Health Resources and Services Administration, they created a theoretical model that attempts to capture all the relevant variables involved in rural nurses' decision to remain with or leave their institutions. Theirs is a massive study, involving more than 3,000 nurses in six states. They included nurses working in hospitals, skilled nursing facilities, and community and public health agencies, and they created models for each of these settings that describe the relationship between job satisfaction and retention. The models provide an extremely helpful way of analyzing the various reasons for nurses leaving or staying in jobs. Their work supports the notion of separating out as many of the complicated variables as possible for analysis.

Many of the rest of the contributions in this appendix also argue for separation of variables so complicated relationships can be better understood. The next three—Adams, Burns Tuck, and McCrea—share a common interest, which is the careful analysis of the degree and type of stress nurses experience as part of their jobs. All three also used a variety of other scales to measure some of the variables involved. Burns Tuck surveyed 127 nurse managers and head nurses working in 14 general acute care hospitals in Pennsylvania, with an overall response rate of 60 percent. Her relatively high response rate and the use of several other validated measurement instruments examining stress and social support contribute to a strong study in a general area in which there are contradictory findings. In her study, high perceived levels of stress were related to lower levels of job satisfaction . Lower levels of social support also contributed to job-related stress.

Adams's research involved all staff RNs in a large, nonprofit urban hospital. Her focus was to analyze the relationship between stress, job satisfaction, and organizational commitment. Like Dunkin, Stratton, and Juhl, Adams created a statistical model to analyze the relative contributions of the several variables in what is a very complicated relationship. In this model, she used each of the six components of the IWS separately, which gave her more sensitive results. The results of her study also demonstrate a relationship between work satisfaction and stress. All of the work satisfaction components except for professional status were negatively influenced by stress, with an especially strong relationship between work stress and task requirements: "The strong inverse association between work stress and satisfaction with task requirements supports work redesign efforts that relieve the nurse of mundane tasks such as paperwork and housekeeping duties. Nurses expect to practice nursing rather than perform tasks better suited to support personnel."

McCrea took a slightly different approach to the relationship of stress and work satisfaction. She studied 90 nurses working in critical care units in four southwestern hospitals. She acknowledges that an important reason for her study is the particularly high cost of training and replacing such specialty nursing staff. Rather than focusing on the nature of the job, which is known for its high stress levels, she chose to concentrate on identifying factors that affect an individual's perception of and response to stress. Her research is anchored in what is known as personality hardiness, and she uses the most recent third-generation measurement tool to assess this factor. (Her literature review on stress and personality factors is an excellent introduction to an important area usually researched by psychologists.) She found high levels of personality hardiness among the nurses she surveyed. She was also able to demonstrate a significant relationship between work satisfaction and personality hardiness, especially for the subscales of nurse-physician interaction, professional status, and autonomy. She concludes that the correlation between work satisfaction and personality hardiness creates a pathway for nursing administrators. . . . Staff may be selected for these attributes as well as programs designed to enhance them. Because of the association with burnout and turnover, the monitoring of work satisfaction is crucial for administrators.

The next three selections—Hlavac, Rush, and Cooley—also discuss stress, but their purpose is primarily to set the context for understanding the level of satisfaction of a variety of specifically trained nurses who practice in high-stress areas, including medical-surgical, telemetry, and critical care nurses (Hlavac); neonatal intensive care unit nurses (Rush); and operating room nurses (Cooley). Hlavac surveyed 93 nurses (with a 75 percent response rate) and compared the responses of those working in a medical-surgical or telemetry unit with those working in a critical care unit. In her study, she could not demonstrate any differences, with the exception of finding that medical-surgical nurses were more dissatisfied than nurses working in a critical care unit. She also discovered that nobody was very satisfied. Her contribution contains an excellent review of the literature on the critical care nurse, which also demonstrates contradictory findings. Her conclusion is to encourage more research on this important work setting for nurses.

Rush and Cooley approached their research from the perspective of identifying possible management responses to a specific type of nursing that may involve a more stressful work environment. Rush studied 100 nurses working in Level III neonatal intensive care units in medical centers in the New York City area. Her emphasis was to relate work satisfaction, conflict management style, clinically assertive behavior, and collegial behavior. The level of satisfaction she found is slightly higher than that of other studies. She was not able to demonstrate many relationships between work satisfaction and the other variables, with the exception of one hospital in which collegiality was significantly related to higher levels of work satisfaction.

Cooley's work involved 49 operating room nurses from two midwestern teaching hospitals, each of which had clinical ladders and a shared-governance type of management. Her study tried to identify differences between the two hospitals on a variety of variables, including several demographic variables. The nurses in her study were most satisfied with autonomy, professional status, and interaction. Their highest level of dissatisfaction was with the role of circulating nurse: the greater the percentage of time spent in the circulator role, the lower the level of overall satisfaction. Cooley speculates on reasons for this, providing some interesting insights on the nature of the operating room nurse. Cooley also found that one hospital was more unhappy with pay than the other. The hospital did a second internal study and documented this, with the result being a change in the pay schedule, especially for on-call operating room nurses. Cooley notes that "conducting this study provided the opportunity to learn the research process and to see how the proper analysis of data can support organizational change."

The next four selections—Ringer et al., Pearson, Joy and Malay, and Prock—focus on using the IWS to measure satisfaction as one way to evaluate organizational change, as did the selections in Chapter 5.

The study by Ringer et al. based at Albany Memorial Hospital, is especially similar to the studies in Chapter 5 in that the IWS is incorporated into an ongoing management system, in this case one used to evaluate the effect of a patient care redesign model involving linking RNs with care partners. The hospital is smaller and not all units were involved at the time of the study, but many of the principles are the same: the investigators used before and after measurements and then annual monitoring over the next three years. Over this period of time, there were statistically significant increases in satisfaction with autonomy and slight increases in satisfaction with professional status.

Pearson also investigated the effect of case management. Her selection focuses on the use of a modification of the case management model, Modified Differentiated Case Management, and provides an excellent review of the literature on the various models of case management. This study is set in a rural hospital in Wisconsin, and, although the sample sizes are small, the response rates are very high, 100 percent and 96 percent. These results provide useful insight into a the ability of a small rural hospital to develop alternatives for the nursing staff. Although there were no clear-cut answers on whether the case management model improved satisfaction, she notes that the process of studying satisfaction enhanced the implementation of the model. Also, as she notes, it may be that not enough time had passed for nurses to feel the effect of the model.

Joy and Malay describe an alternative to case management, a professional practice model developed and implemented at New England Baptist Hospital in Boston. One of the major components of the model is primary nursing. The design to evaluate the model involved before-and-after measurements of nurse and patient satisfaction, the quality of nursing documentation, and interdisciplinary collaboration. Nurse satisfaction and patient satisfaction were high before implementation of the model and remained high. The quality of nursing documentation demonstrated a sharp increase. Like Pearson, Joy and Malay note that this particular study needs to be conducted again after enough time has elapsed to appreciate the effect of the model.

Prock (Selection 14) considers participative management: her study has many similarities to Mancini's (Chapter 5, Selection 4). Both studies compare a hospital with shared governance to another hospital without shared governance. Prock's study had an interesting difference in response rate: only 15 percent responded in the hospital without shared governance, in comparison to 40 percent in the hospital with shared governance. Prock was not able to show any difference in satisfaction between these two hospitals, but she noted both the problem with the response rate and the fact that the shared governance program had just started. In Mancini's study, the hospital with shared governance had had this model for seven years, and in the Gustin et al. study (Chapter 5, Selection 2), the shared-governance model had existed for ten years. In these two studies, the hospital with shared governance had higher levels of nurse satisfaction than the hospital without shared governance. The nurses were especially more satisfied with autonomy, organizational policies, and task requirements. This finding underscores the importance of allowing enough time for the organization to change, as has been noted also by Ingersoll et al. (Chapter 5, Selection 1) and Minnick, Pischke-Winn, and Thomas (Chapter 5, Selection 3), among others.

Although the major theme running through all the contributions in this appendix as well as in Chapter 5 is the importance of the organization in affecting job satisfaction, the study by Koeckeritz (Selection 15) is a reminder that factors outside the organization affect job satisfaction also. Koeckeritz begins her selection with the thought that the job satisfaction of nurses has declined over the past 20 years while working conditions have improved. She concludes with the observation that "Changing the work environment has not alleviated the problems of low satisfaction." She focuses on issues related to the lives of women, especially domestic labor, or what she calls the "second shift." She describes research that surveyed staff nurses at four metropolitan hospitals. Her study measured feminist attitudes and amount of time spent in various areas of domestic labor, including household and child care. The analysis of the several variables is interesting, and, as might be expected, presents a mixed picture. Her contribution is especially valuable in that it enlarges the focus to the lives of the (mostly) women who are nurses and also enlarges the conceptual background of satisfaction to include the theories related to feelings of alienation. Further, her literature review covers several academic disciplines. She includes an excellent review of the domestic labor responsibilities of women and feminist theory as well as job satisfaction and alienation, from a sociological perspective as well as from the nursing perspective.

These 15 contributions provide a window on the research issues that are of significant interest to nursing professionals in the field. It is clear from these studies that an issue of continuing importance is the problem of nurse retention. Each of the contributions addresses this problem in one way or another. However, this is not the only concern: in fact, the contributions are striking in the diversity of issues researched. It is particularly noteworthy that these nurse investigators are willing and able to use concepts and measurement tools from many other of the social and behavioral sciences, as shown in Table 6.1. There is much creative thinking in evidence here. The result is an enlarged view of what should be investigated about nurses.

Many of the studies demonstrate only moderate relationships between nurse satisfaction and the variables in which the investigators are interested. This is primarily a result of trying to measure things that are hard to measure, among them perceived stress, morale or esprit, organizational commitment, personality hardiness, and self-esteem. Although many of the tools used to measure these complex concepts have been used before, many are old or were modified by the investigators, leading to concerns about the validity of the measures. These are important variables, and it is surely worthwhile to develop some accurate measures.

Methodological problems common to many of these studies are small sample size, low response rate, or both. Chapter 6 addresses these problems more fully; they are important limitations to try to overcome. Although two of the studies in this appendix had response rates of 75 percent and 60 percent, they were the exceptions, and several studies cautioned against generalizing their results because of the small number of respondents. Both published and unpublished studies share this problem, which is another reason why more information needs to be shared about the research process. Improving response rates is critical to generating trustworthy results.

Many of the studies focused on the nurse as a member of an organization, which is an increasingly common focus. Dunkin, Stratton, and

Juhl's study is a reminder of how important it is to attempt to capture the "whole nurse," since in their models, one of the most important variables affecting retention was the nurse's level of satisfaction with the community itself. Koeckeritz enlarges that orientation to include the whole life of the nurse outside the organization. Both of these studies serve as not-too-subtle reminders that the problems being investigated are complicated. The problems are complex enough when the organization is the major unit of analysis. When the analysis encompasses factors outside the scope of the organization, it becomes almost overwhelming. We should not be too surprised at the relatively few "sure" answers that seem to be represented in this appendix—or in this whole book, for that matter. The investigators are addressing hard, real-world problems: it may be progress enough to be able to know what to ask and come to an agreement on how to measure it.

1. A Comparative Study of Work Satisfaction of Nurses and the Relationship of Work Satisfaction to Espirit

Carol Sue Schmidt and Patricia Martin

This study compares the overall work satisfaction and component scores of registered nurses at a rural hospital at two points in time, and then examines the relationship between work satisfaction as measured by the IWS and one aspect of organizational climate, esprit. Esprit was measured by items developed from a modified version of the Nurse Organization Climate Description Questionnaire (Duxbury, Henley, and Armstrong 1982).

A rural hospital in northwest Ohio is the setting for the research. This acute care facility is JCAHO-accredited and has a capacity of 130 beds, providing 24-hour emergency care and a broad range of medical-surgical services. Data were collected in 1990 and 1994. Between these two times, the hospital made several management changes. In 1990, 61 nurses responded, and in 1994, 86 nurses responded.

Summary of Major Results

Data analysis describes mean scores for the six components of work satisfaction, which were as follows for Time 1 and Time 2 respectively: pay (3.6 and 3.5); autonomy (4.9 and 4.9); task requirements (3.0 and 3.4); organizational policies (3.2 and 3.1); interaction (5.2 and 5.2); and professional status (5.4 and 5.6). The total scale score in 1990 was 190.9 and in 1994 was 192.5. Correlation of esprit and work satisfaction at Time 2 was $r = .52, p = .001$. Although this study did not reveal an increase in overall work satisfaction, it did find that the group surveyed had a moderately high level of esprit (mean=24.6).

Discussion and Observations

Although there were no significant changes in either overall satisfaction or the component scores between 1990 and 1994, there was a substantive increase in the number of nurses willing to participate in the data collection process.

Carol Sue Schmidt, R.N., C., M.S., is Assistant Professor of Nursing at Lima Technical College, Lima, Ohio. This is part of her master's thesis. Patricia A. Martin, R.N., Ph.D., is Director of Nursing Research at Wright State University–Miami Valley College of Nursing and Health, Dayton, Ohio.

For more information about this study, contact Carol Sue Schmidt at 4240 Campus Drive, Lima, OH 45885. Telephone (419) 394-5914.

The overall satisfaction scores were relatively high, most likely due to the small size of the facility, which has few levels of administration thus facilitating communication between staff and management. Esprit was also relatively high among the nurses in this facility, which is probably also partly due to the small size of the community (8,000) in which the hospital is located. Interaction occurs not only among nurses in the hospital but among their children and spouses in school, area industry, and church and other community activities. Future research in rural settings should incorporate feelings of community, as Dunkin, Stratton, and Juhl suggest in Selection 4.

2. Properties of Work Satisfaction Instrument: Work Satisfaction Relationships with Other Research Instruments

Patricia A. Martin, Phyllis B. Risner, Linda Cox, Tammy
Gustin, Gayle Jordan, and Kimbra Kahle Paden

This study reports on the relationships found between work satisfaction, as measured by the Index of Work Satisfaction, and several other measured organizational dimensions thought to be important to nurse administrators. Descriptive statistics for the IWS over time and the relationship of the IWS to demographics are reported. The main contribution is in terms of how the IWS has been shown to relate to other dimensions in a longitudinal study and in a one-time replication at a second site.

A coalition of hospital nursing and graduate nurse faculty planned the longitudinal study to take place in a midwestern JCAHO-accredited teaching hospital of more than 700 beds. Data were collected from a population of 1,200 nurses seven times between December 1990 and January 1995. The factors measured were: (1) work satisfaction, measured by the IWS; (2) organizational climate, measured by a modification of Duxbury's instrument (Duxbury et al. 1984; Martin 1993); (3) professional practice climate, measured by Miller's Professional Practice Climate Instrument (Martin 1993); (4) professional nursing autonomy, measured by the Schutzenhofer Nursing Activity Scale (Schutzenhofer 1983); and (5) communication satisfaction, measured by a modified version of Downs and Hazen's questionnaire (Cox 1992; Downs and Hazen 1997).

In addition to the longitudinal survey, the investigators administered a one-time survey at a different teaching hospital to establish a baseline for evaluating the effect of a new shared-governance model.

Patricia A. Martin, R.N., Ph.D., is Director of Nursing Research at Wright State University–Miami Valley College of Nursing and Health, Dayton, Ohio. Phyllis B. Risner, R.N., Ph.D., is Professor Emeritus at Wright State University–Miami Valley College of Nursing and Health, Dayton, Ohio. Linda Cox, R.N., M.S., is Nurse Manager at Miami Valley Hospital, Dayton, Ohio. Tammy Gustin, R.N., M.S., is Administrative Officer at Miami Valley Hospital, Dayton, Ohio. Gayle Jordan, R.N., M.S., is Orthopedic Case Manager at Miami Valley Hospital, Dayton, Ohio. Kimbra Kahle Paden, R.N., M.S., is Clinical Nurse Specialist at Miami Valley Hospital, Dayton, Ohio.

Acknowledgment is given to others on the research team: Therese C. Lupo, R.N., M.S., Director of Nursing Administration, and Jean Corron, R.N., B.S.N., Infection Control Nurse, both at Miami Valley Hospital.

Funding for this research was provided by the Miami Valley Hospital Division of Nursing and a Faculty Collaboration Seed Grant from the Wright State University and Miami Valley Hospital Collaborative Agreement.

For more information about this study, contact Patricia A. Martin, 481 Cloverhill Court; Beavercreek, OH 45440. Telephone (513) 873-2579.

Summary of Major Results

Table E.1 shows the overall values for work satisfaction for each of the data collection points. Mean values for each of the components are available from the author. The mean values for each component demonstrated a pattern similar to the overall scores: all values were lower in the second hospital.

Regression models were constructed to analyze the relationship between the various measures. Details of all regression models are available from the author. The IWS shows expected relationships to complementary concepts but clearly differentiates from autonomy ($R^2 = .13$), climate ($R^2 = .45$), and professional practice climate ($R^2 = .35$). The internal consistency measurements for the whole IWS and five of the subscales of the IWS were found to be most satisfactory (total scale alpha = .89, five subscales .71–.88). One IWS subscale, professional status, deserves special attention due to low internal consistency (alpha = .32). (See Appendix B, Section IV for a further discussion of this.)

Discussion and Observations

The IWS can provide organizations with very useful information about level of satisfaction. It is also an instrument that can be used successfully in combination with other measures needed for organizational assessment. The IWS as a measure is complementary to and not repetitive of other organizational dimension measures.

The findings that were produced by this study are similar to those reported by Blegen (1993) in her meta-analysis of work satisfaction.

Table E.1   Total Work Satisfaction, Site One and Site Two

	N	Mean
Total WS: Site One		
December 1990	120	192.3
May 1991	159	198.4
November 1991	143	194.7
September 1992	155	200.1
June 1993	135	196.7
January 1994	184	192.3
January 1995	182	194.1
Site Two	91	184.6

3. Variables Influencing Job Satisfaction in Rural Health Nursing

Jennie M. Klingshirn

The purpose of this study was to identify variables related to the job satisfaction of registered nurses employed in three rural hospitals in northern lower Michigan. The Index of Work Satisfaction tool and a demographic questionnaire were distributed via paycheck to 126 subjects, with a 44 percent response rate. The variables measured included pay, autonomy, professional status, organizational policies, interaction, task requirements, age, years worked at present institution, total years in nursing, and education.

Summary of Major Results

Table E.2 shows the numerical results from this study. As may be seen, pay and autonomy were the most important to this sample, and organizational policies were ranked as least important. This group of rural nurses was most satisfied with professional status and organizational policies and least satisfied with pay. The overall IWS value of 15.94 was higher than the 12.0 value reported by Stamps and Piedmonte (1986).

Several *t*-tests were performed to examine the relationship between the components measured by the IWS and demographic variables including age, length of employment in the hospital, length of time in the

Table E.2 Numerical Scores for Part A, Part B, and Total IWS

Component	Component Weighting Coefficient (Part A)	Component Mean Score (Part B)	Component Total Score (Part B)	Component Adjusted Score (Parts A & B)
Pay	3.44	2.75	16.5	9.46
Autonomy	3.43	5.11	40.9	17.57
Tasks	3.38	4.02	24.1	13.59
Policies	3.07	5.56	38.9	20.41
Status	3.20	5.65	39.6	18.08
Interaction	3.16	5.24	52.4	16.56

IWS Value: 15.94

Jennie M. Klingshirn, M.S.N., R.N., is at Burns Clinic Medical Center in Rogers City, Michigan. This is from her master's thesis.

For more information about this study, contact Jennie Klingshirn at Burns Clinic Medical Center, 573 N. Bradley; Rogers City, MI 49779. Telephone (517) 734-2171; fax (517) 734-2312.

nursing profession, and type of education. None of these *t*-tests was significant.

Discussion and Observations

Job satisfaction for RNs in the rural hospital setting is of concern because of problems with retention along with systemwide healthcare changes. Managers need to learn how factors affect job satisfaction in this unique setting so they can staff the hospital to maximize the meeting of nurses' needs. The IWS provides a way to understand better the different aspects of satisfaction. The overall IWS value obtained in this rural setting was 15.94. The surveyed group were most content with the organizational policies component, indicating they felt a sense of security in their work role. They did not seem to feel the gap between administration and nursing noted in other studies.

Level of satisfaction was also relatively high along with professional status and autonomy, both of which may be perceived differently by rural nurses. For example, within a small rural hospital, RNs are more likely to be viewed as leaders, thus improving their view of their professional status. Also, rural nurses may feel higher levels of autonomy: in a small hospital, physicians or managers are not in the hospital 24 hours a day, so staff nurses are often left to make decisions dealing with emergency situations or other staffing issues. Rural nurses do not rank this component as being as important to their expectations as do urban nurses, but rural nurses feel they are more autonomous. This may be due to the urban hospital having administration around the clock and urban RNs having less decision-making power than rural nurses.

These rural nurses were most dissatisfied with pay, and pay was ranked as most important in terms of expectations. As other studies of rural nurses indicate, there are other rewards important to retention of rural nurses, some of which lie outside the organizational structure. (See Dunkin, Stratton, and Juhl, Selection 4.)

The literature reveals that there are many studies addressing job satisfaction as it relates to nursing. However, additional research needs to be done in the rural setting. It is with these types of studies that nurse managers can learn what makes their staff satisfied so they can retain the staff they have to provide the quality care the rural community needs and expects.

4. Job Satisfaction as a Predictor of Rural Nurse Retention

Jeri W. Dunkin. Terry D. Stratton, and Nyla Juhl

This study was part of a federally funded research project with the general purpose of understanding the job satisfaction of rural nurses, recruitment and retention strategies used by rural directors' of nursing, and the level of vacancies existing in rural healthcare agencies. The study sample involved 3,514 respondents from six states including Vermont, Arkansas, Nebraska, Georgia, Montana, and Colorado. Nurses were working in one of three settings: rural community hospitals, skilled nursing facilities, or community and public health agencies. Level of satisfaction was measured using a shortened version of the IWS. Instead of using the paired-comparisons technique to determine level of importance, the investigators asked respondents to rate each item on a five-point scale of perceived importance.

Summary of Major Results

Several models for explaining retention were developed. A hypothetical model based on the literature was developed, shown in Figure E.1. Then, three setting-specific models were developed based on the data collected from the 3,514 respondents.

Each model revealed somewhat different relationships between the variables; details are available from the authors. In general, the most important "path" to retention was job satisfaction, reinforcing the need for rural nursing administrators to continue to use strategies to increase satisfaction. However, the second most important path affecting retention was the perceived quality of the community in which the nurses live, reinforcing the need for further research into personal factors important in professionals' decision making.

A note of interest regarding using the IWS as a measure of satisfaction is that respondents in this study were asked to rate overall satisfaction

Jeri W. Dunkin, Ph.D., is Coordinator of Research, School of Nursing, Medical College of Georgia. At the time of this research she was Chair, Nursing Division, University of North Dakota Rural Health Research Center (UND RHRC). Terry D. Stratton, M.A., is currently a doctoral student at the University of Kentucky. At the time of the research he was a Research Analyst at the UND RHRC. Nyla Juhl, Ph.D., R.N., C.P.N.P., is Director, Parent Child Nursing at UND and a member of the UND RHRC.

This research was supported by the Office of Rural Health Policy in the Health Resources and Services Administration, U.S. Department of Health and Human Services (Grant No. CSR000005-05-0).

For more information about this study, contact Jeri Dunkin at the Medical College of Georgia; Augusta, GA 30912. Telephone (706) 721-3162; fax (706) 721-0655; E-mail: jdunkin@mail.mcg.edu

Figure E.1   Retention Model for Rural Registered Nurses

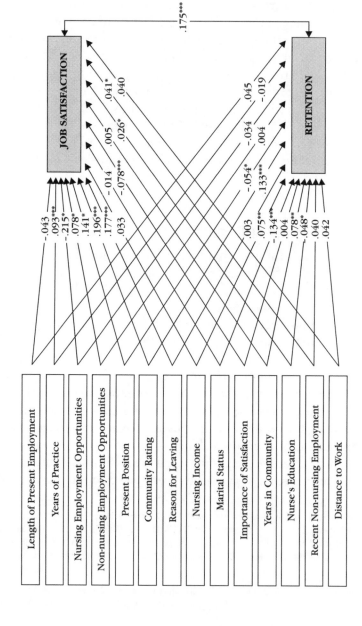

with their job on a five-point scale. The correlation with responses to that item and the overall score on the IWS was greater than .80, reinforcing the structural integrity of the IWS.

Discussion and Observations

Rural nurses in this study were dissatisfied with a number of aspects of their jobs, and many of the points of dissatisfaction were very important to them. However, leaving their current jobs was not part of their plan. This retaining effect is largely the function of community commitments, satisfaction with some parts of the job, and familial ties. In relation to Vroom's (1964) expectancy theory, the importance assigned this "obligation" to one's job may override feelings of dissatisfaction. This is a very different picture than has been found with urban nurses.

Interestingly, a substantial percentage (more than 60%) of rural nurses indicated that job availability played a major role in their decision to take their current position, and lack of availability of alternative jobs played a significant role in their decision to remain in that position. Of course, given the economic condition and geographic location of many rural areas, the fact that little opportunity for employment exists other than a nurse's current employer comes as little surprise. What was somewhat contrary to expectations, however, was the direction of the relationship between employment opportunities and job satisfaction; that is, nurses who reported no such employment options also reported higher levels of job satisfaction. This may reflect dissonance-reducing strategies. Vroom's model states that many factors have an effect on retention and that the importance assigned to a factor depends on the particular situation. This study supports that model and shows that several variables affect retention, including satisfaction with family and community factors as well as satisfaction with a particular job. Another key path was that of reason for leaving. When the nurse listed professional factors that would cause her to leave her position, she was more likely to consider leaving sooner. The identification of this path is important because the nurse administrator has some power to change the work environment to enhance retention, and it is important that this be done.

The acceptability of the community as a place to live (community rating) is another key factor identified in the model for all settings. This finding clearly speaks to the need for nursing administrators to be aware of and possibly involved in community development activities if rural nurses are going to be retained in the rural communities and facilities.

It is important to note that the model differs by practice setting. The model for hospital nurses is fairly complex, with length of present employment entering the model as a significant path. Additionally, the distance to work was critical to hospital nurses but not to skilled nursing facility nurses or community health nurses. Another path that was markedly different between settings was income. Among hospital nurses, it functioned as a path to satisfaction and had an effect on retention in that way, while it was a direct path to retention for community and public health nurses. It was an even stronger predictor of retention than job satisfaction for the community and public health nurses.

Retention literature focuses on management strategies that nursing administrators can use to facilitate the recruitment and the retention of nurses. Considering the shortages or maldistributions of nurses in rural areas, both recruitment and retention are especially pertinent to rural nursing, but the strategies should use rural-based methods rather than urban-based methods. Ironically, it is likely that many of the very same characteristically rural qualities that favor retention in those nurses already socially and professionally integrated into the community, may, simultaneously, hinder recruitment efforts.

This study reinforces the importance of considering organizational variables that are important to level of satisfaction as well as recognizing the importance of variables that are external to the organization.

5. A Casual Model of Work Satisfaction and Organizational Commitment

Donna Adams

This study examined several personal and organizational factors thought to affect job satisfaction, and attempted to create a causal model. Personal variables included self-esteem, and sex-role orientation, as well as length of time in the job. Organizational variables included a measure of organizational commitment and a measure of nursing stress. Information about the measures used is summarized in Table 6.1; additional information is available from the author. The study sample included 43 nurses working in a large, nonprofit hospital in the southwest.

Summary of Major Results

The numerical scores from the IWS are shown in Table E.3. Because of low to moderate Cronbach's alpha for the components of the IWS, the component mean scores were used in the regression model for level of satisfaction rather than one overall score.

The regression analysis showed that work stress was negatively linked to each of the satisfaction components except professional status. The

Table E.3 Component and Adjusted Scores for Index of Work Satisfaction ($N = 143$)

Component	Component Weighting Coefficient (Part A)	Component Total Score (Part B)	Component Mean Score (Part B)	Component Adjusted Score (Parts A & B)
Pay	3.69	15.46	2.58	9.51
Professional Status	3.24	37.61	5.37	17.43
Autonomy	3.18	37.97	4.75	15.11
Interactions	3.07	48.23	4.82	14.81
Physician-Nurse	—	26.56	5.31	—
Nurse-Nurse	—	21.67	4.33	—
Task Requirements	2.78	25.15	4.19	11.66
Organizational Policies	2.37	22.00	3.14	7.46

Index of Work Satisfaction: 12.66
Range: 8.53–19.06
Quartiles: 11.38 - 12.72 - 13.98 - 19.06

Donna Adams, R.N., D.N.Sc., is Assistant Professor at the Arizona State University College of Nursing, Tempe, Arizona. This is part of her doctoral dissertation.

For more information about this study, contact Donna Adams at Arizona State University College of Nursing, Tempe, AZ 85287. Telephone (602) 965-3244; fax (602) 965-0212.

strongest negative relationship was between stress and task requirements, which supports work redesign efforts that relieve the nurse of mundane tasks such as paperwork and housekeeping duties.

The other strong negative linkage existed between stress and the work satisfaction factor of autonomy, a result that may be due to nurses wanting to plan and perform their work without undue interference from the organization. Greater levels of self-esteem mean more satisfaction with autonomy, interaction, and professional status, outcomes supported in past research as well as in the original model. Nurses with high self-esteem may be able to assert their ideas successfully, thus obtaining a more autonomous and professional practice situation for themselves.

Tenure remains a perplexing variable in studies of work environments. In this case, tenure was related to work commitment and not to any of the work satisfaction factors. Similar findings have been reported in past research, but other studies have demonstrated low to high linkages to satisfaction with work. Greater organizational commitment in the more tenured respondents may mean they have learned to operate within the agency to their advantage or may intend to stay in current positions because of economic factors.

Discussion and Observations

Certainly, studies of this nature need to be performed in hospitals, especially since many of the new delivery systems have increased work stress and lessened satisfaction with work. Using the separate component values increased the information available as feedback to an organization about these redesign strategies.

There was a strong connection between organizational policies and organizational commitment in this study, indicating how carefully policies need to be made and interpreted. Satisfaction with pay was another element greatly influencing a nurse's intention to maintain current employment.

Nurses in areas of practice other than hospitals operate with greater autonomy and control over their work. Acute care nurses can function just as independently if more attention is given to providing a working structure that encourages mutual decision making. Professional nurses need to be able to deliver care in an environment that is less encumbered by organizational restraints and more sensitive to their work needs as individuals and professionals.

6. The Relationship Between Stress, Job Satisfaction, and Social Support of Nurse Managers

Marion Burns Tuck

The purpose of this study was to identify areas of work-related stress for nurse managers and to determine the effect of this stress on their level of satisfaction. Nurse managers from 14 general acute care hospitals in Philadelphia and three surrounding counties participated in this study. The hospitals ranged in size from 131 to 747 beds. The nurse managers had to be in their positions for longer than six months. Measures included the Norbeck Social Support Questionnaire, the Caplan Social Support Questionnaire, the Job-Related Tension Index, and the IWS. (Information about these measures can be found in Table 6.1.) Questionnaires were distributed to 210 nurse managers, 127 of whom returned the completed survey, for a 60 percent response rate.

Summary of Major Results

Data analysis focused on the interrelationship of social support, stress, and satisfaction. A lack of support from both supervisors and coworkers was related to lower satisfaction levels. Job-related stress and nurse manager age were negatively related, perhaps due to maturational, personal, or professional development influences. As expected, there was also a significant negative relationship between nurse manager stress and job satisfaction.

There was a significant positive relationship between job experience and management experience and work satisfaction, especially satisfaction with organizational policies and autonomy. As nurse managers in this study gained experience, they became more satisfied with the operational policies that guided the hospital. Also, with increased experience, the nurse managers were encouraged to function in more self-directed ways, which increased their professional autonomy.

Discussion and Observations

Findings from this investigation indicate a close relationship between stress, job satisfaction, and social support, especially from the supervisors of nurse managers. Efforts to enhance the positive effect of supervisor

Marion Burns Tuck, Ph.D., R.N., C.N.A.A., is Vice President of Patient Services, Chestnut Hill Hospital, Philadelphia, Pennsylvania. This is part of her doctoral dissertation.

For more information about this study, contact Marion Burns Tuck at Chestnut Hill Hospital, 8835 Germantown Avenue, Philadelphia, PA 19118.

support have few risks and offer potentially high returns in reducing stress and increasing job satisfaction. Communication channels should be examined with the purpose of identifying effectively functioning elements as well as possible areas for change. Analysis of the methods by which information between supervisors and nurse managers is communicated and discussed, along with problem-solving and decision-making techniques used, could offer indications for potential improvement. Nurse manager involvement in organizational committees and groups that influence policy development should be encouraged. This would not only facilitate a better understanding by the nurse managers of the operation of the organization but would also increase their visibility and demonstrate the contributions that they can and do make. Exposure of nurse managers to a broader range of hospital operations would also enhance their feelings of confidence and satisfaction regarding their work. Nurse managers should be recognized and rewarded for their achievements, and encouraged to function in as autonomous a manner as possible given their varying levels of ability and expertise. Autonomy has been repeatedly linked to work satisfaction, and the wise supervisor will recognize the capabilities of nurse managers and strive to give them the responsibility, control, and decision-making power that they can effectively manage. The role of education and on-the-job training needs to be reexamined in nurses' preparation for the position of nurse manager. Particular attention should be paid to the transition into the nurse manager role.

7. Personality Hardiness and Work Satisfaction of Critical Care Nurses

Mary Anne McCrea

This study explored the personality hardiness and work satisfaction of critical care nurses. Because of the high cost of replacing critical care nurses, the administrators and hospitals should consider them as a capital investment. Moreover, nurse stability is an important part of ensuring quality of care to patients. Both of these factors mean it is very important to retain nurses who work in critical care units. This study investigates whether it is possible to improve retention rates by selecting nurses who have a personality more able to tolerate stress. The measurement for this personality trait is the Personal Views Survey by Kobasa (1982), which provides a measure for what is termed personality hardiness.

One hundred fifty-one questionnaires were distributed to nurses working in critical care units in four hospitals in a southwestern metropolitan area. A total of 92 (61 percent) were returned.

Summary of Major Results

The critical care nurses' scores on the personal views survey indicated high levels of personality hardiness. Table E.4 shows the mean scores for each of the components of the IWS. In comparison to the sample of nurses described by Adams (1991), which included critical care nurses, the respondents in this study were more satisfied with professional status, autonomy, pay, and organizational policies. This sample also reported higher levels of satisfaction with autonomy than those described by Johnston (1991). Table B.6 in Appendix B shows the frequency distribution of responses to each item on the IWS.

There was a linkage between perceived work satisfaction and personality hardiness of critical care nurses. The IWS components of nurse-physician interaction, professional status, and autonomy were positively correlated with the total hardiness score. Information on other correlations with the three subscales on the Personal Views Survey is available from the author.

Mary Anne McCrea, R.N., M.S., C.N.A., is Senior Corporate Director, Inpatient at Carondelet Health Network, Tucson, Arizona.

For more information about this study, contact Mary Anne McCrea at Carondelet St. Mary's Hospital; 1601 W. St. Mary's Road, Tucson, AZ 85745. Telephone (520) 740-2487; fax (520) 740-2452.

Table E.4 Mean Total Scores for Work Satisfaction Components, Ranked from Most Satisfied to Least Satisfied ($N = 92$)

Component	Mean (Range 1–7)
Professional Status	5.8
Autonomy	5.2
Nurse-Nurse Interaction	5.2
Nurse-Physician Interaction	4.5
Task Requirements	4.3
Organizational Policies	3.5
Pay	3.0

Discussion and Observations

The results of this project have been used to create a framework for leadership within one particular critical care service. The entire management team used the process of interviewing and selecting staff for the critical care units based on personality variables. The outcomes associated with the selection process were reduced controllable turnover as well as increased work satisfaction for the staff.

The core principles of personality hardiness include commitment, control, and challenge. These were also the core values that drove a redesign process of the critical care units, as well as some of the educational content for the staff. The buffering aspects of personality hardiness and its correlation with work satisfaction created a framework for change and increased stability within an organization that was experiencing great stress with right-sizing efforts.

The correlation between work satisfaction and personality hardiness creates a pathway for nursing administrators as healthcare and nursing organizations are challenged with demands for increased efficiency within increasingly stressful environments. Staff may be selected for these attributes, and programs may be designed to enhance them. Because of the association with burnout and turnover, the monitoring of work satisfaction is crucial for administrators.

At a more general level, it may be appropriate that hardiness characteristics should be added to basic nursing curriculum as well as orientation programs. Continuing education programs for nurses practicing in highly stressful environments must begin to include the components of hardiness development. Nurses who are characterized by a strong sense of commitment and control over their environment, and who face their profession as a challenge are the employees that will be more satisfied in highly stressful work environments. Consequently, recruitment, selection, and retention strategies for critical care nurses must be directed toward these characteristics. Development of management strategies that support and develop hardiness should be woven throughout the governance models of critical care environments.

8. A Comparison of Job Satisfaction Levels Between Critical Care and Medical-Surgical Nurses

Rosenila B. Hlavac

There has been a substantial amount of research into whether the critical care nurse has a job that is more stressful than the medical-surgical nurse, with the assumption that high stress levels cause low job satisfaction. The results of this research are inconsistent and confusing, with a primary reason being the several types of measurements used. This study compared the level of work satisfaction of nurses working in a medical-surgical unit and an adult critical care unit, using the IWS, which is a more standardized measure of work satisfaction.

A sample of 123 RNs employed in a 361-bed acute care hospital were given IWS questionnaires, with 87 responding for a response rate of 70 percent. Of the 87 respondents, 40 worked in an adult critical care unit, and the other 47 worked in either a telemetry unit or a medical-surgical unit.

Summary of Major Results

Table E.5 shows the mean scores for each of the IWS components for medical-surgical and critical care nurses. Both medical-surgical and criti-

Table 5.E Comparison of Component Mean Scores for Medical-Surgical and Critical Care Nurses

	Component Mean Score	
Component	Medical-Surgical	Critical Care
Professional Status	5.39	5.51
Autonomy	4.14	4.12
Interaction	4.08	4.17
Nurse-Nurse	4.75	4.86
Nurse-Physician	3.40	3.48
Task Requirements	2.91	3.23
Organizational Policies	2.52	2.68
Pay	2.42	2.78

Note. $^{*}p < .05$, Range: 1–7. Quartiles: 2.5-4.0-5.5-7.0

Rosenila B. Hlavac, M.S.N., R.N., is Utilization Review Coordinator at McAllen Medical Center, McAllen, Texas. This is part of her master's thesis.

For more information about this study, contact Rosenila B. Hlavac at McAllen Medical Center, 6112 N. 28th Street, McAllen, TX 78504. Telephone (210) 632-4071.

cal care nurses were most satisfied with professional status. The medical-surgical nurses were least satisfied with pay, while the critical care nurses were least satisfied with organizational policies, closely followed by pay. The only component to achieve statistical significance (by a *t*-test) was task requirements: medical-surgical nurses were significantly less satisfied with this aspect of their job. The IWS value for the medical-surgical group was 11.4, which is just slightly above the twenty-fifth percentile, which reinforces the observation that this is a largely dissatisfied group of nurses.

Data on the frequency distribution of responses to items on Part B of the IWS can be found in Appendix B (Table B.7).

Discussion and Observations

With the exception of task requirements, this study found no differences in level of satisfaction between the RNs working in medical-surgical and telemetry units and those working in a critical care unit. The ranking of the level of importance of the components was similar to that reported by Johnston (1991), who suggested two different groupings of components. The first cluster contains the components of pay, professional status, and autonomy and may represent some values that are similar to professional norms.

In this time of cost constraints in the healthcare industry, increased career opportunities for women and increased types of healthcare work settings for RNs, it is important to know if the type of work setting is a factor that is related to job satisfaction for RNs. It is a common belief that critical care nurses are prone to high levels of stress, resulting in burnout and shortages. For this reason, the institution in which this study was conducted pays critical care nurses 10 percent more than medical-surgical nurses. Yet this investigator's review of studies that compare stress level and job satisfaction of medical-surgical and critical care nurses revealed inconsistent results, with some showing no differences and some concluding that the stress levels of medical-surgical nurses are higher than those of critical care nurses. These inconsistencies make it clear that assuming that critical care nurses experience higher levels of stress than medical-surgical nurses may be a mistake. More studies about this subject need to be done before generalizations can be made. More standardized measures of both perception of stress and job satisfaction are needed.

9. Conflict Management Style, Clinically Assertive Behavior, Collegial Behavior, and Job Satisfaction of Neonatal Intensive Care Nurses

Susan L. Rush

Advances in medical technology have dramatically increased the survival rates of infants born prematurely. The individualized care these infants require has caused an increase in neonatal intensive care units (NICUs), as well as increased demand for nurses skilled in this highly specialized area. Because of the extremely high costs of replacing NICU nurses, it is important to retain them. Nurses frequently cite problems with communication as a primary source of stress and dissatisfaction in their jobs. This study examines the relationship between the use of assertiveness as a communication style, collegial behaviors, and job satisfaction in NICU nurses.

This study involved a convenience sample of 100 RN respondents who had worked full-time for at least six months in a Level III NICU in a medical center in the New York metropolitan area. The five measurement instruments included: the Crowne-Marlowe Social Desirability Scale, the Thomas-Kilmann Conflict Mode Instrument, the NICU Nurses Assertiveness Scale, the NICU Nurses Collegiality Scale, and the IWS. Information about these measures is summarized in Table 6.1.

Summary of Major Results

The IWS was used as a measure of work satisfaction, but the 10 items that make up the interaction component were also used as a measure of collegiality. The scores on these 10 items were compared to scores on the investigator-developed NICU Nurses Collegiality Scale, which is a 12-item instrument measuring communication and collegiality between nurses and between nurses and physicians. The correlation of mean scores between these two was found to be statistically similar.

Discussion and Observations

Overall findings of the study revealed that neither the interaction component of the IWS nor the total IWS score could be reliably predicted from the assertiveness and collegiality scores of all respondents. Analysis of the individual hospitals, however, found that collegiality could predict work

Susan L. Rush, Ed.D., is Assistant Professor in the Division of Nursing at Bloomfield College, Bloomfield, New Jersey.
This is part of her doctoral dissertation.

For more information about this study, contact Susan L. Rush at Bloomfield College, Bloomfield, NJ.

satisfaction for the respondents at one of the hospitals. Some significance was found between collegial behaviors measured by the investigator-developed instrument and the interaction component of the IWS for all respondents.

Further research is needed in this area, especially in developing accurate measures for communication styles.

10. Level of Job Satisfaction of Operating Room Nurses

Nancy A. Cooley

This study used the IWS to determine the factors that relate to job satisfaction of operating room nurses and the factors that relate to tenure. The study was conducted in the operating room departments of two midwestern teaching hospitals. Both hospitals had a clinical ladder system and a shared-governance model. (Specific details on the hospitals are available from the author.) Forty-nine respondents returned questionnaires, for a 48 percent response rate.

Summary of Major Results

The overall mean level of satisfaction of the respondents was 4.1 on a scale of 1 to 7. Table E.6 shows the mean values for each IWS component and for each hospital separately. As can be seen, there were significant differences between the two hospitals in overall job satisfaction, as well as in satisfaction with pay and satisfaction with organizational policies.

Significant negative relationships were noted between job satisfaction and the percentage of time respondents spent in the role of circulating nurse. Stepwise multiple regression was performed. For most of these analyses, the percentage of time spent in the role of circulating nurse was

Table E.6 Differences in Job Satisfaction and Subscales by Hospital

Variable	Total Mean	Hospital 1 Mean	Hospital 2 Mean
Job Satisfaction	4.09	4.33	3.93*
Component			
Pay	3.41	4.16	2.88**
Autonomy	4.70	5.00	4.43
Task Requirements	4.00	4.00	4.03
Organizational Requirements	3.40	3.82	3.20*
Professional Status	4.70	4.84	4.52
Interaction	4.60	4.90	4.70

$*p < .05$ $**p < .01$

Nancy A. Cooley, M.S.N., is Director of Preoperative Services at Memorial Medical Center, Springfield, Illinois. This is part of her master's thesis.

For more information about this study, contact Nancy A. Cooley at Memorial Medical Center, 39 Fairview, Springfield, IL 62707.

the most important variable. The results of the several other statistical analyses are available from the author.

The frequency distribution of responses to the items can be found in Appendix B (Table B.8).

Discussion and Observations

The negative relationship demonstrated between overall job satisfaction and the role of the circulating nurse was especially interesting since the nurse-to-technician ratio at both hospitals demonstrated that the role of the operating room nurse is primarily that of the circulating nurse. The greater the percentage of time spent in the circulator role, the lower the level of overall satisfaction. A possible reason for this might be related to the responsibilities of the circulating nurse, who is in charge of the nursing functions of the operation as well as patient advocacy, use of equipment, instrumentation, and some of the complex interactions that take place throughout the operative procedure. All of these responsibilities may create an increase in the level of stress experienced by nurses spending the majority of their time in the role of the circulator.

The information obtained from this study was presented to the research committee and administrative staff at both hospitals. It was of interest that Hospital 2 had just completed an employee satisfaction survey, which demonstrated the same results relative to level of satisfaction with pay, and had decided to increase the rate of operating room call pay. This study supports continued evaluation of job satisfaction, especially as it relates to the role of the circulator nurse. More research needs to be conducted in the operating room setting.

11. Nurse Satisfaction in Patient Care Redesign

Denise W. Ringer, Amy M. Aliberti, Christine
Ball, Margaret Peruzzi, and Karen A. Tassey

Patient care was redesigned at Albany Memorial Hospital during a three-year project supported by the New York State Department of Health. Major initiatives related to the practice of nursing were a system of case management and reallocation of work to new or expanded roles. A care partner to help the RN with the physical aspects of patient care, caremaps to help the RN manage patient care, and nurse case managers to help with complex patient care situations were patient care model components expected to strengthen the planning, implementation, and evaluation components of the RN role.

Satisfaction, productivity, and clinical indicators were included in the project design. The indicators were analyzed before and after implementation of the new model of patient care. Two units were used in this study: a 36-bed orthopedic-neuroscience unit and a 39-bed surgical unit. The preimplementation survey was done in 1991, and 30 nurses from the orthopedics unit and 18 nurses from the surgical unit responded. The postimplementation survey was done in 1994, at which time 12 nurses from the orthopedics unit and 14 from the surgical unit returned surveys.

Summary of Major Results

Analysis of the results showed an increase in overall satisfaction after implementation of the model. Two specific components also demonstrated an increase: in both units, the increase in the scores on the autonomy component were statistically significant. On both units the scores on professional status also increased, although the difference was not statistically significant. The scores on the interaction component also changed significantly, with scores for the surgical unit increasing and scores for the orthopedics unit decreasing.

Discussion and Observations

The study results were helpful for revising the patient care model as it was developed over a three-year period and useful in determining if the model

Denise W. Ringer, M.S., R.N., C.N.A.A., is Vice President of Patient Services at Albany Memorial Hospital, Albany, New York. Amy M. Aliberti, M.S., R.N., is Nurse Manager at Albany Memorial Hospital, Albany, New York. Christine Ball, M.S., R.N., is Case Manager at Albany Memorial Hospital, Albany, New York. Margaret Peruzzi, M.S., R.N., C.S., is Director of the Workforce Demonstration Project at Albany Memorial Hospital, Albany, New York. Karen A. Tassey, M.S., R.N., C.S., is Assistant Vice President of Patient Services at Albany Memorial Hospital, Albany, New York.

For more information about this study, contact Margaret Peruzzi at Albany Memorial Hospital, 600 Northern Boulevard, Albany, NY 12204. Telephone (518) 447-3552; fax (518) 449-4410.

was associated with an increase in autonomy and professional status as well as an increase in overall satisfaction. The results cannot be generalized to other settings, however. The number of respondents was small, and because of nursing turnover, there was variability in respondents between the two data collection times. Also, it was not possible to hold a constant environment due to the presence of intervening variables that affected the results. For example, there was a work reduction in force in the fall of 1992 that staff saw as a threat to their jobs. There was also a pay scale adjustment increasing salaries in the fall of 1994.

As the project was implemented and revised over a three-year period, complaints about the changes and the process of change itself were often voiced. The IWS was given at approximately yearly intervals to provide valid and reliable data about satisfaction. The yearly scores along with ongoing unit-based focus groups helped distinguish the grumbling that accompanies change from the thoughtful critique provided by the nursing staff in the analysis of the Index results. The IWS scores were presented in the form of bar graphs and made immediately accessible to staff. The IWS was an extremely useful tool in assessing satisfaction during the change process and in providing feedback during the whole period of redesign.

12. Nursing Model and Work Satisfaction

Susan E. Pearson

This study evaluated a new nursing care delivery system implemented in a 51-bed acute care hospital in rural west central Wisconsin. The model, chosen by the hospital in conjunction with a nine-member consortium of west central Wisconsin hospitals, was a variation of the case management model called the Modified Differentiated Case Management (MDCM) model. This is a model driven by "patient needs" rather than "hospital needs." Patients are expected to benefit by improved care and cost-effectiveness, and nurses are expected to benefit by reduced role confusion and frustration and increased responsibility and control.

The IWS was given prior to and one year after the implementation of the model. Because of the small size of the hospital (31 nurses), a goal was set for a 100 percent response rate, which was obtained.

Summary of Major Results

Table E.7 shows the values for component weighing coefficients and the component mean scores obtained from both parts of the IWS. These numbers were also analyzed by looking at nurses hired before the model was implemented (long-term staff) and those hired after the model was implemented (short-term staff). Although the sample sizes were very small, the variation in results between these two groups is interesting. More detailed information about this is available from the author.

The MDCM model is designed to offer each nurse greater autonomy, and it appears that nurses were more satisfied with autonomy after the model was implemented. At the same time, the model forces nurses to concentrate more on patient care activities, resulting in less time to spend interacting with each other. The interaction component did show a decrease in satisfaction over the one-year period.

Discussion and observations

Of course, these results are limited by the small number of respondents, which especially frustrates possible comparisons between the two subgroups. Partly because of the small sample size, no clear-cut answers can be presented about the effect of this model on improving nurse satisfaction.

Susan E. Pearson, M.S.M., is Quality Assurance Coordinator at Black River Memorial Hospital, Black River Falls, Wisconsin. This is part of her master's thesis.

For more information about this study, contact Susan E. Pearson at Black River Memorial Hospital, 711 W. Adams, Black River Falls, WI 54615. Telephone (715) 284-1335, E-mail: pearsons@cuttingedge.net

Table E.7 Summary of Numerical Values from Pre- and Post-MDCM Surveys

Pre-MDCM Survey (N = 31)		Post-MDCM Survey (N = 29)	
Ranking of Components in Part A	Component Weighting Coefficient	Ranking of Components in Part A	Component Weighting Coefficient
Autonomy	3.63	Autonomy	3.70
Interaction	3.48	Interaction	3.40
Professional Status	3.19	Professional Status	3.28
Pay	3.02	Pay	3.16
Task Requirements	2.81	Task Requirements	2.74
Organizational Policies	2.44	Organizational Policies	2.35
Ranking of Components in Part B	Component Score Score	Ranking of Components in Part B	Component Mean Score
Interaction	6.30	Autonomy	5.31
Nurse-Nurse	(5.75)	Interaction overall	5.52
Nurse-Physician	(6.44)	Nurse-Nurse	(5.53)
Autonomy	5.18	Nurse-Physician	(5.50)
Professional Status	5.24	Professional Status	5.62
Pay	3.83	Pay	3.64
Organizational Policies	4.70	Organizational Policies	4.72
Task Requirements	3.95	Task Requirements	3.80
IWS	15.3		15.0

In this study, the most variation in expectations and current satisfaction levels is noted when comparing long- and short-term staff survey results. One such example is in the difference in nurse-physician interaction scores between long- and short-term staff. The long-term staff were more satisfied with their interaction with physicians than with their interaction with each other. It may be useful to compare this difference with the experiences of other facilities and the industry as a whole due to the greater emphasis placed on teamwork skills in the workplace of the 1990s.

Management would be well advised to consider differences in other needs of these two groups of nurses when examining current recruitment and retention efforts. For example, the greatest discrepancy in the entire study was seen in the level of expectation short-term employees had in relation to pay and their level of current satisfaction with that component. Using this information, administration and nursing management could choose to adjust the current pay and benefit package to be more appealing to a prospective employee.

Hospital and nursing administrators need to continue seeking and sharing information and to examine willingly the alternatives to the dilemma of a changing work force and dwindling resources. Groups of hospitals, such as this regional consortium of Wisconsin hospitals, would benefit by sharing information and participating in joint studies relating to recruitment and retention of nurses. It is a certainty that, if nothing changes, everything remains the same.

13. Using the IWS to Evaluate a Change in a Nursing Care Delivery System

Loretta Joy and Marcella Malay

The purpose of the study was to evaluate a change in nursing practice. The objectives were to

1. Demonstrate a cost-effective nursing care delivery system
2. Increase nursing staff satisfaction
3. Demonstrate patient and family satisfaction
4. Improve interdisciplinary collaboration
5. Promote the quality of nursing documentation.

Each objective was evaluated by an instrument specific for that objective.

A professional practice model was developed and implemented at New England Baptist Hospital. Data were collected on two medical-surgical nursing units prior to the initiation of the model and four months later.

Summary of Major Results

Although there was a small positive change in the overall IWS score, examining the components separately proved more helpful. Three of the subscales—autonomy, task requirements, and organizational policies—were unaffected, most likely because of the short period of time between the two data points. Professional status showed a positive change while nurse-nurse interaction showed a slight decrease, probably due to changing the expectations of the staff nurse role. The greatest increase was in physician-nurse interaction.

Discussion and Observations

In addition to the IWS measure of satisfaction, measures were used to evaluate patient satisfaction and interdisciplinary collaboration. Patient satisfaction remained high, and there was an increase in satisfaction with discharge planning among both physicians and other team members.

The major limitation of this study is the short period of time between the two data collection points. However, in a clinical setting, when some

Loretta Joy, M.S.N., R.N., is the Director of Quality Improvement at New England Baptist Hospital, Boston, Massachusetts. Marcella Malay, M.S., R.N., C., is Director of Nursing Education Quality Improvement and Research at New England Baptist Hospital, Boston, Massachusetts.

For more information about this study, contact Loretta Joy or Marcella May at New England Baptist Hospital, 125 Parker Hill Avenue, Boston, MA 02120. Telephone (617) 738-5800.

type of work redesign hinges on the results of an evaluation, a short measurement interval may be desirable to "test the waters."

Objective measures are important for evaluating a clinical redesign. Crucial to a change in practice was the evaluation of nurse satisfaction. The IWS provided an instrument that had been tested, addressed appropriate categories, and was "user friendly."

14. The Effect of Shared Governance on the Job Satisfaction of Hospital Staff Nurses

Stephanie Prock

The purpose of this study was to examine the difference in job satisfaction of hospital staff nurses who practice in a shared-governance model and those who do not. This research took place in two community-based hospitals, one with shared governance and one without. A total of 300 questionnaires were distributed, 150 at each hospital. The response rate was 40 percent from the hospital with shared governance and 15 percent from the hospital without the shared governance, for a total sample size of 83.

Summary of Major Results

An independent *t*-test revealed no significant differences in overall job satisfaction between the two hospitals. The IWS for the shared-governance hospital was 13.3, compared to 13.4 in the hospital without the model. There were also no differences between the hospitals with respect to the components of the scale. Reliability of the IWS was examined by using Cronbach's alpha. The overall alpha for the scale was .79, in comparison to the .82 reported by Stamps and Piedmonte (1986).

Discussion and Observations

The study's inability to show differences in satisfaction between the hospitals may be due to two important factors. The first is the uneven (and small) sample size from the hospital without shared governance. The second is that the shared governance was relatively new, meaning that perhaps enough time had not elapsed to demonstrate changes in satisfaction.

Stephanie Prock, M.S.N., is the Nurse Manager of the Denver Visiting Nurse Association, Denver, Colorado. This is part of her master's thesis.

For more information about this study, contact Stephanie Prock at the Denver Visiting Nurse Association, 3801 E. Florida Avenue, Suite 800, Denver, CO 80210. Telephone (303) 753-7305; fax (303) 782-2573.

15. Domestic Labor Responsibilities, Feminist Attitudes, and Job Satisfaction of Staff Nurses

Jane Large Koeckeritz

Job satisfaction of staff nurses has decreased in spite of increases in pay, autonomy, education, and working conditions. This study investigated variables outside the work environment that may contribute to this lessening of job satisfaction.

The feminist movement and economic realities have resulted in increasing numbers of women, especially women with small children, entering the labor force. Household maintenance historically has been performed by women. The amount of domestic labor required to run a household and who performs the labor have not changed appreciably since the 1970s. This has resulted in women having to work one shift on the job and then a second shift at home. This study examines the relationship between domestic labor responsibilities, feminist attitudes, and job satisfaction.

Data for this study were collected via a self-administered four-part questionnaire distributed to acute care staff nurses working in direct patient care positions in four metropolitan hospitals. Nurses working in a more technology-intensive situation (such as an intensive care or critical care unit) or in an innovative patient care delivery model were excluded from the study because of the extensive literature investigating different levels of satisfaction for nurses working in specialty areas.

Measurements included demographic variables, level of satisfaction measured by the IWS, measures of domestic labor responsibilities, and feminist attitudes. Open-ended questions were also included, especially to gather information about domestic labor arrangements in the respondent's household. Details about these measures are available from the author.

Questionnaires were distributed to 728 RNs. A total of 320 were returned, for an overall response rate of 43 percent. Response rates from each of the hospitals range from 31 percent to 55 percent, depending on the method of distribution used.

Summary of Major Results

Substantial analyses were performed on this data set, all of which are available from the author.

Jane Large Koeckeritz, Ph.D., R.N., is Associate Professor at the School of Nursing at the University of Northern Colorado, Greeley, Colorado. This is part of her doctoral dissertation.

For more information about this study, contact Jane Large Koeckeritz at the School of Nursing, Gunter 3008, Greeley, CO 80631. Telephone (303) 351-2709; fax (303) 351-1707.

The IWS itself was statistically analyzed, both for validity and reliability. The factor analysis produced a factor structure similar to the one reported by Stamps and Piedmont (1986) and can be found in Table B.5 in Appendix B. Cronbach's alphas ranged from .63 to .90 and are given in Table B.3 in Appendix B.

The results of this study support the "second shift" theory put forth by Hochschild (1989). The three aspects of job satisfaction identified as being the least satisfying were task requirements, organizational policies, and pay. These three were all negatively affected by several aspects of domestic labor, especially for nurses with children under age 15.

Domestic labor can be arranged within a household in a flexible or a structured manner. In addition to the quantitative measures used to assess this, respondents were asked to provide open-ended comments about the nature of their domestic labor arrangements. Those who identified their household as being more structured also noted more traditional gender roles. For example:

> Generally we have a structured approach. My husband does all the repairs, shares with cooking and child care. I do most of wash, all cooking, grocery shopping. Generally we have pretty divided male/female roles.

> I perform most household tasks by my own choice, because I believe I care more about these things than my husband, e.g., tidy house, paying bills on time, etc.

Respondents indicating a more flexible approach to household arrangements described a home situation in which whoever had the time or energy completed the tasks on an as-needed bases, with less gender-based roles.

> Tasks are decided in a flexible way in our home and depending on who has time according to their schedule. No one person decides for the other what tasks should be done, and there is a lot of sharing in most tasks in the house.

> Both husband and wife are too busy and share tasks as time allows. When both are too busy, household tasks do not get done. Child care is more important. So the house stays a mess and we eat the same dinner item all week.

None of the comments within either group were inherently positive or negative. Both groups described the situation without a sense of dissatisfaction.

One of the surprising findings in this study was that the respondents who described a more structured distribution of household tasks had significantly higher levels of satisfaction at work, even though they also did a higher percentage of the tasks in their household.

Feminist attitudes did not prove to be statistically significant as a predictor of overall job satisfaction, but were found to be negatively correlated with satisfaction with pay, task requirements, and nurse-physician interaction. The most significant negative relationship was with pay: the stronger the feminist attitudes, the greater the dissatisfaction with pay. This is perhaps not surprising since nurses work in an environment where a gender-based hierarchy and gender-related salary inequities among professions are well documented.

Feminist attitudes were positively related to nurse-nurse interaction, suggesting that nurse-nurse interaction is more satisfying in the presence of a positive feminist attitude.

Discussion and Observations

Job satisfaction in nursing is important primarily because of quality of care and cost-effectiveness issues. Any contribution to further understanding of the variables that create a satisfied nursing staff is important. The findings in this study indicate that, in fact, a nurse's attitude and what happens at home can be one of the factors that determine how one feels at work. An awareness of how home life affects work life, and an increasing level of consciousness among nurses on the effects of the second shift and how it is structured, may help in increasing satisfaction. Satisfaction is a combination of factors within the home situation and the work environment. Change must occur in both arenas in order to improve job satisfaction, but time to pursue changes in the organization may not be available because of the home situation.

Further specific research on the topic of flexible versus structured work and home situations is supported. The findings of this study point to a need for more structured home situations for women in the work force. Early education of nursing students on the relationship between structure and satisfaction may help them work on trying to change their situation at home or design it in the early stages of their relationships and careers. In-service programs for staff nurses presenting the findings of this study may encourage them to evaluate their own current home situations. Ongoing research and dissemination of findings on domestic labor and household-task distribution patterns are important to a profession that is primarily made up of women.

Additional studies on the topic of domestic labor and job satisfaction using alternative research methods are also indicated. The richness of the narrative comments provided by the nurses suggests that a qualitative design looking at the same variables would be useful. Alienation, as it relates to job satisfaction and total work time of nurses, could be better captured through the use of a qualitative approach such as journaling.

In summary, the findings of this research project indicate that some aspects of domestic labor responsibilities and feminist attitudes do affect some facets of job satisfaction as experienced by staff nurses. This relationship is mediated or exacerbated by marital status, children 15 or younger living in the home, and how domestic labor is distributed. The declining satisfaction of nurses, as a group, has not been fully explained by traditional theories of job satisfaction. Changing the work environment has not alleviated the problems of low satisfaction. Each research study moves the field closer to understanding job satisfaction and all of the factors involved. This knowledge will guide the development of educational programs and organizational policies directed at the underlying causes of low job satisfaction.

References

Adams, D. 1991. "A Model of Organizational Commitment in Staff Nurses." Doctoral dissertation, University of San Diego, CA.

Blegen, M. 1993. "Nurses' Job Satisfaction: A Meta-Analysis of Related Variables." *Nursing Research* 42: 36–40.

Cox, L. 1992. "Organizational Communication Factors as Perceived by Nurses in a Metropolitan Hospital." Master's thesis, Wright State University, Dayton, OH.

Downs, C. W., and M. D. Hazen. 1997. "A Factor Analytic Study of Communication Satisfaction." *Journal of Business Communication* 14: 65–73.

Duxbury, M., G. Armstrong, D. Drew, and S. Henly. 1984. "Head Nurse Leadership Style with Staff Nurse Burnout and Job Satisfaction in Neonatal Intensive Care Units." *Nursing Research* 33: 97–101.

Duxbury, M., G. Henley, and D. Armstrong. 1982. "Measurement of the Nurse Organizational Climate of Neonatal Intensive Care Units." *Nursing Research* 31: 83–88.

Hoschild, A. 1989. *The Second Shift*. New York: Avon Books.

Johnston, C. 1991. "Sources of Work Satisfaction/Dissatisfaction for Hospital Registered Nurses." *Western Journal of Nursing Research* 13: 503–15.

Kobasa, S. 1982. "The Hardy Personality: Toward a Social Psychology of Stress and Health." In *Social Psychology of Health and Illness*, edited by G. Sanders and Suls, 3–32. Hillsdale, NJ: Lawrence Erlbaum.

Martin, P. 1983. "Measuring Nursing's Organizational Climate: Instrument Modification and Use in a Large Metropolitan Hospital." Paper presented at the National Instrumentation Workshop, Tuscon, AZ.

Schutzenhofer, K. K. 1983. "The Development of Autonomy in Adult Women." *Journal of Psychosocial Nursing and Mental Health Services* 21: 25–30.

Stamps, P. L., and E. B. Piedmonte. 1986. *Nurses and Work Satisfaction: An Index for Measurement*. Chicago: Health Administration Press.

Vroom, V. H. 1964. *Work and Motivation*. New York: Wiley.

CREATING A NETWORK OF USERS OF THE IWS:
ABSTRACTS OF STUDIES CONTRIBUTING
DATA TO THIS VOLUME

This appendix contains abstracts for 20 examples of research using the IWS as a measure of satisfaction. The authors of all of the studies also contributed their data to the results presented in Chapter 4. Several of these studies have been published. All present interesting examples of using satisfaction as a variable. Space constraints prohibit lengthier descriptions of these studies, but the authors have all agreed to provide more information on request.

The studies are arranged by setting, although this is partially arbitrary. For example, the first five take place in an acute care hospital setting and are primarily descriptive in their emphasis. The next two take place in a psychiatric hospital, one of which is a Veterans Administration hospital. Selection 8 describes a study in which data were collected from 37 different hospitals, as part of the New Jersey Nursing Incentives Reimbursement Awards Program.

Selections 9 through 14 also take place in hospitals, most being set in a single acute care hospital. The distinguishing feature of these six studies is their shared purpose. They are all examples of using the IWS as part of an ongoing management system or as an evaluation of a specific nursing practice intervention. As a result, these studies have been gathered under the category labeled "management and evaluation." Their emphasis is similar to the five practice-based studies included in Chapter 5.

The next four studies focus on specific nursing specialties or settings: a neonatal intensive care unit (Selection 15), intensive care units (Selection 16), and long-term care (Selection 17).

The last two studies in this collection are interesting examples of a different approach to studying nurses. Both use a random-sample approach with a regional mailing list obtained from a state nursing board: one in Arizona (Selection 18) and one in Massachusetts (Selection 19).

1. Acute Care Hospital

General Purpose of Study

This study evaluated the level of satisfaction of nurses working in the medical intensive care unit at Strong Memorial Hospital, a 720-bed acute care hospital in Rochester, New York. The study was conducted in 1989 and involved distributing and retrieving the questionnaires within the organization. The response rate for the sample of 68 nurses was 100 percent.

Summary of Major Results

The analysis included only Part B of the IWS. The components that provided the highest level of satisfaction were nurse-nurse interaction, with a component mean item score of 5.8, and autonomy, with a mean item score of 5.3. The component providing the least satisfaction was pay, with a mean item score of 2.1. The professional status component was not used because of concerns about its reliability.

Person Responsible for Study

Judith Godney Baggs, Ph.D., R.N.
University of Rochester School of Nursing
Box SON
601 Elmwood Avenue
Rochester, NY 14642
Telephone (716) 275-8879

2. Acute Care Hospital

General Purpose of Study

This study examined the effect of collaborative practice on nurses' job satisfaction. The study took place in 1993–94 at St. Mary's Hospital, a 110-bed acute care hospital in Waterbury, Connecticut. Unit supervisors distributed the questionnaires, and respondents returned them to the researcher by interdepartmental mail. Response rate was 67 percent, yielding a sample of 100 nurses. The survey used two measurement tools: Part B of the IWS (Part B) and the Nurse Collaborative Practice Scale, a nine-item item Likert-type scale.

Summary of Major Results

Analysis of the data showed no statistically significant correlation between a collaborative practice model and nurses' overall job satisfaction. There was a significant relationship between scores on the collaboration scale and scores on the nurse-physician subscale of the interaction component of the IWS. More research is continuing on this in an effort to pursue the relationship between a more collaborative practice model and nurse satisfaction.

Person Responsible for Study

Ginny Napiello, R.N.
St. Mary's Hospital
56 Franklin Street
Waterbury, CT 06706

3. Acute Care Hospital

General Purpose of Study

The purpose of the study was to examine job satisfaction and job dissatisfaction among Black nurses, and compare level of satisfaction between Black nurses and nurses in a predominantly Caucasian sample. Ninety-three Black RNs employed at a large medical center received a questionnaire: a total of 42 returned the survey, for a response rate of 45 percent.

Summary of Major Results

There was no significant difference in job satisfaction among Black nurses and job satisfaction among the predominant Caucasian population of nurses studied by Stamps and Piedmonte (1986). The only difference was that the Black nurses found organizational policies to be more job satisfying than task requirements, and the Caucasian nurses ranked the components in the reverse order. Both populations of nurses identified pay as the most dissatisfying job-related component. Black nurses were more likely to remain in lateral positions throughout most of their nursing careers.

The study concluded with implications for nursing administration, nursing education, and nursing research. Implications for nursing administration include: (1) upgrading associate's degree nurses to baccalaureate nurses; (2) examining the method of selection for higher level nursing positions for any discriminatory factors; (3) considering longevity of tenure when promoting staff nurses; and (4) having competitive salaries with differentials for education, experience, and clinical advancement. Nursing education may also want to examine the symbolic rewards given to nurses for their continuing education in nursing.

Person Responsible for Study

Joan Horton, R.N., B.S.N., M.S.
P. O. Box 26367
Dayton, OH 45426

4. Acute Care Hospital

General Purpose of Study

This study compared the level of satisfaction of new nurses with that of more experienced nurses. The new nurses had 18 months or less experience, and the more experienced nurses had at least five years of professional experience. The study took place in a 211-bed healthcare facility in Texas in 1992 and involved a sample of 62, which represented a 57 percent response rate. The questionnaires were distributed and retrieved within the organization, on an individual basis.

Summary of Major Results

The overall IWS for new nurses was 13.7 and for more experienced nurses was 13.5.

There were some small but interesting differences in what new and experienced nurses considered most important (Part A). More experienced nurses valued professional status more highly than new nurses, and new nurses ranked pay more highly than more experienced nurses. Both groups found the most satisfaction from professional status, with new nurses having a component mean score of 6.0 and more experienced nurses having a mean score of 5.5. Both groups found task requirements and organizational policies least satisfying, with more experienced nurses being less satisfied with organizational policies and new nurses being less satisfied with task requirements. On both professional status and pay, there were relatively large differences in mean scores between new and more experienced nurses; and in both cases, experienced nurses were less satisfied.

Person Responsible for Study

Judith Walsh, R.N., M.S.N.
McLennan Community College
Waco, TX 76708
Telephone (817) 752-3320

5. Acute Care Hospital

General Purpose of Study

A 55-bed community hospital in south central Nebraska was experiencing an abnormally high turnover rate of nursing personnel during the summer of 1993. This study sought to quantify and compare level of job satisfaction for nurses who had left the hospital between 1989 and 1993 with satisfaction level for nurses who continued working at the hospital during that period of time.

The sample involved 35 past employees (a 54 percent response rate) and 33 current employees (a 43 percent response rate). Registered nurses, and licensed practical nurses, and nurse aides were included in the sample.

Summary of Major Results

Both groups identified pay, autonomy, and interaction as being most important to them. For both groups, professional status, autonomy, and interaction provided the highest level of satisfaction. The IWS scores for both groups were also similar—12.4 for past employees and 12.1 for current employees.

Person Responsible for Study

Kristin Mitchell, R.N.
2083 Randolph Avenue
St. Paul, MN 55105

6. Psychiatric Hospital

General Purpose of Study

In this study the level of satisfaction of nurses working at a 1,123-bed state psychiatric hospital was related to organizational factors (type of unit, age of patients, rate of nursing turnover, and type of work environment) and personal factors (age, years worked at the facility, years worked on the unit, and years as a nurse). Conducted in 1994, the study was a one-time survey distributed and retrieved by the researcher. Two units were selected for their divergent characteristics, and 48 nurses from these units responded, for a response rate of 58 percent.

Summary of Major Results

Job satisfaction for the respondents was very low. In terms of organizational factors, the nurses on the geriatric unit (older patients, antiquated work environment, high nursing turnover, long patient length of stay) scored significantly lower than the nurses on the medical unit (patients of all ages, modern work environment, low nursing turnover, and short patient length of stay). Job satisfaction was related to the personal factors of age, number of years at the facility, time as a nurse, and years employed on the unit only for the nurses on the geriatric unit. No relationship between job satisfaction and personal factors was found for nurses working on the medical unit.

The analysis included level of expectations and level of satisfaction for all the nurses. The most important components were autonomy and pay, and organizational policies were least important. The component with the highest level of satisfaction was professional status (4.6). Organizational policies (2.6) and pay (2.3) were the least satisfying.

Persons Responsible for Study

Virginie C. Ramsey, M.S.N., A.R.N.P.
Marianna Medical Group
P. O. Box 5836
Marianna, FL 32447-5836

Melinda C. Henderson, Ph.D., A.R.N.P., F.A.A.N.
Emerald Shores Medical Center
5399 Highway 30-A
Seagrove Beach, FL 32459

7. Psychiatric Hospital

General Purpose of Study

This study surveyed the nursing staff in a large (747-bed) neuropsychiatric hospital to determine the factors that contributed to the level of job satisfaction. Nursing staff included registered nurses, licensed practical nurses, and nursing assistants. The theoretical framework for this study was Maslow's hierarchy of needs.

Summary of Major Results

The findings from this study support the data reported in similar studies in the literature. Professional status was the most satisfying component to staff, and interaction was the second most satisfying. Interestingly, interaction ranked highest in terms of importance.

Person Responsible for Study

Amy Anderson, Ph.D., R.N.
Chair, Division of Nursing
235 Wellesley Street
Weston, MA 02193
Telephone (617) 768-7091
Fax (617) 768-8339

8. Multihospital Setting

General Purpose of Study

This study assessed the effect of a variety of nursing care delivery models on nurse satisfaction with work in hospitals that were part of the New Jersey Nursing Incentives Reimbursement Awards Program. During 1990–91 data were collected from 858 nurses at 37 hospitals in New Jersey. This represented a response rate of 60 percent. Questionnaires were mailed directly to the nurses.

Summary of Major Results

Nurses assessed pay as the most important factor, followed by autonomy and professional status. Significant differences existed for level of satisfaction with interactions and task requirements between the nurses on the pilot and control units.

A factor analysis of the IWS was also done. Results are available from the author.

Person Responsible for Study

Christine Kovner, Ph.D., R.N., F.A.A.N.
Associate Professor
School of Education, Division of Nursing
New York University
429 Shimkin Hall
50 West Fourth Street
New York, NY 10012-1165
Telephone (212) 998-5300
Fax (212) 995-3143

9. Management and Evaluation

General Purpose of Study

The major purpose of this study was to compare nurse satisfaction factors before and after implementation of a case management model. The study took place at OSF Saint Francis Medical Center, an acute care hospital of over 500 beds, during 1992–93. It involved 100 percent of the 75 nurses on a progressive cardiac care unit. The questionnaires were distributed and retrieved in a group setting.

Summary of Major Results

The use of the IWS was helpful in evaluating the implementation of the case management model. Nurses were most satisfied with professional status (mean score of 3.9), interaction (mean score of 3.8), and autonomy (mean score of 3.7). The nurses were most dissatisfied with pay and task requirements. (Both had means scores of 2.4 at the time of the pretest.) Mean scores on components with the lowest level of satisfaction (task requirements, pay, and organizational policies) increased after implementing the case management model. Satisfaction with organizational policies increased from a mean of 2.8 to a mean of 3.2.

Person Responsible for Study

Linda J. Joos, M.S., R.N.
Patient Care Manager
OSF Saint Francis Medical Center
530 NE Glen Oak
Peoria, IL 61627
Telephone (309) 655-2684
Fax (309) 655-2532

10. Management and Evaluation

General Purpose of Study

This study gathered baseline data from the nursing staff to assist in evaluating the need for organizational restructuring. The survey also helped identify areas that, from the nurses' perspective, needed change.

The sample consisted of 254 nurses, with a 52 percent response rate. Included in the survey, which took place in 1994, were registered nurses with various educational backgrounds, as well as licensed practical nurses. All staff were invited to participate, including full-time, part-time, and per diem. The survey setting was Huntington Hospital, a 378-bed acute care, nonprofit community hospital in Huntington, New York.

Summary of Major Results

Values were calculated for both parts of the IWS, along with a frequency distribution of responses and a factor analysis of Part B. The overall IWS score was 12.96, with nurses being most satisfied with the components measuring professional status (mean score of 5.7), interaction (mean score of 4.9), and autonomy (mean score of 4.6).

These results were used to improve and redesign the communication mechanisms with the nursing staff and to increase the overall understanding of what is most and least satisfying to the nursing staff. The results from this study were also used to redesign methods of nursing care delivery and prioritize long-term departmental goals.

Person Responsible for Study

Lucy D. Alexander, Ph.D., R.N., C.N.A.
Assistant Director of Nursing
Huntington Hospital
270 Park Avenue
Huntington, NY 11743
Telephone (516) 351-2312

11. Management and Evaluation

General Purpose of Study

In the state of New Jersey, the advent of deregulation of the healthcare system in 1993 and the infiltration of managed care resulted in a dramatic change in care delivery systems, with a refocus on outpatient services and a decrease in the use of acute care beds. As a result, the occupancy of acute care beds declined, as did the number of staff required to care for inpatients, resulting in a decrease in the use of agency nurses as well as change in the practice of assigning staff.

At Somerset Medical Center, there was a realization that the professional rewards and recognition achieved by nurses during the late 1980s and early 1990s should continue, as the level of staff excellence is critical to the implementation of nursing reengineering processes, as well as a commitment to Total Quality Management. Expecting that staff would be involved in many types of innovations, a decision was made to assess the level of nursing staff satisfaction prior to implementing any change project.

The IWS was chosen as the measure of nurse satisfaction because it provides information for nursing management to use in developing strategies to address areas of dissatisfaction. Also, the IWS has been used by the state of New Jersey in evaluating the success of its Nursing Incentives Reimbursement Awards program. A demographic data form was also developed so that level of satisfaction could be analyzed by clinical area and skill level.

Following the nursing management restructuring in 1993, the IWS was first administered to all nursing management staff at an annual retreat. Two weeks after the management retreat, the IWS was distributed to all categories of nursing staff on all units. All nursing staff were included because of Somerset Medical Center's commitment to teamwork, although subsequent analysis revealed that the IWS as currently designed is not as relevant to all team members.

Each nursing care coordinator selected a unit representative to assist in the distribution and collection of the surveys in order to maintain the anonymity and confidentiality of participants. Participation was voluntary; however, each member of the nursing staff was strongly encouraged to complete a survey. As an added incentive, survey participants were eligible to take part in a raffle for a gift certificate at a local department store. Surveys were distributed to each member of the nursing staff, and time was allotted for staff to complete the survey on on-duty time. Collection boxes were positioned on each nursing unit, and in the nursing office for float and per diem staff. A two-week time frame was given for the distribution and collection of all surveys, to give weekend and per diem staff the opportunity to participate. Unit representatives were responsible for returning all surveys to the nursing office by the deadline.

Response rate was 95 percent, probably due in part to the fact that on-duty time was given to complete the surveys and that unit representatives took great responsibility to see that as many surveys as possible were completed. In addition, the relationship between nursing administration and nursing staff had been characterized by open communication and a desire on the part of staff to make their opinions known. The influence of the raffle is difficult to weigh, but the opportunity for a bonus appealed to staff.

Summary of Major Results

The results for the total nursing staff, as reflected by the adjusted scores, showed that professional status and autonomy ranked highest in level of satisfaction, and that pay and organizational policies ranked lowest. Pay, autonomy, and professional status were highest in priority ranking, indicating that these factors had the largest effect on level of satisfaction for all staff.

The adjusted scores for RNs only were slightly different from those of the total staff. Professional status and autonomy again ranked highest in level of satisfaction; however, task requirements and organizational policies ranked lowest. The priority rankings for RNs only were the same as for the total staff.

The outcome of the Index of Work Satisfaction survey was shared with nursing staff on each patient care unit. The nursing care coordinator, nurse manager, and the manager of nursing systems conducted staff meetings and presented the data to the staff on each unit. The areas of dissatisfaction were highlighted, and unit-specific issues related to those factors were identified. Action plans were formulated to address the issues identified as having the greatest effect on staff dissatisfaction. Follow-up on resolving the unit-specific issues was the responsibility of the nursing care coordinator.

In addition, one goal established prior to administration of the Index of Work Satisfaction was that the outcomes of the survey would be used as a baseline to measure the effect of organizational changes. Dramatic changes at both the organizational and nursing department levels have occurred since the initial survey, with plans to reassess the level of satisfaction for nursing staff members in two years. Outcomes of both surveys will be compared to identify changes in satisfaction levels, trends, and opportunities for further research and improvement.

Persons Responsible for Study

Anne Auerbach, M.S., R.N., C.N.A.
Manager, Nursing Systems
Somerset Medical Center
110 Rehill Avenue
Somerville, NJ 08876
Telephone (908) 685-2200

Lois Dornan, M.S.N., R.N., C.N.A.
Director, Resource Management
Somerset Medical Center
110 Rehill Avenue
Somerville, NJ 08876
Telephone (908) 685-2200

12. Management and Evaluation

General Purpose of Study

This study evaluated a nursing clinical advancement system (CAS). CAS Level I nurses were still at an entry level; nurses at CAS Level II and above had been promoted into advanced CAS positions.

The study took place in 1990 at Strong Memorial Hospital, a 741-bed acute care university hospital located in Rochester, New York. The sample size was 355, and the response rate was 58 percent. The questionnaires, using only Part B of the IWS, were distributed and retrieved by mail.

Summary of Major Results

For entry-level (CAS Level I) nurses, the most satisfying components were professional status (with a component mean score of 5.4) and nurse-nurse interaction (with a component mean score of 5.3). By far, the least satisfying component was pay (with a component mean score of 2.4). The advanced (CAS Level II and above) nurses showed a similar pattern, although their numerical scores were somewhat higher. Professional status (5.6) and nurse-nurse interaction (5.5) were most satisfying, and pay was least satisfying with a component mean score for the advanced nurses of 2.74. The mean total score for advanced nurses (4.3) was slightly higher than for entry-level nurses (4.2).

Complete results of this study are available in the *Journal of Nursing Administration* 23 (2): 13–19.

Person Responsible for Study

Alison Schultz, Ed.D., R.N.C.
University of Rochester School of Nursing
601 Elmwood Avenue
Rochester, NY 14642

13. Management and Evaluation

General Purpose of Study

This study evaluated nurse satisfaction as part of an overall management strategy that involved concerns about several issues, including Total Quality Management, strategic planning, and nurse retention programs. The study took place in 1993 at Foote Hospital, a 488-bed acute care hospital in Jackson, Michigan. The sample involved 650 respondents, which was a 48 percent response rate. The questionnaire was distributed and retrieved by mail.

Summary of Major Results

The data generated by this study were analyzed in several ways, including by specialty group (medical, surgical, maternal and child health, critical care, mental health, ambulatory care, and floating). Overall results indicated that the components providing the highest level of satisfaction were professional status (mean score of 5.5) and nurse-nurse interaction (mean score of 5.2). Components providing the least amount of satisfaction were organizational policies (mean score of 3.1) and pay (mean score of 3.2).

The benchmarks that were most useful for incorporation into the management strategies were both the component weighting coefficients and the component mean scores, rather than a total score. Results were broken into four possible categories: (1) respondents are satisfied; (2) respondents don't place much importance because expectations are met; (3) respondents feel that satisfaction is unattainable; and (4) respondents feel that improvement is needed and can be achieved.

Based on this study, a comprehensive salary study and compensation program analysis was undertaken. The IWS proved useful in addressing several management concerns.

Person Responsible for Study

Barbara Christy, R.N.
V.P. for Patient Care Services
Foote Hospital
205 N. East Avenue
Jackson, MI 49201
Telephone (517) 788-4890

14. Management and Evaluation

General Purpose of Study

Evaluation of whether a nursing care delivery model would affect level of nurse satisfaction was the major purpose of this study. It was conducted at Good Samaritan Hospital, a 600-bed acute care hospital in Cincinnati, Ohio. The survey took place between June 1992 and December 1993.

The IWS was administered two separate times. The initial administration involved 134 nurses (a 79 percent response rate). The second administration six months later involved 57 respondents (a 16 percent response rate). Both surveys were distributed and retrieved by mail.

Summary of Major Results

At the time of the pretest, the overall Index of Work Satisfaction was 12.3. The components that provided the most satisfaction were professional status (with a component mean score of 5.3) and autonomy (4.5). The components that provided the least satisfaction were pay (2.8) and organizational policies (3.1). At the end of one year, the IWS was 12.7, and the level of satisfaction with autonomy increased slightly (to 4.8), as did the level of satisfaction with organizational policies (to 3.5). The largest change was with satisfaction with organizational policies, although this largely contributed to dissatisfaction rather than satisfaction. Overall, the changes made in the nursing care delivery system produced less change in level of satisfaction than had been hoped for and anticipated.

Person Responsible for Study

Beatrice Huss Hodovanic, R.N., M.S., C.C.R.N.
Good Samaritan Hospital
375 Dixmyth Avenue
Cincinnati, OH 45220
Telephone (513) 872-4080

15. Neonatal Intensive Care Unit

General Purpose of Study

The major purpose of this study was to determine the effect of participation in research on the level of satisfaction among neonatal intensive care nurses. The study took place in 1994 at Kingston General Hospital, a 379-bed acute care hospital in Kingston, Ontario. The sample consisted of 64 registered nurses in the neonatal intensive care unit. Questionnaires were distributed and retrieved in a group setting within the hospital. The study involved two administrations—a pretest and a posttest.

Summary of Major Results

Results involving component scores showed that, for most components, scores increased at the posttest. The components with the highest level of satisfaction were professional status and autonomy. The component with the lowest level of satisfaction was organizational policies.

Person Responsible for Study

Joan Tranmer, R.N.
Director, Nursing Research
Kingston General Hospital
76 Stuart Street
Kingston, Ontario
Canada K7L 2V7
Telephone (613) 548-3232 ext. 4952

16. Intensive Care Units

General Purpose of Study

This study explored work satisfaction of nurses working in intensive care units. Of particular interest were variables related to longevity of employment in the same intensive care unit (more or less than three years) and level of nursing education (M.S.N., B.S.N., A.D.N., diploma). The study was done in 1994 and took place in three Veterans Administrations teaching hospitals: a 400-bed medical center in Kansas City, Missouri; a 700-bed medical center in St. Louis, Missouri; and a 280-bed medical center in Columbia, Missouri. The questionnaires were distributed and retrieved by mail. A total of 70 nurses responded, for a 47 percent response rate. Comparisons were made between length of employment and level of education.

Summary of Major Results

For all groups, nurses were most satisfied with professional status (component mean scores between 5.3 and 5.5). Autonomy (component mean scores between 4.3 and 4.5) and interaction (component mean scores between 4.1 and 4.6) were the next most satisfying. For all groups, the component with the lowest level of satisfaction was organizational policies. Nurses with less than three years of experience were the most dissatisfied with this component, regardless of educational level.

For all the groups compared, the components that were of highest importance were pay and autonomy. The components of least importance were task requirements and organizational policies.

Person Responsible for Study

Sara J. McCauley, R.N.
Moses H. Cone Memorial Hospital
615 Summerwalk
Greensboro, NC 27455

17. Long-Term Care

General Purpose of Study

This 1994 study took place in a rural 165-bed acute care hospital in eastern North Carolina and included a 40-bed long-term care unit associated with the hospital.

The study involved 118 nurses—both RNs and licensed practical nurses—for a response rate of 67 percent. Questionnaires were distributed and retrieved in a group setting within the organization.

Summary of Major Results

The IWS for the nurses was 12.75. The components that were most satisfying were professional status (with a component mean score of 5.4), nurse-nurse interaction (with a component mean score of 5.1), and autonomy and task requirements (both of which had component mean scores of 4.8). The component providing the least satisfaction was organizational policies (with a component mean score of 3.1).

Persons Responsible for Study

Sue Wagner, R.N., M.S.N.
P. O. Box 486
Maxton, NC 28364
Telephone (910) 844-5227

Carole Gibson, R.N., M.S.N.
Telephone (910) 462-2802
9340 Morgan Street
Laurel Hill, NC 28351

18. State Mailing List

General Purpose of Study

Concern about nursing availability has prompted much research in the area of retention, turnover, and job satisfaction. Professional nursing organizations focus on many issues of concern to nurses and the profession, including issues related to job satisfaction. The purpose of this study was to determine if there is a difference in self-perceived job satisfaction between nurses who belong to a professional nursing organization and those who do not.

Summary of Major Results

The sample for this study was drawn from a mailing list provided by the Arizona State Board of Nursing. Out of the 265 people in the list, 149 were contacted by mail; a total of 39 responded.

The findings from this study did not demonstrate a significant difference in job satisfaction between nurses who reported belonging to a professional organization and those who did not. However, several important problems in this study indicate the need for more research in this area. One of the most important problems is a low response rate (26 percent) that resulted in a small number of nurses (16) who reported belonging to a professional organization. Based on what is expected from the literature in this area, it is important to do this study with a larger sample size.

Person Responsible for Study

Sheryl A. Peteuil, R.N., M.N.A.
Director of Admissions/Case Manager
Handmaker Jewish Services for the Aging
P.O. Box 13090
Tucson, AZ 85732
Telephone (520) 322-7004

19. State Mailing List

General Purpose of Study

This study was undertaken to investigate whether certain reward strategies within nursing lead to greater job satisfaction, resulting in the retention of nurses. Motivation plays an important role in providing job satisfaction; job satisfaction results in people remaining in their jobs.

Summary of Major Results

The membership list of the Massachusetts Nurses Association was used to select a sample of respondents stratified by age, geographical area, and educational preparation.

The IWS was used to measure job satisfaction. Other data were collected by means of a case study approach in which nurses were asked to choose which of three possible reward strategies—salary, primary nursing, a clinical ladder—would be most likely to be viewed as an important reward strategy.

Of the six components of job satisfaction, respondents were most satisfied with professional status, autonomy, and interaction. Lower levels of satisfaction were found for pay, task requirements, and organizational policies. The professional status component scored the highest for all nurses, regardless of education, availability of reward strategy, or length of time in a job.

In terms of reward strategies, salary was viewed as being most influential in choosing a job, although nurses who worked in settings with a clinical ladder had a significantly higher level of job satisfaction than those who did not.

Person Responsible for Study

Joan A. Bruce, R.N., C.S., Ed.D.
43 Glen Road
Westwood, MA 02090
Telephone (617) 769-5171

INDEX

study, *281*; ranking comparisons, 79, *82*, 83; validation study, 201, *202*

Content theory, 11–12

Continuing education, 33

Cooley, N.A.: operating room nurse study, 167, 266–67, 292–93, *292*; on professional experience, 167

Corcoran, N.M., 51

Coward, R.T.: long-term care nurses, 38, 56; modified IWS, 173, 174–75, 209, 212

Cox, L., 273–74

Critical care nurse: comparisons, 168; research studies, 265–66, 285–89, *286*, *288*; retention strategies, 51

Cronbach's alpha coefficient, 173, 192, 193, 196, 201

Cultural values, 37

Czajka, J.M.: downsizing organization, 53–54; measurement tools, 56; on organizational climate, 46; stress measurement, 52

Darr, K., 11

Data analysis: guidelines, 248–50; technical assistance, 259

Database, 94–98, 260; creation of, 91, 94–96; issues, 91–96; quality assurance, 94–96; use of, 96–98, 102

Data collection: care delivery system study, 299; enhanced professional practice model study, 111, 112–13, 114; external influences study, 302; methods of, 162; organizational assessment study, 273; paired-comparisons, 253–54; perception monitoring study, 107, 118, 119, 122; quality improvement activities study, 131–32; shared-governance study, 134–35

Decentralized management, 46–47

Decision making, 44; participation in, 171; research study, 108, 140–52

Defenses, lines of, 17

Delegation, 22, 25, 47, 131

Demographic variables, 245, 254–55; enhanced professional practice model study, 114–15; perception monitoring study, 119–20; satisfaction levels and, 107, 165–68; shared-governance study, 134–35; types of, 33–36

Dienemann, J., 24

Discrepancy theory, 14–15

Dissatisfaction, 12, 92; job-related factors, 27; as motivator, 14; organizational factors, 46; rewards and, 16; sources of, 14, 31–32, 40, 51; stress and, 52; turnover and, 50, 51, 52; as variable, 18

Diversity, 5

Domestic labor, 303, 304–5

Downsizing, 53–54

Drews, T.T., 45, 170

Dual-factor theory, 14, 31–32, 232

Dunkin, J.W.: on external influences, 178; IWS modifications, 175; measurement tools, 173; on professional experience, 166; rural nurse study, 264–65, 277–80, *278*; on whole nurse, 269–70

D'Amico, M., 43

Education, 34–35; level of, 167; workshops, 54

Edwards, A.L., 190, 238

Effort-net return model, 18

Empowerment, 4, 5, 10; communication and, 19, 21; components of, 20; concept of, 20; definition of, 20; effects of, 25; job redesign and, 23–24; measurement tools, 47; organizational effectiveness and, 20–21; organizational theories and, 16–19; productivity and,

53; measurement tools, 56; retention strategies, 50–51; turnover model, 35
Snyderman, B.: on dissatisfaction, 27; on external influences, 109; on motivation, 12; satisfaction factors, 138
Social integration, 40
Social reference group theory, 15–16
Social support, *159–60*, 283–84
Somerset Medical Center, 319
Staff development, 33
Standards, 93, 97–98, 207, 251
Statistical analysis, 192–94, 201–2
Steffy, B.D., 59
Stillwaggon, C.A., 21
Stratton, T.D.: on external influences, 178; IWS modifications, 175; measurement tools, 173; on professional experience, 166; rural nurse study, 264–65, 277–80, *278*; on whole nurse, 269–70
Stress, 66; behavior and, 17; levels of, 92; measuring, 52; negative effect of, 51–52; perceptions of, 92; positive, 52; research studies, 265–67, 281–93, *281, 286, 288, 292*; response to, 36; satisfaction levels and, 176
Strong Memorial Hospital, 309, 322
Structural power, 48
Subtractive theory, 14–15
Systems model, 16–17
Szilaggi, A.D., 40

Task requirements component: alpha values, 173; mean score distribution, *88, 90*; modifications, 200; ranking, *82*, 83; response distribution, *204, 217, 221, 225, 229*; tau values, 200; total score distribution, *83, 84*, 86, 87; value distribution, *80*
Task-role power, 48
Tassey, K.A., 294–95

Taylor, F., 11–12, 134
Team building, 20–21
Team nursing, 22
Tebbitt, B.V., 20, 23
Tenure, 146, 149
Theory "M," 44
Thomas, C.: data collection methods, 162; professional practice model, 170–71; quality improvement activities study, 107–8, 124–32; reliability estimates, 208; timelines, 268
Timmesman, G.M., 49
Total mean score, 77, 79, 249
Total quality management, 23, 24, 169, 323
Total scale score, 77, 79, 249
TQM. *See* Total quality management
Tucson Medical Center, 24
Tumulty, G., 38, 40, 45
Turnover: anticipated, 53; costs of, 49–50; definition of, 49; dissatisfaction and, 50, 51, 52; education and, 35; factors affecting, 50; intention studies, 53–54; internal transfers, 49; measurement of, 48, 53–55; rate, 3, 25–26, 32; research study, 313; shared governance and, 140–41

Unit outcomes, 38
Unit service manager, 129
University of Massachusetts, 188
Urban nurses, 38
User survey, 65–94, 207–8; comments, 215, 232; field use, 70–74, *73*; item analysis, 212, 215, *216–31;* process, 68–70; questionnaire development, 68–69; reliability analysis, 208–9, *209*; response rate, 70–71; sample criteria, 69–70; validity analysis, 209, *210–11*, 212, *213–14*
USM. *See* Unit service manager

Vacancy rates, 49